**World Yearbook
of Education 1989**

World Yearbook of Education 1989

HEALTH EDUCATION

Edited by Chris James, John Balding
and Duncan Harris (Series Editor)

Kogan Page, London/Nichols Publishing Company, New York

Previous titles in this series

World Yearbook of Education 1982/83
Computers and Education
Edited by Jacquetta Megarry, David R. F. Walker,
Stanley Nisbet and Eric Hoyle

World Yearbook of Education 1984
Women and Education
Edited by Sandra Acker, Jacquetta Megarry,
Stanley Nisbet and Eric Hoyle

World Yearbook of Education 1985
Research, Policy and Practice
Edited by John Nisbet, Jacquetta Megarry and Stanley Nisbet

World Yearbook of Education 1986
The Management of Schools
Edited by Eric Hoyle and Agnes McMahon

World Yearbook of Education 1987
Vocational Education
Edited by John Twining, Stanley Nisbet and Jacquetta Megarry

World Yearbook of Education 1988
Education for the New Technologies
Edited by Duncan Harris (Series Editor)

First published in Great Britain in 1989 by Kogan Page Limited
120 Pentonville Road, London N1 9JN

British Library Cataloguing in Publication Data

World yearbook of education – 1989
  1. Education – Periodicals
  370'.5   L16

  ISSN 0084–2508
  ISBN 1–85091–735 3

First published in the USA in 1988
by Nichols Publishing,
an imprint of GP Publishing Inc,
PO Box 96, New York, NY 10024

Library of Congress Cataloguing in Publication Data

Main entry under title:
World Yearbook of Education: 1989
1. Education – Periodicals
  ISBN 0-89397-334-3
  LC Catalog No.. 32-18413

Typeset at The Spartan Press Ltd, Lymington, Hants
Printed and bound in Great Britain
by Biddles Ltd, Guildford

Contents

6   **CONTENTS**

List of Contributors

Nilda Segura Cid, Nuble Health Education Committee, Chile   *Chapter 10*
Keith Tones, Leeds Polytechnic, England   *Chapter 25*
Jean Tulloch-Reid, University of the West Indies,
   Jamaica   *Chapters 11 & 12*
Harry Vertio, Department of Health Promotion, Finland   *Chapter 22*
Beverley Walker, La Trobe University, Australia   *Chapter 16*
Rodney Wellard, La Trobe University, Australia   *Chapter 16*
Christopher Wood, African Medical and Research Foundation,
   Kenya   *Chapter 18*
Ian Young, Scottish Health Education Group, Scotland   *Chapter 28*

Introduction
Health education worldwide: the state of the art in 1989

Chris James and John Balding

This edition of the World Yearbook of Education has health education as its theme. This is particularly appropriate with the continual increase in population in so many countries and its associated problems. Many important health themes are common to most nations, if not all, and other major issues can no longer be seen as the particular concern of just one nation or culture nor will they remain so. The pursuit of good health for all and the need for health education cuts across all international frontiers.

The yearbook sets out to illustrate the diverse and fascinating nature of health education around the world. It was too much to hope that the yearbook would be a systematic portrayal of health education in particular nations chosen because they were in some way typical of a particular geographical region or political grouping. Rather, the intention is that this yearbook should illuminate health education in a wide range of settings.

Potential contributors were approached via personal contacts, or by means of contacts identified for us by the World Health Organization (WHO) and the British Council. We are indebted to these bodies for identifying appropriate people for us to contact, and to those people who responded when contacted for making such valuable and interesting contributions.

Contacts were identified in 40 countries and we eventually received papers from 16 of them before the deadline set by the publishers. In each country we attempted to discover two appropriate authors, who would both provide one article. The first article, **the overview**, is intended to give a picture of health education in that country. We suggested that contributors might consider questions such as: How is health education perceived? What professions are involved in its delivery? How is central government involved in controlling and resourcing health education? What are the major health issues and what aspects of health education are currently being promoted? What is the influence of external factors? How politically important is health education? What are the future trends? Authors responded to this framework of prompts according to the different emphases they perceived in their own country. Taken together the overview articles reveal a very wide range of health education structures and processes.

The second article from each country is intended to complement the first by describing a particular aspect of health education in practice. This article, which we have described as a **case study**, is intended to illustrate health education in practice so that the reader can gain an insight into the reality of the health education described in the overview chapter. The case studies are accounts of particular programmes, developments or initiatives. We suggested to the writers of the case study articles that they might address questions such as:

☐ What is the background?
☐ What was the need?
☐ What are the purposes and aims?
☐ What is the target group or population?
☐ What is the nature of the programme, development or initiative?
☐ Did the programme face any particular difficulties and how were these overcome?
☐ What did the evaluation of the activities and outcomes reveal?
☐ Are any future activities planned?

As with the overview article, we offered a framework of prompts against which each author could respond.

The contributions from around the world

The chapters in the yearbook reveal a very wide range of issues, trends, health education programmes and strategies, structures, and modes of organization and operation. We have chosen the sequence to demonstrate this diversity while at the same time pointing up links and common themes.

The contributions from the **Netherlands** show clearly a level of sophistication and development in health education which has resulted from it being the subject of explicit government policy and the fact that much attention has been paid to structure and funding including training and research. The development of health education in the Netherlands seems to be very advanced in commerce, industry and schools. This is reflected in the smoking prevention programme which is described in the case study. It is a video peer-led programme which uses a wide variety of educational methods. It is based on a study of determinants of smoking behaviour, prevention research and theories of social psychology.

In **Denmark**, health education has a very diverse pattern which is referred to by Jens Mathieson in his chapter as 'a puzzle without a picture'. Mathieson suggests that this may have arisen from the fact that there is no one word or phrase for health education in Danish. The case study chapter describes a comprehensive and detailed project aimed at influencing the diet-related behaviour of young people by means of a very wide range of educational and health promotional strategies.

The transition from the prevention of illness as the central issue, through health education to do with life style, to health promotion is a feature of the chapter by Eugene Donoghue and Anna-May Harkin which gives an overview of health education in **Eire**. This transition is reflected in the control and administration of health education and health promotion. The case study from Eire is an account of the lifeskills programme in the north west region. From the description, the programme has clearly been well thought through and has been carefully and systematically implemented. It has generated considerable interest and commitment among teachers in the schools.

The overview of health education in **Spain** is both interesting and illuminating. The decentralization of control of many public services with the creation of 17 autonomous communities has been taking place since 1979, and many of these now provide a service in health education. Since the early 1960s, health education activities have been expanding and these are now identified with many different agencies. The case study is a colourful and exciting description of a programme which took place within a university school of nursing to create, for the first time, a 'non-smoking school'. The students in the school designed and ran the programme which was aimed at all the members: students, professors and staff. We suspect that in the translation the article may have lost some of the impact that the article would have had in Spanish. We hope that the translation has not significantly distorted the picture.

In **Chile**, where health and education activities are integrated through national policy-making structures, the overview chapter asserts that health education has played an important part in improving the nation's health. The practice of health education is illustrated by Nilda Segura Cid's chapter which describes the part health education plays in the activities of the health service in the province of Nuble. From this informative article it is clear that a team approach is considered essential. In this way, health and education expertise and practice are integrated at the level of delivery which reflects the planning process at national level.

The detailed and comprehensive chapter by Jean Tulloch-Reid, Ivy McGhie and Cathrine Lyttle, describes how health education has been recognized as an important component in public health programmes in **Jamaica** since the early part of the century. Indeed, there have been formal health education structures in place since the mid-1920s albeit with limited resources. The long history of health education development is clearly reflected in the case study. It is a fascinating description of a community development project which combined very practical measures with strategies designed to develop the interpersonal skills essential for the development's success. The account of the project illustrates the beneficial outcome of different agencies co-operating on a particular initiative – an issue raised elsewhere in the yearbook. The case study also stresses how important it is that health education initiatives take account of existing cultural norms in the community, again an issue raised elsewhere in the yearbook.

The overview of health education in **Canada** describes, with great clarity, trends in health education and the significant part health education now plays in the wider strategy of health promotion. It is clear from Ken Allison's chapter that the status of health education has is based on strategies that are well thought through and soundly based. Part of this sound basis has arisen from the surveys of health knowledge and the surveys of health-related attitudes and behaviour which are described in the chapter by Beazley and

King. This chapter also gives renewed emphasis to the power that data gained by means of surveys can have in bringing about change.

The clearly presented overview from **Australia** deals succinctly with the organization, differences between states and major pressure groups amongst other issues. It concludes in a very positive fashion by stating that health educators in Australia are expecting to learn from other countries in some areas but are proud of the number and extent of 'our community development programmes, our consumer action groups, and the willingness to keep our policy and theory grounded in practice'. The case study concerns the development of a post-graduate course in health education. The course attracts participants from most health disciplines and has evolved against a changing background of political factors, structural factors within organizations, broad developments in the field of knowledge and the interpretations the staff have put upon this complex evolutionary process. It reflects in a practical way the concluding sentiments of the overview statement.

The importance of taking the community context into account in the implementation of health education initiatives is re-emphasized in the chapter giving an overview of health education in **Kenya**. One of the ways this is achieved in Kenya is by having a range of trained personnel involved at a variety of levels. The case study from Kenya gives an insight into the role of one particular agency, the African Medical Research Foundations (AMREF), in delivering health education through a variety of programmes. The chapter also raises an issue common elsewhere in the yearbook, namely the challenge of matching the intended health education messages to the cultural background and the level of understanding of the target group.

Important issues in health education in **Nigeria** are raised in the chapter which describes the setting up of 'comfort stations'. These are combined toilets, laundries, and buildings for the communal use of social groups comprising several families. Again, the success of this venture has resulted from an understanding and awareness of the context, in this case the existing social structure and culture within the group. The fascinating article by Professor Z. A. Ademuwagun describes how significant improvements in health were achieved not through the imparting of health messages but through 'motivators' which were connected with deeply held values of privacy and cleanliness.

In **Italy**, the case study illustrates some of the challenges facing those wishing to implement changes in health education with a view to changing health-related behaviour. The article by Archangela Mongelli describes her own impressive endeavours to bring about change. It is clear from the chapter how much energy and enthusiasm are required to achieve community involvement, an essential ingredient for the success of any health education initiative.

A very clear and detailed picture from **Norway** of the health of the people is given by Eli Endresen in her chapter with the intriguing title 'Norwegians – as fit as fiddles?'. The chapter describes the findings of a national health survey carried out in 1985. It covered a range of health issues and the findings give a vivid backdrop to the description of the administration and organization of the public health system, the education system, and non-governmental organizations.

The overview of health education in **Finland** indicates that health education is heavily influenced by the activities of various non-governmental organizations in common with other accounts.

There is a youthful vigour in the account of health education in Wales. It looks forward from a point in time in the 1980s with the birth of the health promotion authority for Wales. It is uncluttered with a confusion of historical origins and perhaps this provides the current vitality of its efforts. Within the account of the case study, 'Lose Weight Wales', the campaign details and progress are examined and the involvement of industry and commerce as well as the health sector shows particular promise in the long term.

The overview from **England** shows the width and complexity resulting from an evolution of health education and health promotion over many years. The account is carefully presented and, as with all the overview chapters, will form an authoritative statement from the viewpoint of an informed professional about the stage of development as seen in 1988. Two overlapping case studies have been provided. Gill Combes' account gives a wide ranging and perceptive description of parental involvement; it is very practical and is firmly rooted in the experiences of teachers pupils and parents. John Balding's contribution portrays the effects of consultation with pupils/ students, parents, teachers, governors and health care professionals through survey work on the status of health education in the school curriculum. Some very interesting, and differing, points of view, emerge.

The overview from **Scotland** portrays a high level of organization of health education which has had substantial influence for many years. The role of the Scottish Health Education Group (SHEG) is clearly significant involving a multi-disciplinary staff team and close liaison with central government, universities and the media. The health education activities it promotes are wide ranging and clearly highly co-ordinated. The case study is a reflection of this level of development and demonstrates careful co-ordination and monitoring of a multi media intervention aimed at influencing drug use by young people.

Conclusions

As editors we found we were on occasion rewriting parts of the English translations, usually at the invitation of the author concerned. We were always fearful that we might be altering the sense of the message that had been intended, and hope that this was not too often the case. We hope too, that we did not soften any of the impact that some of the 'translated' statements would have had when presented in their own language. We anticipate that readers who are interested in following up any of the chapters will communicate directly with the authors concerned.

The international 'health market' is highly political and in reading this book comparisons between countries are bound to be made. We are proud to be associated with the contributions that we have been enabled to gather together. They are wide ranging in character from those based on highly sophisticated research methodology to the down to earth accounts of working in the field with disadvantaged communities with meagre resources.

We had hoped to receive contributions from all major geographical divisions of the globe; inspection of the content shows that there are some notable omissions which is unfortunate. The collection that has emerged is varied and exciting; it represents an authoritative statement from many countries on the state of the art of health education in 1988.

We have enjoyed the support of many people in creating this collection of accounts. We are particularly grateful to those who provided names of others in countries throughout the world from whom we could then discover the identities of health care professionals of appropriate status to approach to write the chapters. This information came from Dr Desmond O'Byrne, World Health Organization, Copenhagen; Marilyn Rice, Pan American Health Organization, Washington, USA; and numerous British Council Representatives around the world who gave care and attention to our requests.

1. Health education in the Netherlands – AN OVERVIEW

J. Hagendoorn

Summary: In the early 1960s health education was made a subject of explicit government policy and since that time attention has been paid to structure and funding including training and research. A National Institute of Health Education has been set up. The Dutch health care system is composed of three sub-systems; the first tier is preventive in character, the second, mainly concerns general practitioners and the delivery of home care and the third tier involves specialists, clinics and hospitals.

Health education is delivered both within the health care system and outside it. There are many government campaigns, health education is compulsory in primary schools and emphasized in secondary schools where it is not yet obligatory. Health education is also an important element of occupational health. There is a well structured support system for the promotion of health education including a special unit within the Ministry of Health. The Dutch Health Education Centre was set up in 1981 and has proved an effective force in accumulating background knowledge and in supporting people in carrying out health education activities. Future trends suggest an emphasis on the work place, the elderly, sports and secondary schools.

The Netherlands have a surface area of 41,160 square kilometres with a population of 14,600,000 whose density is 355 people per square kilometre with an annual rate of increase of 0.4 per cent. Infant mortality rate is 8.0 per 1,000 live births with a life expectancy at birth of 76 years. The urban population is 89 per cent of the total.

Introduction

For many decades, health education has been an activity carried out by several organizations in and outside the health care system in the Netherlands with organizations for mother and child care, anti-smoking organizations, a heart foundation, anti-alcohol organizations, and such like.

In the early 1960s health education became the subject of explicit governmental policy, and gradually it was introduced, first as an important element in the work of health care workers, then later, as an essential aspect of health care and health care policy, and in the 1980s it became a cornerstone of the health promotion policy to the year 2000.

Along with this political development, attention was paid to the structure and financing of health education, including training and research.

Government policy

In 1976 the government set up a committee to establish a National Health

Education Plan. Its recommendations, which were published in a final report in 1981 have been of crucial importance in the development of health education in the following years. The committee recommended the establishment of a special unit for health education in the Ministry of Health, the creation of a National Institute of Health Education, the development of a regional support structure for the country, with recommendations on training and education, financing and research. Many of these recommendations were implemented in the following years. In the national health policy, although health care was limited by resources, health education was given high priority. In several government white papers, for example those on public health, mental health and patient education, much emphasis was put on health education. In 1985 health education was introduced as a compulsory subject in primary schools in the Netherlands. In 1986 a reorientation of health care policy put its central focus on a large variety of elements to improve health. Health education is considered to be an important tool in reaching the targets set by the WHO-Euro Health for All Policy by the year 2000.

Health education in the health care system

The Dutch health care system is composed of three sub-systems. The first tier is that of public health, preventive in character, not curative, and funded by local or regional government. In this sector health education is an important element, and in most public health services, specialists in health education are appointed to carry out activities or to support the activities of other organizations in their region. The second tier consists of the mainly curative care by general practitioners, mother-and-child care and home delivery care. In this sector the general philosophy is that the curative work also has important preventive, health education elements. These elements of the work are supported by a network of specialists in health education, most of whom are engaged in carrying out population-oriented health education activities, either at local or regional level. With curative care, health education in the form of patient education is provided as a daily routine. The third tier is the care provided by specialists, mostly in the setting of a clinic or hospital. In this sector patient education is of special importance. A new development is to appoint specialists in patient education in hospitals.

Another important area of health education is the out-patient mental health clinics. In each of these 60 institutes prevention specialists are appointed to carry out programmes aimed at the prevention of mental problems. The health care system in Holland is the subject of much debate as is the system of financing it, because of ever increasing costs. Of course this is unfavourable for the development of health education in all the above mentioned sectors. Nevertheless, there has been a gradual increase in the potential for health education activities in the care system itself.

Health education outside the health care system

As mentioned before, health education is traditionally carried out by a large number of specialized institutes. Their activities are mostly directed at the general public, or to special target groups. Their activities range in method from large television campaigns to the distribution of leaflets and stickers. Topics of their specialization are for example, sex education, heart disease, nutrition, smoking, asthma, accident prevention, safety in sports. These organizations, some privately funded, others funded by the government, are an important element of health education in the Netherlands. There is no centralized institute in the Netherlands that provides different sorts of health education on a variety of topics.

The government launches special campaigns, mostly aimed at the public at large, on topics of major importance to the health of the nation: AIDS, alcohol, smoking, and so forth.

Health education has been compulsory in primary schools for the past two years. A general introductory stratagem has developed to provide schools with adequate materials, training and practical support.

In secondary schools health education is not obligatory yet, though there is currently much discussion as to whether there should be a special curriculum for health education; the AIDS issue makes this particularly urgent. Health education as such is not a generally accepted issue yet in most secondary schools.

Although labour laws aim to achieve good working conditions, health education, which is an important element of occupational health is at the moment only introduced through them occasionally. This will probably be a key issue in the development of health education in the Netherlands in the near future.

Support of the development of health education

An important element in the development of health education in the Netherlands has been the central idea of a new approach to health, in which the healthy behaviour of individuals and groups is important. A support structure should be set up to promote health education at a policy level; it will have to accumulate knowledge about health education and stimulate its quality.

There is a special unit in the Dutch ministry of health, whose task is to promote and integrate health education in legislation and to stimulate governmental policy by creating favourable conditions for its development. Since its creation in 1981 the unit has proved to be of the utmost importance in expediting the development of health education in Holland. Another element of support was the creation of a network of small institutes at regional level, to promote and co-ordinate health education at that level. This structure is still in the process of evolving, and surrounded by uncertainty over the national restructuring of its funding system and pay structure. Nevertheless, many of these institutes have worked for several years in a very creative and positive way in both forming regional platforms for co-operation and carrying out innovative projects.

A third aspect of the support system was the creation of a national service institute for the accumulation of knowledge, the improvement of the quality of health education and the stimulation of new initiatives. The Dutch Health Education Centre (DHEC) was founded in 1981 and has proved to be a very effective institute in building a body of knowledge and supporting the people who carry out health education activities. In the seven years of its existence it has become a central point for workers, scientists and policy makers in the field of health education.

In 1988 it became a collaborating institute of the World Health Organization (WHO) for health promotion and health education. Its present functions are: documentation, training, research, development of methods and registration of activities. An important part of any new scientific approach is the academic support that is invested in its development. In Holland there is one university where health education is an academic specialization: the University of Limburg. Graduates find their way, as specialists, to many organizations for health education. Many of the appointed specialists in health education are graduates in social psychology, communication, sociology. Up till now most of the health educators in the Netherlands had an academic training. Many health care workers and teachers involved in health education attended a post graduate course. Gradually, more research is being done in health education, either by universities, or by research institutes. Although much remains to be done, research shows that health education can be a very effective approach. The DHEC published a comprehensive study on the 'Effectiveness of health education' in 1988.

Future trends

At present much of the structure of health education is still being developed. In the last few years there has been a rapid increase of resources, people and activities. Undoubtedly, reductions in the budget of many healthcare institutes will affect their evolution. On the other hand the general policy is favourable to the long-term development of health education. New areas such as health education in the working place, the elderly, sport, and secondary schools, will attract political and public attention, as will the general contribution of health education in the global strategy of the WHO for health promotion. The promotion of health without attention to human behaviour is unthinkable.

With respect to the future of health education it is of the utmost importance to carry out all health education activities in a systematic, scientific way, accompanied by research, to evaluate the results and demonstrate that health education is worth its money. As the future will show, no health education programme is viable without sufficient scientific support. At the moment health education can be seen to be cost efficient, and many companies and institutes will probably be founded in this field to the extent even of its becoming big business. That could be another trend.

Conclusion

In Holland health education had a good start under favourable conditions. It is gradually developing as an activity that is essential to the health of people.

However, much has still to be done in politics, in actual support of the health workers, in amassing knowledge, in training and research. One thing is clear: if there are no people that actively promote health education, if there are no supportive structures, if there is no general awareness and support and if there is not a policy of raising funds continuously, health education will always be a noble goal but one that is never achieved.

2. Non-smoking: your choice, a Dutch smoking prevention programme – A CASE STUDY

Hein de Vries and Margo Dijkstra

Summary: In 1986 a Dutch smoking prevention programme was developed. It was based upon the results of a study of the determinants of smoking behaviour in Dutch children, the insights from prevention research mainly from the United States, and social psychological theories. The Dutch smoking prevention programme 'non-smoking: your choice' is a video peer-led programme. This means that the current content and structure is explained on video by adolescents. The programme uses several educational methods such as active participation and active learning. It consists of five lessons and is supplied with manuals. Both the content and the structure are explained and discussed in this case study.

Introduction

This paper discusses the development, the implementation and the evaluation of the Dutch smoking prevention programme 'Non-smoking: your choice'. First, the research on smoking prevention will be reviewed briefly. Second, the determinants of smoking in Dutch children will be discussed. Third, the structure and content of the Dutch smoking prevention programme will be described. Finally, the results of the project will be discussed.

History of smoking prevention

Some decades ago research indicated that smoking is harmful to health. This resulted in the development of smoking cessation programmes for smokers. However, cessation of smoking is difficult and only partly successful (Leventhal and Cleary, 1980). Preventive activities aimed at non-smoking children probably constitute a more successful approach to the smoking problem. Many adolescents have a negative attitude towards smoking. Nevertheless, as they grow older a substantial percentage of them starts to smoke. An important explanation of this phenomenon has been given by Evans (1976), who stresses the role of direct social pressure. Adolescents start to smoke due to the pressure of their parents, the media and, most importantly their smoking peers. Direct pressure refers to a variety of behaviours, such as the offering of cigarettes, persuasion, challenging, and pestering. However, indirect social influences are important as well. Indirect pressure refers to the impact of smoking models on the attitude of a non-smoker. By observing positive outcomes from smoking, a non-smoker may start to believe that smoking has some advantages. This process, which is also called vicarious learning (Bandura, 1986), can initiate changes within the belief system of non-smokers. The impact of indirect pressure is nevertheless hard to demonstrate. Adolescents won't feel pressure to smoke from seeing other people smoke, or by observing cigarette advertisements but this may, however influence beliefs about smoking. Some studies support the idea of indirect pressure: as non-smoking adolescents grow older they associate more advantages with smoking (De Vries and Kok, 1989). Observing a friend smoking without noticing any observable disadvantages, causes a non-smoker to perceive himself as less vulnerable to the negative effects of smoking (Urberg and Robbins, 1984). Friedman et al (1985) show that adolescents do not report pressure to smoke, although the onset of smoking does take place within a social context. Therefore, a smoking prevention programme should focus on both direct and indirect pressure. Initial smoking can lead to regular smoking. Although at least 90 per cent of the population has at one time tried smoking a cigarette, this does not necessarily imply regular smoking. The likelihood of becoming a regular smoker increases if initial smoking is repeated more than four or five times. Studies suggest that this may cause addiction in 70 to 90 per cent of the initial smokers. The chances of addiction further increase if the time interval between the first cigarettes is short (Hirschman et al, 1984; McKennel and Thomas, 1967; Salber et al, 1968).

Since Evans and his colleagues (Evans et al, 1978) developed a successful smoking prevention scheme in 1976, a smoking prevention tradition has developed in the United States. According to Evans's assumption, health, personal and social factors are important in explaining the development of smoking behaviour in an individual. Smoking prevention programmes should focus more on short-term effects of smoking, because the traditional long-term effects like cancer, appear to be less relevant and salient for adolescents. Another major contribution of this approach is the focus on social pressure. Therefore, anti-smoking programmes should focus on increasing resistance in non-smoking adolescents towards these pressures. In order to increase resistance Evans applied McGuire's inoculation theory (McGuire, 1964) by confronting non-smoking students with arguments of smokers to start smoking. This confrontation triggers resistance and counter-arguments in non-smokers that will make them cope more effectively with the pressure to smoke.

Inspired by Evans's work many researchers have developed successful prevention programmes which have included important innovations (Aaro et al, 1983; Best et al, 1984; Biglan et al, 1983; Botvin and Eng, 1982; Flay et al, 1983; Hurd et al, 1980; McAlister et al, 1979; Murray et al, 1984; Schinke et al, 1985; Telch et al 1982). Many programmes comprise a training of refusal skills which are practised by role-playing. Several students use a peer-led system in which an adolescent of comparable age introduces the programme. The advantages of a peer-led system are increased attractiveness and comprehensibility of the programme and increased changes of imitation of the non-smoking behaviour of the peer-leader (Klepp, *et al*, 1986). Some programmes incorporate active learning techniques: instead of providing students with information, they are stimulated to search for relevant information. This will lead them to discover gaps in their own knowledge, which will make them more open to new information (Flay *et al*, 1983). Some programmes provide booster sessions in which the major issues of the programme are repeated several months later. Other studies use commitment techniques to increase chances of behaviour maintenance. Students are asked to commit themselves (publicly or anonymously) to their non-smoking behaviour. A crucial factor in the evaluation is the self-report of adolescents. To increase self-report validity, smoking prevention studies use biochemical measures, such as saliva thiocyanate, expired carbon monoxide or cotinine samples. Another method is the bogus-pipeline procedure (Horning *et al*, 1973) by which students are made to believe that their self-reports will be checked by biochemical validation. Although an actual validation does not occur, this method may increase self-report validity (Evans *et al*, 1978; Mittelmark *et al*, 1982). A more extensive overview of the innovations and the (methodological) problems has been given by Flay *et al*, 1983 and recently by Best *et al*, 1988.

Smoking prevention and health education: four basic questions

When attempting to solve a health problem (for instance smoking) by education, applied behavioural research has to deal with four different questions (De Vries and Kok, 1986):

1. the analysis of the problem, which regards the relationship between a health problem and human behaviour;
2. the analysis of determinants of health behaviour and why people start to smoke;
3. the development of an intervention;
4. the evaluation of the intervention.

This framework has been used by the Dutch smoking prevention project to develop and to implement a smoking prevention programme.

Problem analysis

Dutch figures show that as a result of smoking 18,000 people die every year of lung cancer, coronary heart diseases, asthma and bronchitis (Smoking and Health Foundation, 1986). Although the percentage of children smoking between the ages of 10 and 15 has decreased (1979: 22 per cent; 1983: 11 per cent; 1986: 10 per cent), this decline seems to have come to an end. Moreover, in excess of a third of the Dutch adult population still smokes. Therefore, smoking remains a serious problem and its prevention is an important issue. As the incidence of smoking increases sharply between the ages of 13 and 14 in the Netherlands, smoking prevention may have great impact at the age of 13. Many try smoking (90 per cent), but this does not always lead to regular smoking. Therefore, preventing initial and experimental smoking is probably hard to realize and may be unwise as experimenting with behaviour is a normal phenomenon during adolescence. The goal of the Dutch programme is to prevent the transition from initial and experimental smoking to regular smoking. Regular smoking is defined as smoking at least one cigarette a week.

Determinants of smoking in Dutch children

Research in the Netherlands did not sufficiently indicate the determinants of smoking in adolescents. Generalizing data from studies from other countries may be dangerous as determinants of smoking may differ between countries (Newman and Martin, 1982). Moreover, little was known as to differences between beliefs of initial and regular smoking. Therefore, we have started with an analysis of determinants of initial and regular smoking in Dutch children. As the prevention programme is based on this study, its results and conclusions will be discussed briefly (for more information see De Vries and Kok, 1986).

The Fishbein and Ajzen (1975) model was used in analysing the determinants (see Figure 2.1). This model permits a careful analysis of both attitudinal and social factors that influence behaviour (see for example Bauman and Chenoweth, 1984; Newman and Martin, 1982; Loken, 1982; Page and Gold, 1983).

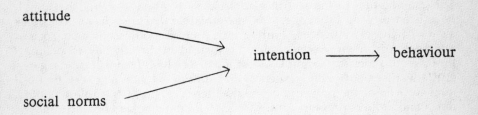

Figure 2.1: *Model for explaining behaviour*

The results of the analysis of determinants show that non-smokers had a stronger negative attitude towards smoking because they connected smoking more strongly with negative outcomes, such as health hazards (for example bad health, damage to the lungs, cancer, bad physical condition, coughing, irritated eyes, nausea, breathing problems) and personal hazards (addiction, expense). Non-smokers were also more convinced that smoking caused passive smoking and was noxious to others. Although smokers did recognize these drawbacks, they minimized their significance. Smokers associated more advantages with smoking: sociability, nice to do, showing off, relaxing, a good taste, and it relieved boredom. Non-smokers, however, related smoking to opposite effects: they regarded smoking as unsociable, not nice to do, not relaxing, distasteful and causing nervousness. There are two important implications. First, smokers are capable of influencing non-smokers by minimizing the seriousness of the disadvantages. Second, smokers report advantages while non-smokers merely see disadvantages. This discrepancy may create a challenge for non-smokers to initiate smoking, in order to discover which party is right.

Consequently a prevention programme has to reinforce the non-smoking attitude of non-smokers. The advantages of non-smoking and the disadvantages of smoking should be stressed, and special attention has to be paid to the short-term effects of smoking, because these are more salient for children. The results indicated which consequences are connected with smoking. They also indicated that the prevention programme should protect non-smokers from pressure to change their attitudes, by demonstrating the inaccuracy of some preceived advantages of smoking (for example, that it is relaxing), and by indicating that the advantages of smoking can also be realized by other activities (for example dancing, discussion and sport) or personal attributes (such as clothes). The challenging effects of the discrepancy between the positive beliefs of smokers and the negative opinions of non-smokers should be clearly indicated.

Non-smokers experienced a more negative social norm towards smoking from their parents, brothers, sisters, relatives, the general practitioner, non-smokers, non-smoking friends, the Smoking and Health Foundation, and the public health department. Smokers experienced pressure to smoke from friends and classmates. Both smokers and non-smokers experienced pressure to smoke from smokers, cigarette industries and cigarette advertisements. The reported pressure, however, was not as large as expected. This may be due to the fact that adolescents hesitate to admit that they have been pressed to smoke. It is also possible that they have not been aware of these influences. Furthermore, our hypothesis is that social influences are often exerted indirectly instead of directly. By modelling positive outcomes (for example, adulthood, sociability) smokers and cigarette advertisements will influence the attitude of non-smokers in the long run. Smoking prevention should therefore stress the role of both direct and indirect pressure, and should train non-smokers how to handle these pressures. Resisting direct pressure can be learned by skill-training, as other programmes already have indicated. Coping with indirect pressure may be harder to learn, as this type of pressure is less visible. Training should focus on recognizing these pressures and on eliciting copying responses.

Regular smoking was mostly associated with long-term consequences, such as increased risk of cancer, addiction, and passive smoking. Initial smoking was associated more with short-term disadvantages, such as nausea and breathing problems, and with short-term advantages, like discovering the taste and satisfying curiosity. Initial smoking was seen as less addictive to adolescents than regular smoking. As indicated before, studies show that addiction can occur for 70 to 90 per cent of those who have smoked only three or four cigarettes, and that the chance of becoming a regular smoker increases when the interval between the first cigarettes is short. Moreover, the preceived norms of parents, relatives and the general practitioner, were also less negative on initial smoking than on regular smoking. Smoking prevention programmes should therefore clearly indicate that although initial smoking is linked with advantages, it may easily lead to addiction.

In some situations non-smokers were less negative towards their intention not to smoke. Besides situations in which they experiment with cigarettes (when nobody sees them), other situations seem to have a social function (being outside, in discos and cafes, in the street, with friends and at parties). Smoking prevention programmes should discuss these at-risk situations. Skill-training sessions can focus on these situations and on how to cope with their challenges.

The Dutch smoking prevention programme

Based on these results, and using information from other smoking prevention research and applying psychological theories (McGuire, 1985), a smoking prevention programme, 'Non-smoking, your choice', has been developed. It is a video peer-led programme for adolescents aged thirteen and fourteen (8th grade). The structure and the content of the lessons can be summarized as follows: (a) introduction of the theme on video, presented by two adolescents (seven minutes); (b) peer-led activities in small groups (fifteen minutes); (c) continuation of the lesson and presentation of real-life situations by adolescents on video (eight minutes); (d) peer-led activities in small groups (fifteen minutes); (e) home-activities.

The activities which focused on the theme of the lesson, were realized in groups of four or five students and were led by a non-smoking student of their own class. This peer-leader explained the activities to the other students in his group and stimulated them to work seriously. The peer-leaders received a special one-hour training, which consisted of following the first lesson and discussing their tasks. Some activities focused on skill-training to practise refusal techniques. These techniques were modelled on video, and were trained afterwards during activities. Active participation of students was stimulated. Moreover, instead of providing information, students were encouraged to discover information (active learning).

Every student received a manual in which the major information of the lessons was summarized by cartoons. Activities were explained in the manual as well. Peer-leaders and teachers received their own manual in which additional information was given about their specific tasks. The teacher's task was to co-ordinate the lessons, to assist the peer-leaders, and to encourage the students. As the structure of the programme is simple, the teacher only needed to have a short special training of one hour.

The programme consisted of five lessons of forty-five minutes. The first lesson gave a general introduction. During the activities students discussed why people begin to stop smoking, and indicated possible ways to refuse cigarettes. The second lesson concentrated on the short-term effects of smoking, which were demonstrated on video as well. The activities focused on the knowledge of students about these effects and on passive smoking. The third lesson discussed peer pressure. Refusal skills were trained during role-plays. The fourth lesson analysed indirect pressure from adults and advertisements. The activities focused on interpreting advertisements and on alternative behaviours for realizing positive outcomes associated with smoking. The last lesson provided a summary. The activities focused on skill-training, on decision making and on commitment to students' non-smoking behaviour. To increase commitment, non-smoking adolescents were asked to conclude a non-smoking contract (anonymous commitment), and to write their name on a non-smoking poster which could be clearly noticed in the school, and thus by other students (public commitment). As a reward for their decision non-smokers could receive a non-smoking poster and a non-smoking button.

The structure and content of the lessons were explained on video by youngsters. This method has several advantages. First, the teacher only needs a short training and the programme can be used in different classes (biology, English, and so forth). Second, by using adolescents to introduce the lessons on video the attraction of the programme and its comprehension by students is improved. Third, the comparability between schools is higher, as all schools using the experimental programme do so in the same way.

The development

The actual development of the programme took one year, and included the following activities: script-writing, production, screening players for the video film, pre-testing and adapting the programme, and contacting schools to participate (see Figure 2.2).

The script-writing and the production of the film was accomplished by the two researchers of the project. When necessary, experts were consulted, for

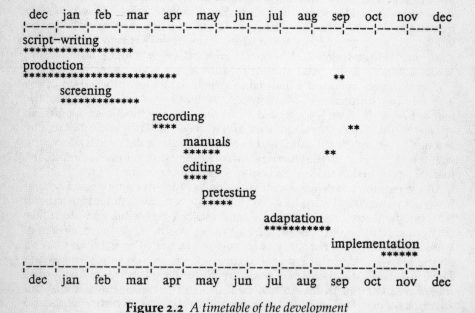

Figure 2.2 *A timetable of the development*

example, for the lesson dealing with the physical effects of smoking. Several teachers checked the script and the manuals on the reading level of the target group. The production included a variety of activities, such as procuring the equipment (for example equipment to measure the degree of trembling), analysing animation films, selection of tunes, and discussion with the crew (further consisting of a director, an assistant director, a cameraman, a designer, a photographer, and technicians for light, sound, editing, and decor). Players for the film had to be selected as well. More than 300 people, mostly adolescents, participated in the video. From a screen-test for 60 people, four adolescents were selected to introduce the video and explain the activities. Others were selected for roles in real-life scenes. Another purpose of the screen-test was to check whether these scenes corresponded with the real-life situations of adolescents, and whether the language of the script corresponded with the language of the target group. The recording of the programme took 16 days. The programme was pre-tested in two classes, one at a vocational school, the other at a high school. This resulted in some revisions.

Evaluation of the Dutch smoking prevention programme

The programme was implemented in November 1986 in four vocational schools and five high schools. The pre-test was in September 1986 and a post-test took place one year later. The programme was evaluated by questionnaires and by group discussions. The results indicated that students rated the video, the activities and the peer-led approach positively. The manuals with the cartoons were also positively rated. The group discussions revealed that the students liked the alternation of video and activities which prevented loss of attention. The activities were positively rated because of their content, and because of the possibility of bringing out individual experience. Most students liked the peer-led approach. The peer-leaders and teachers found that their training was clear, didn't consume too much time and was sufficient. Some of the vocational school teachers indicated that they had to help the peer-leaders with organizing their groups. High school teachers hardly mentioned any problems with the peer-leaders. The success of the peer-led approach was surprising, because hitherto this method has been unknown in the Netherlands. Some high school students concluded that the programme was rather easy, and indicated a need for more information and discussion. This was not surprising as the educational base-line level of the programme focused on vocational schools.

To evaluate the programme's effects two different outcomes were measured. The first outcome included both experimental smokers (smoking from time to time, but not every week), and regular smokers (weekly and daily smokers). The measured outcomes reported here refer to the differences in increase in smoking that occurred within one year.

Figure 2.3 shows that the programme successfully prevented smoking in general. Smoking increased by 4.3 per cent in the experimental group, while increasing by 6.0 per cent in the control group. Although this difference is not significant, the increase was less than the national increase of 12

N=1031	item	mean (+2;−2)
VIDEO	programme	.80
	lessons on video	.74
	watching the video's	.93
ACTIVITIES	activities in general	.70
	(Σ activities)/16	.80
	home activities	.75
	activities during lessons	.81
	manual	.68
PEER–LED SYSTEM	working in groups	1.27
	having a peer–leader	.85
	assistance by peer–leader	.49
	assistance by teacher	.78

+2 = good; −2 = bad

Figure 2.3 *Evaluation of the programme*

per cent. The programme appeared to be especially effective with vocational school students. For these students smoking increased by 1.5 per cent in the experimental schools, and by 8.4 per cent in the control schools (p<0.05). The differences in increase among the high school students for the experimental and the control group were not significant.

The former results refer to smoking in general, including those who smoke from time to time although not regularly each week. If we focus on regular smoking (those who smoke at least one cigarette per week), it appears that the prevention programme was especially effective in reducing regular smoking. Regular smoking increased by 4.8 per cent in the experimental group and by 7.4 per cent in the control group (p<0.05). Again, the programme was most successful for students at vocational schools. Regular smoking increased by 6.7 per cent in the experimental group and by 15.8 per cent in the control group (p<0.005). The results may seem somewhat contradictory as the increase in smoking in general seems smaller than the increase in regular smoking. This is due to the fact that many experimental smokers (who are in the category of 'smoking in general', but are not in the category of 'regular smokers') have started to smoke regularly. This transition from experimental to regular smoking cannot be observed in the category 'smoking in general', because both experimental and regular smokers are regarded as smokers. Many experimental smokers start to smoke regularly. However, as can be seen from the results for regular smoking, the prevention programme often prevented the transition from experimental to regular smoking in the experimental group (see De Vries et al, 1989 for more details).

Conclusions and discussion

A systematic approach in which attention is paid to the analysis of the problem, the determinants of behaviour, the intervention and the evaluation of the results is important. It increases the likelihood of a clear analysis of the problem, it indicates what is known and which topics need more attention or specific analysis, and which theories and results are relevant.

The analysis of the determinants indicated both for smokers and for non-smokers the consequences that were connected with initial and regular smoking. It also suggests how smokers may influence non-smokers. Non-smokers merely saw disadvantages, while smokers associated advantages too with smoking. This discrepancy between the two groups may initiate initial smoking in non-smokers. Smokers experienced stronger direct and indirect pressure to smoke. Both groups experienced direct pressure to smoke from cigarette advertisements. However, the impact of these advertisements is probably even stronger, because advertisements represent a form of indirect pressure that may (slowly) influence the attitude to smoking in adolescents. Recently De Vries *et al* (1988) found that self-efficacy is an important factor in predicting behaviour. Further research on determinants should include this factor as well.

The video peer-led aproach was attractive for both students and teachers. The alternation of videos and activities prevented boredom and lack of attention. The video-led nature of the programme increased the chances of implementation, because teachers did not have to follow time-consuming training sessions. This also made it possible to implement the programme during for example, mathematics, biology, history or a combination of different classes. By introducing activities adolescents can integrate information with their lifestyle.

The programme appeared to be especially effective for students at vocational schools. Therefore, a nation-wide implementation is recommended (some small refinements are suggested). Although the programme was successful, the recent data and the recent theoretical insights stress the need for additional developments in smoking prevention programmes and further research, to increase the likelihood of the successful prevention of smoking. These programmes should be developed according to the needs and characteristics of the different target groups. Therefore additional research on the following questions is recommended:

1. Smoking prevalence is already high in Dutch vocational schools at grade two. Therefore, a careful analysis has to indicate whether the social pressure programme can also be effective at grade one of vocational schools.
2. High school students of the experimental and the control groups did not differ significantly with regard to the increase in regular smoking (although the increase in both groups was rather small). An explanation for the small increase in the control group is that the carbon

monoxide test had a preventive effect on students of the control group. A second explanation is that the programme, primarily focusing on resisting social pressures, did not have enough impact on high school children, because these children at age 13 do not experience severe social pressure to smoke. A third explanation is that high school students needed a more cognitive oriented prevention programme (as some students indicated during the process evaluation), because they may have a stronger need for cognitive schemata and discussion (see for example Petty and Cacioppo, 1986). More research is necessary to develop prevention programmes for specific groups and on how to adapt messages to the needs of the target group.

An attractive and effective programme, however, does not guarantee the successful prevention of smoking. Schools often have different and conflicting priorities. Health education should therefore become an important subject within the curriculum, which is not the case in the Netherlands and in Europe. Even then one may wonder if smoking prevention can be maximally effective. Smoking prevention is more credible if it takes place within a society that takes a clear stand on health and health promotion. Smoking prevention may be less credible in a society which stimulates health but at the same time promotes advertisements that are noxious to health. Within such a context smoking prevention and health education cannot have an optimal impact. Moreover, adolescents will have a difficult problem to solve namely, that if smoking really is bad, why aren't cigarettes and especially cigarette advertisements forbidden?

References

Aarö, L E, Bruland, E, Hauknes, A, Lochsen, P M (1983) Smoking among Norwegian schoolchildren 1975–1980. III. The effect of antismoking campaigns *Scandinavian Journal of Psychology* **24**, 277–283

Bandura, A (1986) *Social Foundations of Thought and Action: a Social Cognitive Theory* Prentice-Hall: New York

Bauman, K E and Chenoweth, R L (1984) The relationship between the consequences adolescents expect from smoking and their behaviour: a factor analysis with panel data *Journal of Applied Social Psychology* **14**, 28–41

Best, J A, Flay, B R, Towson, S M J, Ryan, K B, Perry, C L, Brown, K S, Kersell, M W, D'Avernas, J (1984) Smoking prevention and the concept of risk *Journal of Applied Social Psychology* **14**, 257–273

Best, J A, Thomson, S J, Santi, S M, Smith E A, Brown K S (1988) Preventing cigarette smoking among school children *Annual Review of Public Health* **9**, 161–201

Biglan, A, Severson, H, Bavry, J, McConnel S, (1983) Social influence and adolescent smoking: A first look behind the barn *Health Education* **14**, 14–18

Botvin, G J, Eng, A (1982) The efficacy of a multicomponent approach to the prevention of cigarette smoking *Preventive Medicine* **11**, 199–211

De Vries, H and Kok, G J (1986) From determinants of smoking behaviour to the implications for a prevention programme *Health Education Research* **1**, 85–94

De Vries, H, Dijkstra, M and Kuhlman P (1988) Self-efficacy: the third factor besides attitude and subjective norm as a predictor of behavioral intentions *Health Education Research* **3**, (in press)

De Vries, H and Kok, G J (1989) *Adolescents' Beliefs on Smoking: Age and Sex Differences* (in preparation)

De Vries, H, Dijkstra, M, Kok G J (1989) *Results of the Dutch Smoking Prevention Programme* (in preparation)

Evans, R I (1976) Smoking in children: developing a social psychological strategy of deterrence *Journal of Preventive Medicine* **5**, 122–127

Evans, R I, Rozelle, R M, Mittelmark, M B, Hansen, W B, Bane, A L and Havis, J (1978) Deterring the onset of smoking in children: knowledge of immediate physiological effects and coping with peer pressure, media pressure and parent modeling *Journal of Applied Social Psychology* **8**, 126–135

Fishbein, M and Ajzen I (1975) *Belief, Attitude, Intention and Behavior: an Introduction to the Theory and Research* Addison Wesley, Reading, Mass.

Flay, B R, D'Avernas, J R, Best, J A, Kersell, M W, Ryan, K B (1983) Cigarette smoking: why young people do it and ways of preventing it. In: P J McGrath and P Firestone (eds) *Pediatric and Adolescent Behavioral Medicine* Springer, New York, 132–183

Friedman, L S, Lichtenstein, E, Biglan, A (1985) Smoking onset among teens: an empirical analysis of initial situations *Addictive Behaviors* **10**, 1–13

Hirschman, R S, Leventhal, H and Glynn, K (1984) The development of smoking behavior: conceptualization and supportive cross-sectional survey data *Journal of Applied Social Psychology* **14**, 184–206

Horning, E C, Horning, M G, Caroll, D I, Stillwell, R N, Dzidic, I (1973) Nicotine in smokers, non-smokers and room air *Life Science* **13**, 1331–1346

Hurd, P D, Johnson, C A, Pechacek, T, Bast, L P, Jacobs, P R, Luepker, R V (1980) Prevention of cigarette smoking in seventh grade students *Journal of behavioral Medicine* **3**, 15–28

Klepp, K I, Halper, A, Perry, C L (1986) The efficacy of peerleaders in drug abuse prevention *Journal of School Health* **56**, 407–411

Leventhal, H and Cleary, P D (1980) The smoking problem: a review of the research and theory in behavioral risk modification *Psychological Bulletin* **88**, 370–405

Loken, B (1982) Heavy smokers', light smokers' and non-smokers' beliefs about cigarette smoking *Journal of Applied Psychology* **67**, 616–622

McAlister, A L, Perry, C, Maccoby, N (1979) Adolescent smoking: onset and prevention *Pediatrics* **63**, 650–658

McGuire, W J (1964) Inducing resistance to persuasion. In: L Berkowitz, (ed) *Advances in Experimental Social Psychology* I Acad. Press, New York

McGuire, W J (1985) Attitudes and attitude change. In G Lindzey and E Aronson *Handbook of Social Psychology* (Vol 2), Lawrence Erlbaum Associates, New York

McKennel, A C and Thomas R K (1967) Adults and adolescents' smoking habits and attitudes *Government Social Survey* Ministry of Health, London

Mittelmark, M B, Murray, D M, Luepker, R V, Pechacek, T F (1982) Cigarette smoking among adolescents: is the rate declining? *Preventive Medicine* **11**, 708–712

Murray, D M, Johnson, C A, Luepker, R V, Mittelmark, M B (1984) The prevention of cigarette smoking in children: a comparison of four strategies *Journal of Applied Social Psychology* **14**, 274–288

Newman, I M and Martin, G L (1982) Attitudinal and normative factors associated with adolescent cigarette smoking in Australia and the United States of America: a methodology to assist health education planning *Community Health Studies* **6**, 47–56

Page, R M and Gold, R S (1983) Assessing gender differences in college cigarette smoking: intenders and non-intenders *Journal of School health* **53**, 531–535

Petty, R E and Cacioppo, J R (1986) The elaboration likelihood model of persuasion in L Berkowitz (ed) *Advances in Experimental Social Psychology* (Vol 19), Academic Press, London

Salber, E J, Freeman, H E and Abelin, T (1968) Needed research on smoking: lessons from the Newton study, in E F Borgatta and R R Evans (eds) *Smoking, Health, and Behavior* Aldine, Chicago

Schinke, S P, Gilchrist, L D, Snow, W H (1985) Skills intervention to prevent cigarette smoking among adolescents *American Journal of Public Health* **76**, 665–667

Smoking and Health Foundation (1986) *Annual Report* The Hague

Telch, M J, Killen, J D, McAlister, A L, Perry, C L, Maccoby, N (1982) Long-term follow-up of a pilot project on smoking prevention with adolescents *Journal of Behavioral Medicine* **5**, 1–7

Urberg, K & Robbins R (1984) Perceived vulnerability in adolescents to the health consequences of cigarette smoking *Preventive Smoking* **13**, 367–376

3. Health education in Denmark: a puzzle without a picture – AN OVERVIEW

Jens Mathiesen

Summary: There is no single word or phrase in Danish to describe health education. This has resulted in a very diverse pattern of activities and agencies related to health education. Early strategies focused on disease rather than health. The Danish Committee for Health Education was formed in 1964. It organized a series of seminars from which the 'Health pedagogic movement' emerged. This gave a broader context to health education. The National Prevention Council, formed in 1979, has a health promotion function and works in conjunction with other agencies. The AIDS campaign from the National Board of Health is described. Since 1976, health education has increased in importance politically. Future trends, which indicate an increasingly important role for health education, are outlined.

Introduction

There is no equivalent in the Danish language for the English concept of Health Education. This would not be a problem, if there were a generally accepted term that could cover the same field. Unfortunately, this is not the case. Due to this lack of a unifying concept, the field of Health Education as it developed in Denmark is a story filled with examples of the problems and advantages that have arisen because there has never been an agreed terminology.

The most serious consequence of this conceptual confusion has been the difficulty in getting health education recognized as an important priority requiring government attention. There has been no one word or for that matter catch phrase that ambitious politicians could be given in order to start a political debate. Various words and concepts have been introduced by different conceptual schools and by various pressure groups in recent decades, but there is still no 'winner' in sight.

Although it has been difficult to make the state responsible for health education, there have been certain advantages in this conceptual confusion. The competition between conceptual pressure groups has produced much descriptive material and a rich variety of qualified proposals for action.

Parallel to the sometimes quite heated debates over concepts and content, a great number of activities, both traditional and innovative, have been initiated. These activities have been carried out enthusiastically by people with little or no theoretical knowledge but with great practical experience. The result however, is that although many interesting lessons can be learned from practical work and the history of conceptual discussions, rather than a conceptual framework to present them to the world in – there is still only a richly coloured 'puzzle without a picture'. In this chapter some of the more typical and more interesting developments will be described and commented on. Some of the work described (including analyses) are common knowledge in the field of health education in Denmark, while there will be more personal observations and comments by the author.

Background and History

In the final decades of the last century, there was widespread debate concerning public health issues in Denmark, mostly as a result of new knowledge of the origins of bacteria and of how epidemics spread. The results of this debate could be seen in the enormous investments that were made in developing sanitation systems and clean water supplies in major Danish cities. The first phases of Denmark's industrialization took place at this time and the urban areas expanded rapidly. There was a general belief that many health problems could be solved by moving people out of the medieval city centres which were overpopulated and were constantly threatened by fire and cholera.

The Danish folk high-school movement also began at this time. Inspired by the famous poet, priest and historian Grundtvig, the unique tradition of a general adult education available to all citizens, was developed. It was here that one of the basic components of Danish health education was born: the idea of providing a basic education encompassing different humanistic and technical disciplines, to otherwise educationally deprived segments of the population.

One of the first medical resource books for the general public was published in Denmark in 1883 under the title *Huslægen* (The House Doctor). This book contained detailed advice about lifestyle, diseases and the promotion of good health.

A similar publication from the beginning of this century is also worth mentioning. The Danish physician Alfred B Olsen, (who was the director of Caterham Sanatorium near London, UK), published a 200 page book of medical advice with the visionary title 'Sundhed for alle' (Health for All) and thereby preceded the WHO programme title by more than 60 years. Including the fifth printing in 1916, the book sold more than 50,000 copies in Denmark alone. The book was also published in England and Ireland prior to the Danish edition.

The publication of disease-oriented encyclopedias for home use expanded during the 1940s and 1950s. These were often written by the country's most prominent medical experts. These volumes could best be described as books about disease information rather than health education.

In 1955 an innovative economist, E Toft Nielsen, began publishing the family magazine *Helse* (a traditional word for health), supported by the Danish Medical Association and financed by the Federation of Sick-benefits

Associations. For the past 33 years this magazine has been distributed free of charge to the Danish public and circulation has grown from 300,000 to 480,000 copies per volume. Today *Helse* is published six to eight times a year. As a consequence of the nationalization of the health insurances system in the early 1970s, the magazine is now financed by the local authorities and the Pharmacists Association. The magazine keeps the public up to date on relevant aspects of health and disease. Although the style is popular, the content is based on reliable information provided by qualified professionals.

In 1964, a national organization was formed to promote, develop and produce health education materials and to co-ordinate health education activities: The Danish Committee for Health Education (DCHE). This is sponsored by the major professional unions within the health field, as well as the association of local authorities and counties. The Ministries of Health, Social Affairs and Education (including their relevant boards) are represented on the board of advisors.

In the early 1970s, the DCHE organized a number of seminars in co-operation with the Ministry of Education. Between 1971 and 1977, professionals from the health and education sectors attended these seminars. From this activity new concepts of health education developed, the so-called 'Health pedagogic movement'.

The basic principle of the 'Health pedagogic movement' was to view health education within a broader context than before. More specifically the inclusion of social factors was emphasized, for example – working conditions, housing and lifestyles. The goal of activities based on this principle was to improve environmental and social factors and make them healthy. The idea was to provide target groups and individuals with knowledge about health, as well as familiarizing them with strategies for change. The motivation for change was to be obtained through a change in 'consciousness' resulting from the newly acquired knowledge.

The 'Health pedagogic movement' accused the traditional health education effort of being too individualistic in its approach as well as for its' tendency to focus on disease rather than health. Many of the ideas and proposals from the movement are similar to the content of the health promotion programme put forth by the World Health Organization (WHO) as exemplified in the Ottawa Charter. The 'Health pedagogic movement' succeeded in arousing new interest in health education, but many people found the methodological elements too vague and had difficulties in formulating concrete projects.

In 1976, under the influence of key members in the movement, a government commission proposed the formation of a National Prevention Council (NPC). The Danish parliament approved the proposal and The NPC was established by law in 1979. The NPC is that governmental body within the public administration (under the Ministry of Health) whose purpose is to promote health education in general. The activities of the council are best covered by the term 'health promotion' rather than the more traditional medical term prevention, which has been promoted in Denmark by enthusiastic politicians giving rise to the unintended and unfortunate phrase 'health prevention'.

Since 1984, the DCHE and the NPC have jointly published a newsletter resource journal for professionals and administrators *News on Prevention*. This joint publication reports on relevant initiatives in health promotion in Denmark. A recent survey conducted by the two organizations has revealed that even though there is a very high frequency of health education activities among public bodies and private organizations, there still exists a considerable lack of co-ordination and co-operation in the field.

Apart from the general responsibilities for health education and health promotion activities, which come under the NPC, a number of state councils, research institutions and administrative boards under the responsibility of their respective ministries, conduct health education campaigns for example: Working Environment Council (Ministry of Labour), Danish Road Safety Council (Ministry of Justice), Danish Government Home Economics Council (National Consumer Board and Ministry of Industry), Danish Council on Alcohol and Narcotics (Ministry of Health), National Board of Health (Ministry of Health), and National Board of Food (Ministry of Health).

Another campaign is worth mentioning here, as an example of an outstanding health education effort in Denmark: the AIDS campaign from the National Board of Health 1986 to 1988. This campaign is not only the most costly to date (with a budget of more than five million Danish crowns) it is also the first campaign using all available media including pamphlets, radio, television, newspaper and bus advertising, newsletters, posters and so forth. The campaign has succeeded in combining effective propaganda for condom use with very charming propaganda for a satisfying sexual life while at the same time avoiding HIV (AIDS) infection.

The AIDS campaign has played a major role in health education becoming recognized as having as much relevance as the treatment system in the eyes of the political-administrative system. A decisive factor in obtaining this political acceptance was first and foremost the potential threat of astronomic costs in treating future AIDS patients within the hospital system, which has had very little success so far in the treatment of AIDS for which there is no cure in sight. This rather bleak situation has forced politicians to invest money (more whole-heartedly than ever before) into prevention and information. It makes a strong impression, when, on national television, the most distinguished medical experts (who otherwise regard health education as desirable but not important) advocate health education as the *only* way to save the nation.

Professions active in health education

In Denmark various professions are involved in health education. Two groups are especially active, those involved in the health care system and those involved in primary school education. Their activity in the field is unfortunately too dependent on their own personal talents and interest as health education is seldom a regular part of their main job functions. In fact, it is often described as 'a very important thing to do, but we are so busy, that we seldom do it the way we would like to'.

Two exceptions are worth mentioning: health visitors and the public preventive child dentistry system.

The health visitors (nurses with specialist post-graduate training) visit, mothers with babies and small children. Their job consists of advisory and control functions and they are very active and often quite experienced in health education.

During the past 10 to 15 years the public preventive child dentistry system has demonstrated a remarkable success in that they have nearly eradicated caries among children.

The personnel employed in the preventive child dentistry clinics are dentists and dental hygienists. In Denmark, dental hygienists are the only professionals with extensive health education training as part of their basic education. The preventive child dentistry system is financed by the local authorities and the system has been so effective that the dental profession has had to focus its treatment services on the older population as the basis for its future income.

Aside from the training of dental hygienists and the health visitors, there are no formal training programmes for people interested in health education, either as basic training or as postgraduate education. Consequently, there are no jobs that require formal qualifications in health education.

There is a large variety of professions represented among people working full time in health education within the different agencies and institutions. Journalists, psychologists, sociologists (especially cultural sociologists), nurses and academics specializing in several languages – these are the most common professions represented. Physicians are relatively rare.

Many people working in health education try to improve their background by attending various courses in, for example: health planning; health economics; epidemology; use of different media and so on. There is always great interest whenever a special course in health education is offered. Many qualified applicants respond whenever a full time job in the field of health education is posted.

There is a big and rapidly growing need for specialist training in health education. The traditional university system however is very rigid, and usually takes decades to respond to emerging social needs. Some of the newer university centres are however planning courses where candidates can combine disciplines. These efforts are geared towards jobs in the rapidly expanding information sector. We can therefore expect, that before long, many relevant training programmes for health educators will be offered.

In Denmark, there are very few places where one can find more than a handful of people working together on a daily basis in the field of health education. Those who do are occupied with day to day problems and have little time for extra professional activities, which include international co-operation, that takes a lot of time and effort and gives few benefits in the short term. Some of the large associations such as the Heart Association and the Cancer Society have good international co-operation within their own fields no doubt. These contacts however are never shared with others outside their immediate circle and can hardly be considered as co-operation in the field of health education.

Among the Nordic countries co-operation exists between the national and state organizations for health education but contacts to Europe and the rest of the world are sporadic and are quite personal in character.

A great deal of interest was created by the introduction of the WHO programme 'Health for All by the Year 2000' and especially after the publication of the target document in 1984. The Health for All (HFA) Programme has inspired many new projects which contain health education elements. A Danish version of the European target document was published by the Danish Committee for Health Education in April 1985 which included recommendations by the Minister of the Interior (who at that time had responsibility for the health sector). Until now more than 18,000 copies of the book have been distributed. The ideas put forth in the HFA programme have penetrated ever deeper into the thinking of health professionals as well as becoming a part of the public debate. The HFA programme is now the common frame of reference for co-operative efforts between disciplines and sectors.

Two Danish cities have been invited to participate in the WHO 'Healthy cities' programme: Horsens (a small city with approximately 40,000 inhabitants, the smallest city in the programme) and the city of Copenhagen (the central municipality with approximately 500,000 inhabitants). As cities are difficult to reorganize within the framework of the five-year programme, most of the activities will be of a health education character involving very extensive co-operation with other cities in Europe and Denmark as part of the project.

One example of the widespread interest in HFA, is the one-day conference organized by the Danish Committee for Health Education held in February 1988. This meeting attracted more than 600 participants including professionals, politicians and administrators from all over the country. The purpose of the conference was to evaluate the effect of the HFA programme in Denmark and the result was that over 100 major initiatives were identified.

Health education as a national political issue

Health education moved from the professional scene to the political scene in 1976. There is little doubt about the motives of the politicians involved which can be seen in a report from a governmental commission on future priorities in the health sector. The rapid growth of the hospital sector had become a threat to the national economy. Health education (or prevention) served as an acceptable slogan for the unpopular cuts in the health budget. Cheap pamphlets instead of expensive hospitals. Suddenly politicians rediscovered the old phrase: 'prevention is better than cure'.

During the years that followed hypocrisy became more obvious: hospital budgets were cut, but the health education and prevention budgets were cut even more, probably because the preventive sector is so weak and therefore offers less resistance.

The widespread use of various words associated with health promotion, health education and prevention during the past decade that appeared in numerous important political speeches, has had an interesting effect on the political debate. At the beginning of this period it was obvious that the demand for health education meant budget cuts. During the 1980s an ever more sincere atmosphere developed around health education as politicians found that the theme was popular with their voters.

In the last years health education measures and health promotion projects are slowly moving from the theoretical level to the practical one. Experimentation and innovation has been encouraged by the political-administrative system and unusually large amounts of money have been made available through special administrative funds from the Ministries of Education, Social Affairs and Health. As health in Denmark is perceived in the broadest WHO definition – as a state of complete physical, psychological and social well-being – it is difficult to distinguish between adult education in general – projects promoting social well-being and health education in its widest sense. The background for the public funding of experiments on such a large scale is partly due to the fact that the public sector has been too large and costly. Politically it is very difficult to reduce it without pointing out new ways for community development based on people's *own* activity and not on public service.

Another reason for the expected growth in health education is worthy of mention. The disease pattern in Denmark, (a highly industrialized society) is dominated by accidents (mainly traffic), chronic disease (heart, cancer) and psychological-psychiatric disorders. These health problems are all very expensive and difficult to treat within the health care system. They are, however, possible to influence by strong and long-term health education, which politicians are beginning to understand. The only problem is that treatment has to continue until prevention starts to work.

Danish health education in the future

There is no doubt that health education will become a more important issue in our society. Consumer viewpoints will be given more space and the traditional authoritarian attitudes among health professionals will be substituted by more service-oriented attitudes which include better informing of patient or clients in the health care system.

There is a strong need for more and better co-ordination, co-operation and theoretical development. Research and evaluation will become a necessity as increased investment in the sector will require cost-effectiveness analysis.

The extent of future development will depend on the activities of a rather limited group of people, their goodwill and intelligent behaviour. If we succeed, we might be able to 'give the puzzle a picture'.

4. The Danish Government Home Economics Council's School Campaign 1986 to 1987: 'You become what you get to eat' – A CASE STUDY

Anelise Bredholt

Summary: The article describes a campaign aimed at school children to disseminate information about diet and nutrition. A wide range of campaign materials was produced. The campaign was split into two phases: a 6 to 12 year-old age group and a 12 to 17 year-old age group. Materials developed for both phases are described. Teacher training was an important element of the project. Promotion of the campaign through the media proved valuable.

Background

In 1984, the Danish Folketing (Parliament) adopted a resolution that established a national food policy. The resolution specified increased dissemination of information about diet and nutrition as one of several means of action.

The reason for promoting a Danish national food policy was the increasing understanding of the correlation between a wrong diet and certain diseases. More specifically, the large energy content, the biased energy distribution and the fibre deficiency of the national diet correlated with obesity, heart and vascular diseases, certain forms of cancer, and gastrointestinal diseases.

In connection with the parliamentary resolution, the Danish government Home Economics Council, which is the body responsible for public food information in Denmark, was asked to conduct a food information campaign aimed at school children (nursery school class up to, and including the tenth form). The campaign was called 'You become what you get to eat'.

Target group of the campaign

The reasons for selecting school children as the target group were as follows:

- ☐ The preventive effect of giving food information to children and young people was expected to be higher than the effect of giving information to adults.
- ☐ Children and young people represent a risk group as far as food is concerned because they are major consumers of inferior products (sweets, refreshing drinks, certain types of fast food).
- ☐ Hardly any schools in Denmark provide school meals.

☐ Teachers and health personnel in the educational system could spread the messages of the campaign during lessons and through other forms of contact with the pupils.

Campaign objectives

The Danish Government Home Economics Council established the following objectives for the campaign:

☐ to make children and young people feel like eating wholesome food;
☐ to make them interested in eating wholesome food;
☐ to increase their activity in relation to wholesome food;
☐ to make them feel responsible for their own eating habits.

The overall objective of the campaign was to influence young people's health-related behaviour in relation to nutrition. The campaign material was therefore developed for use in the practical as well as the theoretical parts of teaching subjects and was related to home meals, food at school, and food outside the home or the school.
The nutritional messages in the campaign were:

☐ wholesome meals;
☐ less sugar;
☐ less fat;
☐ coarser diets.

Campaign materials

Materials for the message conveyors

Teacher's guides were developed for teachers and the health staff (for example, the school doctor, the school nurse, and municipal dental service personnel) who would convey the campaign messages. In addition, pamphlets were prepared that gave basic knowledge on nutrition and on nutritional problems experienced by children and young people.

Materials for the pupils

In the teaching material for younger pupils, the main emphasis was on topics relating to nutritional and food studies and on the dietary recommendations of the Home Economics Council. The main emphasis in the teaching materials for older pupils was on eating habits and the psychological, socio-psychological, and sociological factors that determine them.
Both sets of materials had been developed as a varied collection of specific teaching ideas. These materials offer all teachers inspiration, guidance and plans for lessons on wholesome food, regardless of teachers' experience, the teaching time they have available for the teachers' preferred method of instruction.

For practical reasons the campaign was split into two phases: phase one, in April 1986, was the distribution of material for the 6 to 12 year-old age group (the nursery school class to the fifth form). Phase two was in December 1986 and was for the distribution of material to pupils in the sixth to tenth forms (12 to 17 year-olds). The material was circulated to all Danish schools, which are approximately 3000 in number.

Materials for nursery school class to fifth form (6 to 12 years)

Posters

The campaign poster was developed entitled 'You become what you get to eat'. It showed a selection of wholesome and unwholesome foods running a race. The food that comes first of the wholesome and unwholesome foods is purely incidental and should not be considered as an indication of the comparative wholesomeness of the particular food. Rather, the idea was that the poster would help the children to realize that wholesome food is best for them.

The balloon poster was also developed showing food divided into wholesome food (green balloon), 'watch-out' food (yellow balloon) and unwholesome food (red balloon).

Leaflets

A leaflet with the title 'You become what you get to eat' was prepared for the children. The leaflet could be read aloud to the youngest classes, and the pupils of the third to fifth forms could read it on their own. The leaflet story is about two boys. One is called 'Krumme' the other is called 'Snaske'. The name 'Krumme' is derived from crumby bread which has a connotation of energy. 'Krumme' is portrayed as a boy with good eating habits and a perfectly sound attitude to food. The name 'Snaske' has a connotation with an unappetizing mix of sweets. He has a less than sound attitude to food but starts reflecting as the story goes on. 'Krumme' is drawn as a coarse bun with cheese and 'Snaske' is a piece of pastry with chocolate.

A further leaflet with the title 'Your child becomes what it gets to eat' has been prepared for parents. This leaflet is also available in English, Arabic, Urdu–Parkisani, Yugoslav–Sebo-Croat and Turkish. It is about wholesome meals and gives general advice on diets.

Classroom Materials

Materials for use in class have been developed. The materials cover a number of issues including:

- meals of the day;
- sugar and sweets;
- fat;
- nutrition;
- recipes.

All the classroom materials are numbered – there are some 40 sheets altogether – and they come in a folder with a survey sheet. On the back of each work-sheet there are instructions as to how to use the particular sheet as well as teaching ideas. All classroom materials can freely be copied by the school.

The teacher's guide

The teacher's guide provides the necessary basic nutritional knowledge, teaching ideas, teaching programmes, a description of the campaign material, a list of media, an evaluation sheet and a materials requisition form.

The video film

The video film, 'You become what you get to eat – I' can be used as an introduction to lessons or discussions. It is about an ordinary Danish family's problems in deciding what to eat for breakfast, school-lunch, and so on. It shows how the two children in the film take the matter into their own hands.

Weight problems

The material 'Obesity in children' has been worked out on behalf of the school health service to be used in connection with children from nursery school age up to fifth form age who are moderately overweight. It consists of: material for handing to parents, material for the child and a weight records scheme (appointment card).

Material for sixth to tenth forms (12 to 17 years)

Poster

The campaign poster 'You become what you get to eat' shows a red mouth and a fork; it is designed to provoke the thought that the food which you put into your mouth will decide how you feel.

Pamphlets and leaflets

The pamphlet 'Young on a healthy diet' has been developed for the pupils and the leaflet 'Your child becomes what it gets to eat' is for parents and deals with the dietary problems of the young.

Classroom materials

Materials comprising a total of 35 worksheets are used for teaching purposes. They have the following themes:

- [ ] eating habits;
- [ ] hunger;
- [ ] school camp/overnight excursion;
- [ ] school magazine health journal.

Teacher's guide

The teacher's guide provides teaching ideas and teaching programmes on the basis of the four themes described above. In addition, suggestions are made for subject areas under which the respective topics may be raised. A list of media, a description of the campaign material, an evaluation sheet, and a materials requisition form are included in the teacher's guide.

The video film

The video film 'You become what you get to eat – II' can be used as a basis for discussion. It is about four youngsters and their views on food and eating habits.

School sales booths and school canteens

The pamphlet 'School sales booth or canteen' describes how to go about setting up a canteen or a sales booth. The pamphlet also gives ideas for increasing the variety of foods that might be sold. The purpose of including this pamphlet in the campaign material was to emphasize the importance of giving pupils the opportunity of buying wholesome food at school as an alternative to sweets, cakes and so forth from the local kiosks or bakers' shops.

Weight problems

'Reduce your weight' is a pamphlet for young people with a weight problem and for young people who imagine they have such problems. The pamphlet gives specific information and good advice on diet.

Computer-assisted learning

The Home Economics Council is engaged in developing a computer programme entitled 'You become what you get to eat' which was due to be distributed in October, 1988.

The programme design allows the pupil – and others aged 10 and over – to select a person, who may be the pupil himself or herself, and to indicate age, sex, weight and height. Food and drinks are then selected for one day. The pupil also lists the activities performed during the day. This one day then becomes the exponent of all the days in the following year.

Against the background of these choices, the pupil will see what is going to happen to the subject's body and whether there are any tendencies towards conditions such as obesity, heart or vascular diseases, cancer and constipation.

If the pupil wants a diet and a life-style different from the one first chosen, he or she may change food and activity selections. It is this phase of the programme that should give the pupil a sense of the correlation between diet, exercise and good health.

The programme also contains an information section which allows the pupil to retrieve information on food and nutrition, exercise and diet-related diseases as he or she goes along.

Circulation of campaign material

The Home Economics Council had originally fixed as their target that at least 50 per cent of the schools would use all or part of the campaign materials in their instruction. Nutrition teaching is only incorporated into the syllabuses for domestic studies, which has two or three weekly periods at the sixth form level (12 to 13 year-olds). In addition, the subject of domestic studies is optional in the eighth to tenth forms.

In the event, the demand exceeded all expectation. By 1 July 1987, over 85 per cent of schools had ordered supplementary material from the Home Economics Council after receiving the 'Free materials package – I' in April and the 'Free materials package – II' in December 1986.

Use of campaign materials in teaching

No systematic investigation has been conducted into how schools have used the campaign materials. Feedback from schools suggests that the materials have been used in very different ways and that they adapt easily to the methods of instruction used in the individual schools, in the individual classes, and by the individual teacher. The following are examples of ways in which the campaign materials have been used. They have been used:

- ☐ in connection with projects dealing with pupils' immediate environment;
- ☐ in theme courses, theme days and theme weeks on subjects relating to health;
- ☐ during examinations of their eating habits and those of their friends with subsequent evaluation of diets and guidance on diets;
- ☐ to examine the food on offer in the school sales booth, the school canteen and in local shops;
- ☐ during the preparation of wholesome food;
- ☐ during visits to factories;
- ☐ in exhibitions of wholesome foods;
- ☐ during parents' meetings;
- ☐ in dramatic activities to do with food and diet.

Home Economics Council's campaign marketing courses for teachers and others

At the time of sending out the material, the Home Economics Council offered short-term courses for teachers and the schools' health staff. These courses have received nation-wide interest from many related groups and agencies, such as teachers of domestic studies, other teachers, school doctors, school nurses, personnel with the municipal children's dental service and canteen staff.

Cultivating the media

In connection with the circulation of the two sets of classroom materials, the Home Economics Council sent out press releases and held press conferences. Professional and trade journals have received campaign material or articles on the campaign. Radio and television stations have been offered interviews or other contributions to programmes.

The campaign was broadcast by Radio Denmark's TV section in January 1988. The duration of broadcast was approximately one hour.

The Home Economics Council has paid for two features on the campaign in the OBS (an acronym for information to the citizens about society) spots on Denmark's Radio. These have been broadcast approximately ten times.

Such cultivation of the media has resulted in positive coverage of the campaign. This has been partly in the form of publicity before the material was circulated, and partly as features describing the work at the schools in the local communities.

Measuring the effect

In 1985, prior to launching the campaign, the target group was subjected to a base-line measurement of their nutritional knowledge and activities in connection with food. The effect of the campaign was to be measured during the Autumn of 1988.

Carrying the campaign further

In order to follow up on the campaign, the Home Economics Council distributed supplementary material to schools during the Autumn of 1987.

Early in 1988 the campaign was extended with the production of materials for the sports and athletics sector.

5. A transition from health education to health promotion – AN OVERVIEW

Eugene Donoghue and Anna-May Harkin

Summary: Early emphasis was on the prevention of illness. The Health Act (1970) constituted health boards which took on the responsibility for health education. In 1970, the Minister of Health established the Health Education Bureau (HEB) which was given eight specific functions. In 1982, the HEB adopted a life cycle model of health education as a framework for future developments. The HEB's main areas of activity are: positive health promotion and public education; formal education, training and development programmes; and research, evaluation and information services. The transition from health education to health promotion during the mid-1980s is described. The new health promotion structure consists of: a health promotion unit to be located in the Department of Health; a cabinet sub-committee on health promotion; and an advisory council on health promotion. This structure gives explicit recognition to the multiplicity of factors underlying health problems.

Introduction

The opportunity to document the history and development of health education in Ireland is timely. The newly established health promotion unit in the Department of Health is one year in existence. Its creation is the culmination of a progressive movement towards integrating health education activities into the broad considerations involved in health promotion.

In this chapter we will consider the history and development of health education by examining: the underlying policies; the operational structures for delivery; the issues and activities dealt with and the main target groups. The intention is to give the reader some insight into the rationale informing and guiding current developments in health promotion.

Historical overview

In common with other countries in the western world, Ireland traditionally dealt with health education under the general heading of prevention of illness. Ireland gave a priority to services of a curative nature aimed at the alleviation or cure of symptoms and signs of physical or mental illness in individuals. Services were also in place aimed at preventing the development of illness, through provision of antenatal care, immunization, inspections of food and water, and in more recent years the provision of health education and information to individuals, groups and the public in general.

Since 1970, the provision of health services in Ireland has been entrusted to eight regional health boards, responsible for providing services at local level and overseen by elected local representatives under the general direction of the Minister for Health. The Health Act of 1970, which constituted the health boards, also entrusted them with statutory responsibility for the dissemination of health information which has broadly been interpreted as a responsiblity for health education (Health Act 1970). From the early 1980s many of the health boards employed personnel in the capacity of health education officers/co-ordinators. Health boards identified their own priority areas for health education and many of them have put in place services aimed at schools, community groups, industry, youth and such like. The development of these local initiatives resulted in giving access to health education to families and individuals in an immediate personal way.

The voluntary sector has traditionally played an important role in health education in Ireland. A number of major organizations, for example The Irish Heart Foundation, The Irish Cancer Society, The Mental Health Association of Ireland, The Dental Health Foundation and the Irish National Council on Alcoholism, have been active nationally and in local communities (through schools, women's groups, youth organizations and so on) in education and training activities aimed at prevention of illness related to their own interest area.

The National Health Education Bureau (HEB)

Formal recognition of the need at national level for health education came in February 1975 when the Minister for Health established the HEB, under the Health Corporate Bodies Act of 1961. The HEB was set up principally in response to recommendations of the Committee on Drug Education made in April 1974. This committee recommended that 'a health education authority be set up as a matter of urgency to supply the needs of health education and to co-ordinate the existing efforts'. This body was responsible for advising the Minister on the formulation of policy in relation to health education and for co-ordinating the development and provision of health education programmes.

The particular functions of the HEB were:

a. to advise the Minister on the aspects of health education that should have priority at national level;

b. to draw up, in accordance with the agreed national priorities, programmes of health education for promotion at national and local level;

c. to carry out such programmes with the co-operation of the statutory and voluntary bodies engaged in health education;

d. to maintain contact with voluntary bodies engaged in particular aspects of health education and, in accordance with the agreed national priorities, to give financial assistance to such bodies as appropriate and to the extent that the resources of the Bureau will permit;

e. to provide statutory and voluntary bodies engaged in health education with help in carrying out their local programmes, including the production and distribution of educational material;

f. to promote and conduct research and to evaluate health education activities;

g. to act as a national centre of expertise and knowledge in all aspects of health education;

h. to promote greater concern for health education generally in the community.

By the early 1980s the HEB recognized the need for a more comprehensive framework within which to carry out its work. In 1982, staying within its remit for health education, it adopted a life-cycle model of health education as a framework for the future development of programmes. This model identified key issues, phases and needs at each stage from pre-birth to old age. It facilitated identification of priority target groups. The overall aim was to provide means/opportunities for people to protect, maintain and improve their health as far as educational methods permit. The main areas of activities were:

a. positive health promotion and public education;
b. formal education, training and development programmes;
c. research, evaluation and information services.

Positive health promotion and public education

Television, radio, press, pamphlets and public relations were the main educational media used under this heading. Publicity campaigns were organized generally as part of an overall educational strategy to alert the general public to messages advocating healthy behaviour. The subject matter was based on priorities identified by the Minister for Health and the HEB and included such issues as smoking; responsibility in alcohol use; healthy eating; hygiene; health in later life; dental health; immunization against childhood illnesses such as measles and whooping cough, AIDS, healthy lifestyles and safety.

Formal education, training and development programmes

The education and training division was mainly responsible for the initiation, development and implementation of health education program- mes aimed at particular target audiences. These included; primary and second level schools, teacher training colleges, universities, technical colleges, and professional groups including teachers, general practitioners, nurses, social workers and dentists. This division also worked closely with youth groups, women's groups and self help groups. Much of the work was carried out in co-operation with health boards. Educational packs were developed on particular health issues and targeted at special audiences, for example packs for schools on hygiene, alcohol, drugs, nutrition, smoking and packs for community groups – for example on drugs and women's issues. As part of the process of mobilizing support for health education, the

HEB brought groups together from time to time, to discuss issues and share ideas in seminars and conferences.

A major in-service teacher training initiative was developed and implemented by the HEB in 1983. This training programme was designed to introduce teachers to the concepts and methods appropriate to teaching health education. The course was an in-service one over a four year period, and was attended by over 2,000 teachers from schools throughout the country. This programme of training was one of a number of training courses on offer at that time. Some health boards had also initiated teacher training courses to support teachers in their work in schools. Some of these schemes have gained prominence nationally and their personnel are involved in helping developments in other regions. Recently many of the teachers involved in these training programmes have been meeting with a view to forming a national school health education association.

The HEB also undertook education and training activities jointly with the many voluntary organizations who had been traditionally active in health education. Together they produced numerous booklets, leaflets, videos and organized training courses. The voluntary sector provided the HEB with invaluable expertise and knowledge as well as access to relevant target groups.

Research, evaluation and information services

To provide an informed base from which to carry out its work, the HEB engaged in a variety of research and evaluation activities. Among major national research studies carried out were the following:

1. smoking and drinking behaviour;
2. people's beliefs and practices in relation to health and illness;
3. attitudes to mental handicap;
4. nutrition beliefs and practices – including regular surveys of the level of breast-feeding.

Research was also conducted into aspects of school programmes, lifestyle patterns related to work and leisure, sociological factors associated with depression in women and selected aspects of health in a rural Irish community. Literature research was conducted on a number of health education topics. Pilot studies were conducted on several educational packs. Pre-testing, monitoring and evaluation formed an integral part of several mass media campaigns.

The HEB Library and Information Service was developed as a national resource centre for health education materials including books and videos which were available on loan to health education workers. Up-to-date resource lists were prepared on particular health education topics and provided information on relevant books, articles and organizations.

The transition from health education to health promotion

By the mid-1980s the HEB, on the basis of its own experience in an Irish context and from its contacts with international agencies in the field, became increasingly aware of the need for the development of healthier public policies. However responsibility for this wider dimension of health promotion lay outside its own remit. It decided to adopt an advocacy role and began a process of informing and educating health and education workers and policy makers with regard to health promotion. To this end a series of meetings, seminars and conferences were organized. Many of these meetings included participants and colleagues from other countries, from the International Union for Health Education and from the WHO Euro Office.

One of the first of the conferences which the HEB organized in late 1984 was on the theme of 'Value for effort – social and economic aspects of health education/health promotion'. This conference was the first major airing of health promotion issues in the health services in Ireland. In his opening address, the Minister for Health referred to the need for a health promotion approach:

> There are many types of situations which require changes in organizational structures to ensure that each government department becomes aware that almost every aspect of government policy contains a critical health element. (Health Education Bureau, 1984) .

Many of the issues and dilemmas involved in the transition from education of individuals and groups to the wider approach of promoting healthy public policy were discussed at the 12th World Conference on Health Education which was sponsored by the International Union for Health Education and hosted in Dublin by the HEB in 1985. Subsequent to that conference, the HEB sought and obtained approval from the then Minister to prepare a report on the issues to be addressed in setting out to promote health through public policy. The HEB then established an intersectoral group with the following terms of reference:

1. to demonstrate the need for a health promotion policy for the health and well being of the people on both economic and epidemiological grounds;
2. to draw up a model for a multi-sectoral approach to health issues at national level;
3. to illustrate the application of this model through selected issues.

In January 1987 the findings of the group were released in the report 'Promoting Health through Public Policy' (Health Education Bureau, 1987). The report examined the considerations involved in health promotion; it pointed to compelling arguments for it and outlined its main implications. It recommended structural arrangements as esssential elements in the initiation of a health promotion policy.

The Department of Health itself published a document 'Health – the wider dimensions' (Department of Health, 1986) which dealt with similar considerations but was different in that it examined the implications of a new health promotion policy on the health services as a whole. Both reports were supportive of the need for a shift in policy towards promotion of health and prevention of illness.

New delivery structure for health promotion

In 1987 the Minister for Health, following considerable discussion (Health Education Bureau, 1987, Department of Health, 1986) took on board the broader issues of a healthy public policy and announced that he proposed to set up a new health promotion structure. This consisted of a health promotion unit to be located within the Department of Health, a cabinet sub-committee on health promotion and an advisory council on health promotion.

The Health Promotion Unit

An executive unit located within the Department of Health, replaced the HEB with effect from January 1988. The functions and activities of the HEB were transferred to this new unit which was also given a broader remit for the development of an inter-sectoral policy on health promotion.

The Cabinet Sub-Committee on Health Promotion

This is chaired by the Minister for Health and consists of the Ministers for Agriculture, Education, Energy, Environment and Labour. This sub-committee facilitates the discussion of intersectoral health issues at the highest level.

The Health Promotion Advisory Council

This has a membership drawn from a wide cross section of interests impinging on the health of people: agriculture, nutrition, environment, life insurance, local authorities, youth, sport, women's groups, voluntary organizations, and suchlike. The Council's function is to examine the various influences that determine the quality of people's health, to identify priority areas for action and to recommend measures that are likely to advance the health of the individual.

An Academic Base

This is recognized by the Department of Health as an important complement to the work of the Health Promotion Unit. The Department is currently examining how best this should be structured. The establishment of this academic base will represent a further significant phase in the development of Ireland's health promotion structure.

The Health Promotion Unit, already mentioned, is the national executive unit for health promotion. Its work programme reflects a broad inter-sectoral orientation. In addition to health service-based programmes such as immunization, the Unit is currently involved in developing policies on a range of issues including nutrition; smoking; alcohol; safety and exercise. In this process the Unit is involving other government departments and a range of interested groups in the voluntary commercial, professional and educational sectors.

The new structure of health promotion in Ireland gives explicit recognition to the multiple factors underlying contemporary health problems and the need for the co-ordination of health promoting policies on an intersectoral basis. The development outlined in this chapter takes cognizance of the fact that education, for health or any other aspect of life, does not take place in a vacuum and can scarcely hope to be effective if its messages are being ignored or undermined by the policies and activities of other sectors of society. It is implicit in the developments that a more coherent and integrated approach will lead to greater acceptance and effectiveness when policies are implemented.

References

Department of Health (1986) *Health – The Wider Dimensions* Dublin

Health Act (1970) Government Publications Office, Molesworth Street, Dublin 2.

Health Education Bureau (1984) *Value for effort – social and economic aspects of health education health promotion,* proceedings of a conference held in Athlone in 1984

Health Education Bureau (1987) *Promoting Health Through Public Policy* Dublin

6. North Western Health Board of the Republic of Ireland: lifeskills programme for schools – A CASE STUDY

Brian McAuley

Summary: In 1978, the North Western Health Board set up a health promotion programme in their schools to promote the health of young people in the region. The project team responsible decided to adopt a 'lifeskills' approach and key skills were identified. In 1981, the programme was piloted in 11 of the 50 second level schools in the region. Over the following five years the programme was introduced into all the schools. Since 1986, the project has been in a 'maintenance' phase supporting schools and promoting fresh developments. Typically, in the first three years of the programme, the emphasis is on health topics. In the final two years, the approach is more skills-based. Active learning strategies predominate in the programme and the in-service teacher training has reflected this. Parental involvement has been a feature of school developments. Evaluations of the programme have been positive although further work is needed to build on the programme's achievements.

Introduction

The North Western Health Board is one of eight health boards in the Republic of Ireland and serves a population of some 212,000 people in three counties – Donegal, Sligo and Leitrim. Over the past ten years, the board has been active in setting up a programme of health education for the 20,000 second level students in the region.

Establishing the programme

At a seminar on school health education in 1978, teachers in second level schools in the area called on the health board to set up health education programmes in their schools. The chief executive officer of the board responded to the teachers' request by setting up a working party in 1979 under the chairmanship of an area medical officer. The working party was made up of teachers, school administrators and health board personnel, and produced a report in 1980 under the title 'Report on health education in second level schools' (Brenner, 1980). This working party report was immediately adopted as board policy.

Working party report

The working party report advocated the establishment of 'a programme of health education that would minimize the risks of disease and injury resulting wholly or in part from ignorance, habits and ways of living'. The programme should promote human relationships, the lessening of stress, a more effective use of leisure, and an ability to adapt to the problems arising from technological and scientific developments. It should be shared by schools, parents and the community and would have as its objective the development of 'a person with enough knowledge of health, among other things, to promote a reasonable chance of leading a healthy and responsible life'.

The report recognized that education for health needs to take place not only in the cognitive area, through information-giving, but also through the development of personal attributes that will facilitate health-promoting habits and ways of living. It included 22 recommendations covering teacher training, programme content, parental involvement and methods of implementing a programme.

The community care division of the health board was given responsibility for organizing the resources necessary to implement the recommendations of the working party, and in 1981 a project team was established consisting of a school guidance counsellor and a social worker.

Objective

The underlying objective of the North Western Health Board's intervention in schools is to promote the health of the young people in the region. It is generally accepted that much of the illness that occurs in later life is the result of decisions made earlier, often during school years, for example cancers brought on by smoking. Consequently the health board was anxious to intervene at an early stage in promoting the health of the population.

The lifeskills approach

The project team adopted the lifeskills approach (see Hopson and Scally 1981) as an appropriate model of health education. Implicit in this approach is the notion that it is not sufficient simply to have information about health matters in order to adopt a healthy lifestyle. People need to develop positive attitudes to health and to use a range of personal skills so that they can take responsibility for themselves. This approach stresses action in relation to health behaviours which is based on knowledge, critical analysis, and the ability to make decisions and choices and to act on them. The lifeskills approach also recognizes that any individual can be hampered in acting in this way by a range of constraints which make it difficult to assess a situation, or to have access to information that is relevant to the situation, or indeed to possess the confidence and ability to cope with it. The fundamental objective of the lifeskills approach is to overcome these constraints by developing self-empowerment in the individual. This self-empowerment (Hopson and Scally 1981) is enabled by combining relevant information with the development of a range of attributes and skills which include self-acceptance, an ability to question, analyse, and clarify, and to exercise choice. Particular stress is placed on recognizing and integrating value systems and informed effective decision-making and action in relation to values.

The teaching approach emphasizes the development of self-esteem and of an internal locus of control, the promotion of healthy values and their expression in healthy action through skill development and informed decision making (McLooner and McAuley, 1985).

Key skills

The following seven key skills were identified by the North Western Health Board Project as particularly relevant to the promotion of health and well-being:

☐ communication skills;
☐ relationship building skills;
☐ self-esteem skills;
☐ time management skills;
☐ the skills of maintaining physical well-being;
☐ decision-making skills;
☐ assertiveness skills.

Implementing the programme

The target group for the project was all 50 second level schools in the region. It was envisaged that the schools would undertake the work themselves and that the project team would provide training, materials and consultancy. There is a number of geographical and organizational challenges in providing support to schools in the north western region. An area of great natural beauty, it is nevertheless mountainous for the most part and sparsely populated. Outlying schools are separated by a distance of nearly two hundred miles and they range in size from 1300 pupils to just 95 pupils. In addition, there are four different management structures ranging from local authority control through central government control to private ownership.

Assumptions

In setting out to establish the programme the project team made a number of assumptions, namely, that:

☐ The primary task was to create conditions so that health education programmes would be taught in all schools.
☐ A coherent rationale would be communicated to teachers so that they might be motivated to take on, what was in effect, a voluntary programme.
☐ The major resource input from the board would be teacher training and that this would be done on a gradual basis over a number of years.
☐ Teachers have a range of teaching skills and these could be extended by introducing new teaching methods.
☐ The many excellent curricula in health education and lifeskills that had

been developed would be made available to schools which would provide a starting point for the work.

☐ Teachers should have an important say in the planning and organization of the work.

Introducing the programme

In early 1981, all the second level schools in the North Western Health Board's area were invited by letter to participate in a health education curriculum initiative on a pilot basis. Of the 50 schools approached, 11 responded positively at that time, and a meeting was held with the principals and some teachers from these schools. In the following format for introducing a health education programme it was decided that:

1. The programme would begin in the new school year.
2. The programme would be timetabled for one class period per week.
3. There would be a co-ordinator of the programme in each school.
4. The health board would provide teacher training and teaching materials.
5. The programme would begin with first year students and, in succeeding years, progress to all other classes in the school.

The programme began with a series of two-day in-service training sessions for teachers. These introductory courses included workshops on a rationale for health education in schools, detailed programme planning for the coming year, and experiential work on methods and teaching approaches. The training continued at weekends during the first year with sessions on specific personal skills and topic areas such as drugs, first aid, and relationships and sex education.

A five-year programme was developed for introducing the programme to all schools on a phased basis and through all classes within those schools. The programme was introduced to schools in a series of clearly defined steps:

1. The principal teacher was contacted or an inquiry was received from the school.
2. A member of the project team visited the school and informed the head teacher of the programme rationale and the requirements for implementing it within the school.
3. The head teacher would then discuss the matter with the staff and later invite a member of the project to explain the programme to the staff.
4. Teachers volunteered to teach the programme and a school co-ordinator was appointed.
5. An in-service training course was organized and the programme started with the first year group in the school.

During this period the health board, through the project team offered support to schools in:

1. assisting schools in setting up and organizing a programme;
2. training teachers;
3. providing teaching materials in health education;
4. setting up resource centres for teachers;

5. producing a newsletter;
6. planning evaluation;
7. providing a consultancy and problem-solving service to schools;
8. facilitating 'staff days' for all the staff in schools.

Towards school autonomy

By 1986, all schools in the region had introduced a lifeskills programme and the project team embarked on the third phase of the work – helping schools to become autonomous in running their own programmes. During this period, government cutbacks in education seemed set to marginalize the lifeskills programme which was a local initiative in an otherwise nationally directed curriculum. The project team developed a strategic plan with the main aim of making schools take on responsibility for their own programme. The main features of the plan were as follows:

1. the development of a school policy in each school in relation to health education;
2. the establishment of an informal contract between each school and the board in relation to the provision of services and the delivery of a health education programme;
3. the development of the role of school co-ordinators as managers of the programme within their schools;
4. the establishment of a syllabus planning committee in each school;
5. the development of suitable teaching materials;
6. the establishment of a training group among the teachers themselves;
7. the development of closer links between home and school;
8. the establishment of a health education programme in primary schools;
9. the development of the concept of 'the health promoting school'.

A series of meetings was held between school principals and senior health board management during 1987 and each school agreed to the new proposals. An agreement between each school and the board was drawn up and most schools have set up a health education committee to plan a suitable syllabus, organize teacher training and to monitor the programme within the school. Training workshops for co-ordinators have been held and will continue during the next two years. Teaching manuals are in preparation and draft copies are in use in schools for the past two years. A training group was set up in 1985 and was given an intensive course in teacher training. This group has undertaken much of the additional training which takes place during the school year. Working groups on primary school health education and on the 'health-promoting school' concept will be set up in 1988.

As the programme moves into a 'maintenance phase' the health board is committed to maintaining its support and to stimulating new approaches and developments in school health education.

The programme

As noted above the working party suggested a number of subject areas which could be included in a health education programme. These included relationships, smoking, drugs, alcohol, personal hygiene, accident prevention and first aid. The subject areas provided a context for classwork in the early stages of the project. However, as teachers' understanding of the nature of lifeskills and health education developed there was a move towards a more skills-based approach. This included direct teaching of such personal skills as assertiveness, working in groups, developing self-esteem and stress management and also the use of skills in developing health topics like drugs, accident prevention and body maintenance. For example when dealing with the issue of 'smoking', attention would be paid to the development of such skills as making decisions about tobacco use and assertiveness in managing peer pressure as well as to actual information about the dangers to health of tobacco as illustrated in Figure 6.1.

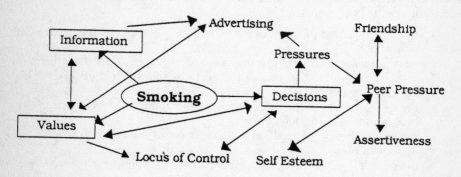

Figure 6.1 *The issue of smoking*

The programme has developed a more skills-based approach with senior classes. In teaching the lifeskill 'how to be assertive', the subject matter relates to the age and stage of development of the student and his or her real life experiences:

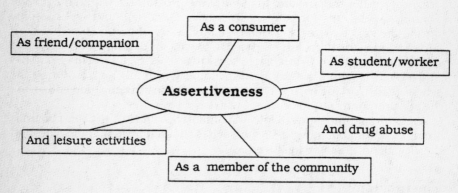

Figure 6.2 *Assertiveness and related contexts*

The time provided in schools for lifeskills teaching is admittedly small. Teachers, consequently, must make careful decisions about the priorities for their classwork. The project team worked with teachers on a number of frameworks of skill development such as the 'lifeskills model' (Hopson and Scally 1981), the 'life career approach' (Super, 1975), and the 'Foroige personal effectiveness model' (Cleary, unpublished). Teachers were also trained in undertaking 'needs assessment' surveys with their classes using a

Year	Subject area	Skills involved in...
First Year	Change to a new school	Transition making
		Problem solving
		Study skills
	Relationships	Working in groups
		Self esteem
	Hygiene	Body Cleanliness
		Dental Hygiene
		Social Implications
	Drug Education	Smoking
		Alcohol
		Assertiveness
		Decision making
	Safety	Pedestrian skills
		Basic First Aid skills
	Growth and Development	Self Esteem
		Changes at Puberty
	Environmental Health	Litter
		Community Action
Second Year	Relationships	Building self confidence
		Making friends
	Safety	Accident skills
		First Aid Skills
	Leisure Education	Time management
		Community analysis
	Drug Education	Alcohol
		Assertiveness
		Substance abuse
	Environmental Health	Pollution
		Community work
Third Year	Decision Making	Career options
		Drugs
	Relationships	Friendships
		Sex Education
	Body Maintenance	Nutrition
		Fitness
	Safety	First Aid skills
		Swimming accidents

Table 6.1 *A typical programme for years 1–3*

variety of methods such as student questionnaires, specially designed classes and open-ended interest surveys. Parents were often involved in this process.

When designing appropriate learning experiences, teachers were trained to take into account the age and stage of development of the pupil; issues of local concern such as: alcohol abuse or farm accidents; their own perceptions of students' needs; the stated interests of the students and relevant epidemiological research. In theory, each teacher then develops a syllabus suited to his or her own class group. In practice, year groups within schools co-ordinate their work. A spiral curriculum has been developed which deals with similar topics and skills in different years taking into account the ability and maturity of students. Over the years it has been possible to discern a general trend in the work undertaken by the majority of teachers (See Tables 6.1 and 6.2).

Table 6.2 *A typical programme for years 4 and 5*

Year	Subject area	Skills involved in...
Fourth Year	Transitions	Managing transitions New relationships Career education
	Relationships	Communication skills Negative emotions
	Working in Groups	Leadership skills Cooperation
	Drug Education	
Fifth Year	Stress Management Study skills Home making skills Job Finding skills Goal setting Relationships	 Parenting Sex education AIDS education

Teaching materials

The North Western Health Board has made available to schools a wide range of teaching materials from which teachers could plan their lessons. Over the past number of years members of the project team have developed classroom materials suited to the particular approach and needs of teachers in the north west region. These will be published over the next few years.

Methodology and training

The methods appropriate to health education are those commonly used in personal and social education in schools. Small group discussion is widely used and informal teaching techniques such as role play, artwork, visualization and drama are among the teaching methods employed. The majority of teachers working on the programme reported that the methods and approach consistent with the health education ethos differ significantly from those traditionally used in the teaching of other school subjects. Consequently a heavy emphasis has been placed by the lifeskills project on training for teachers who are to participate in the programme. In the course of the evaluation research it was found that the vast majority of teachers felt that training was of the utmost significance for the satisfactory implementation of the programme (Hilliard, 1986). The importance of training was also appreciated by the majority of school principals, although not as fully as it is by those who actually take lifeskills classes. Each teacher attends a two-day introductory in-service course at the beginning of each school year which includes workshops on planning, teaching methods and the teaching of specific skills. During the school year, workshops are provided outside of school time on a range of topics, usually requested by the teachers, such as relationships and sex education, drug education, communication skills, consumer skills, environment education, personal development, drama, role play, study skills, creative techniques, and so on. Training for lifeskills teaching is widely regarded by teachers as making a major contribution both to their classroom performance and to individual development. Some of the benefits noted are as follows:

□ improvement in classroom management;
□ improvement in ability to relate to pupils;
□ development of preparation skills in relation to teaching;
□ development of confidence as teachers and in one's own life;
□ improved relationships in general;
□ more tolerance of others;
□ greater ability to analyse situations;
□ more respect for pupils and for others in general;
□ more questioning of own attitudes, values and behaviour.

Parental involvement

The working party report emphasized the role of parents in health education. The project team has encouraged schools to involve parents in their programmes and members of the team have attended meetings of parents in a large number of schools.

Programmes for parents have been organized in a number of schools and training workshops for teachers to help them run such programmes have been developed. These 'lifeskills for parents' programmes usually take place once a week in the evening time over a period of six weeks and are facilitated by teachers. The common themes at the meetings have been:

a. communication with teenagers;
b. fostering self esteem in my children;
c. values;

d. sex education;
e. dealing with conflicts;
f. decision making.

Parents have evaluated the sessions and they have found them very useful. They report increased awareness of their own and their children's situations. Parents have also reported that they develop more confidence through sharing ideas with other parents and that the sessions have provided them with insights into how they might be of assistance in dealing with the children's problems.

In some schools parents have participated in devising the syllabus for health education within the school under the guidance of the lifeskills teachers. Special seminars for parents are being devised for each year group so that the work of the programme in school can be more closely linked to the home.

Evaluation

An external evaluator was appointed to the programme in 1984. Using an illuminative and qualitative approach, the evaluator selected six schools for special attention and studied work in 23 other schools. A wide range of evaluation techniques were used including: classroom observation; semi-structured interviews with teachers and principals; group discussions with pupils; students' essays; standardized tests and participant observation at training sessions. In all, 92 interviews were held with teachers and principals over a ten-week period in the school year 1985 to 1986. An evaluation report was presented to the Board in 1987. The findings indicated that outcomes from the programme have been both significant and positive for the vast majority of teachers at a personal as well as at a professional level. The programme also had an identifiable impact on pupils in six specific lifeskills areas. There is also a growing awareness among school personnel of the implications of the philosophy of empowerment for the school as an institution. The evaluator identified a number of factors especially relevant to the successful implementation of the programme. These include an awareness of the need for such an educational innovation, 'voluntarism' in undertaking lifeskills teaching, the active support of the school management and participation in training. The evaluator concluded by commending the lifeskills programme as:

> having a significant and beneficial impact in the educational world of not only the north western region, but also in other health education quarters. None the less, while goodwill certainly exists towards the lifeskills programme in the schools visited in the course of the evaluation research, it would be misleading to equate goodwill with commitment. Considerable work continues to be needed to build on what is emerging as an important and successful educational innovation (Hilliard, 1986).

References

Brenner, H (1980) *Report on Health Education Second Level Schools* North Western Health Board, Manorhamilton

Cleary, M B (Unpublished) *The Foroige Personal Effectiveness Model* Foroige, Dublin

Hilliard, B (1986) *NWHB Lifeskills Programme for Schools –. External Evaluation* Health Education Office, Donegal

Hopson, B and Scally, M (1981) *Lifeskills Teaching* McGraw-Hill, London

McLoone, S and McAuley, B (1985) *The Lifeskills Programme for Schools in the North Western Health Board Region* North Western Health Board, Manorhamilton.

Super, D E (1975) Vocational Guidance: Emergent Decision Making in a Changing Society *Bulletin of the International Association for Educational and Vocational Guidance* **29.**

7. Health Education in Spain – AN OVERVIEW

Pilar Najera

Summary: In Spain, the movement towards decentralization of control of many public services, including health, with the creation of 17 autonomous communities and their own governmental structure, has been taking place since 1978 and is still proceeding. Fourteen of the 17 communities now provide a service in Health Education.

Historically, health propaganda can first be identified in 1934 in the government 'public health structure' and important work between 1940 and 1960 in the 'Mother and child' preventive programme is well recognized. A programme of 'Food and nutrition education' commencing in 1961 is suggested as marking the beginning of an expanding health education programme which now involves its identification within many different agencies.

A law passed in 1986 includes a statement on the systematic adoption of action for health education and each of the 17 autonomous communities acknowledges this in a similar way. The first health education training course of 80 hours was run in 1978 for provincial health service personnel. Since this date, more time and stature has been given to health education courses but, as yet, there is no separate profession of health educators. Health education remains a component of professional training within the health care and teaching professions.

Collaboration with other countries and the support of the WHO are benefits felt within the country. The aims of health education in Spain are far reaching. The main health problems are those common to developed countries.

The country

Spain, with a surface area of 504.782 square kilometres has a population of 38 million inhabitants with a life expectancy at birth of 76 years and a natality rate of 13.58, a general mortality rate of 7.8. and an infant mortality rate of 9.0 per 1000 live births.

From the 1978 Constitution: Spain is passing through a process of decentralization to 17 autonomous communities with their respective governments that are progressively receiving responsiblities in different fields. For instance, four of them are autonomous on health matters and six on educational matters.

Historical data

From 1934, in the governmental public health structure, there was a section on health propaganda. Health education played an important role in the mother and child preventive programme, especially during the difficult years of the 1940s and 1950s. But to find health education as the essence and main objective of a programme we have to turn to the Programme for Food and Nutrition Education, started in 1961.

In 1962 an attempt was made, with the technical assistance of WHO to create a health education section within the National School of Public Health but it was not established until 1973 and given the practical means to function only in 1975. Also the health education section of the General Directorate of Health was created in 1974 and began its work in July 1975.

In the meantime a Spanish committee on health education, established by the tenacity of some health professionals, worked and held The Sixth International Conference of the International Union of Health Education in 1976.

With the political change in the following years, the new constitution of 1978, the creation of the Ministry of Health, the decentralization of the country to autonomous communities and the progressive transfer of responsibilities to them, health education has been developed to its present status.

Concepts of health education

Although for some Spaniards, even some doctors, health education is perceived as the transmission of knowledge about health, prevention of disease and acceptance of doctor's prescriptions, the concept of health education has changed because its main objectives have also expanded from a focus on individual responsibility for health and the corresponding change of behaviour to include a consideration of conditions of living and socio-cultural factors on health and lifestyles related to health.

Health education then, is mainly directed at developing a critical judgement of the physical and socio-cultural environment where people live and at creating the knowledge, attitudes and abilities that the population needs to improve its living conditions. This capacity will be acquired with the help of health educators, who have the task of enabling people to achieve their fullest health potential, of advocating good health and of mediating with other sectors of society, governmental or not, to create supportive environments for lifestyles conducive to health.

These ideas, taken from the documents of the conferences of Alma Ata, Ottawa and Adelaide and spread to Spanish health educators and personnel responsible for health services, are theoretically accepted but not yet developed in practice, due to the inertia of working attitudes and the rigidity of administrative structures.

The new General Health Law, passed in April 1986, enumerates the goals of public health administrations. Article 6 intends: 'To produce individual and social interest in health by means of the appropriate health education of the population'. Article 18 puts the first requirement of the health system as: 'Systematic adoption of action for health education as the main element for the improvement of individual and community health'.

All the legislative health texts of the autonomous communities acknow-ledge health education in a similar way.

A change has also taken place in the attitude of the people, who in recent years have moved from being passive and receptive to being responsible and participant in all aspects of life and also in the specific field of health education. The participation of the community in the formulation of health policy and the control of its implementation is a prerequisite demanded by the General Health Law. The rights of the users of the health system, the criteria and the bodies for the democratic participation of the people are clearly specified by law. But still the implementation of participation is in its early stages.

Professions involved in the delivery of health education

According to the traditional medical model of health education, doctors, and consequently nurses, are the professionals mainly involved in the delivery of health education. They are considered by the population and by themselves as the source of knowledge about health matters. The widen-ing of the view from medical practice to include social aspects related to the care of patients, mainly chronic ones, has involved in the practice of health education a number of other professionals working as a team, especially in primary health care services: social workers, psychologists, physiotherap-ists, and others.

Pharmacists have been engaged in health education for many years in several ways but mainly through the relationship that they establish over the counter with the people who buy medicines. Their implication in aspects of food hygiene and nutrition is another field in which they provide information and influence the attitudes of the population.

In a country where the problems of zoonoses (Malta fever, hydatic cysts, and so on) are still important, veterinarians also play an important role in education about these health risks especially in rural areas. Since their work involves food hygiene and the control of the health aspects of services such as slaughterhouses, food industries, markets, restaurants, and so forth they have an important role in the health education of food handlers and of the general population.

Teachers, as general educators, are another professional group usually involved in health education activities. Most of the programmes developed in this field in Spain are either health-service centred or school based and these ones generally are the result of a collaborative effort of school personnel and professionals of the health service, mainly school doctors and nurses. At the moment, and related to an important reform of primary and secondary education in Spain, the Ministry of Education, with the collaboration of the Ministry of Health is implementing the integration of health education both in primary and secondary general education. Some of the autonomous communities, such as Cataluna, Andalucia and Ara-gon, have already implemented programmes of integration of this subject in their school curricula. Teachers then become responsible for this en-deavour.

Some other professionals are engaged in health education in the health aspects of their work. For instance, the agricultural extension services, depending on the Ministry of Agricultural have field personnel working in rural areas especially to help in the production, preservation and use of foods. They are trained as health educators in food and nutrition by the Ministry of Health. Some others, such as community development professionals, journalists, and suchlike also collaborate sporadically in health education programmes.

Training in health education

For many years training in health education has been reduced to its integration in the general training of public health personnel (doctors, pharmacists, veterinarians, health visitors and sanitation agents and hospital administrators) through the National School of Health. The first health education course (80 hours) was run in 1978 to train provincial health service personnel to integrate health education in their activities.

With democratization and decentralization, interest in health education increased and the number of jobs for professionals specialized in this field also increased quickly. Many of these people were trained abroad, especially at the Experimental Centre for Health Education of Perugia, Italy.

At present many courses for health personnel and for teachers are organized at central and regional levels by governmental and private institutions, but this is still totally insufficient for the demand and the needs of training. The National Institute of Health in collaboration with the Experimental Centre for Health Education of Perugia is organizing a high course on health education for the next school year (315 hours) especially devoted to personnel responsible for health education at area level.

Training in health education is always a specialization for professionals in other fields, as already stated. There is no individual profession of 'health educator'. Career prospects are very unclear.

Health education structure

The administrative structure is now developing but still far from complete. At central level there are two groups of people responsible for health education:

a. at the Ministry of Health, 3 university level people, 2 medium level and 4 auxiliaries, with planning and management activities;
b. at the National Institute of Health, 3 university level, 2 medium level and 2 auxiliaries, with training and research responsibilities.

At the regional level 14 of the 17 autonomous communities have a service of health education, in the remaining three, health education is one of the components of another service such as promotion of health or primary health care. The number of people working as health educators in these services varies from 1 to 12 and their professions are: doctors 21, psychologists 2, sociologists 2, pedagogues 3, teachers 4, nurses 11, journalists 1 and biologists 1.

At local level there are some people entirely devoted to health education especially in the municipalities of the main towns. In the private sector and NGOS there are also jobs for persons trained in health education.

Health education is a matter already transferred to the autonomous communities and for this reason control by central government is reduced to the co-ordination of planning and high level inspection.

For health education co-ordination, an annual seminar began in 1985, uniting the people responsible for this subject from the autonomous communities and from the state services in order to join efforts and share experiences. The seminar has WHO sponsorship and the advice of the Experimental Centre for Health Education of Perugia.

Main aspects of health education

The main aims of health education in Spain, both at state and community level, are:

1. Integration of health education in the education system, previously mentioned, that will start in 1990 in the eleven regions still dependent in educational matters on central government and which has been already integrated by law in Cataluna and will very soon be in another two regions.
2. Integration of health education in the health care system, particularly in primary health care. After the Alma Ata Declaration, the General Health Law gives high priority to the improvement of primary health care services, where care must be practised in a comprehensive way integrating curative and rehabilitation care with preventive practices, health education and promotion of health. With this perspective, the existing primary health care services are being converted into health centres in which education is taking an increasingly important part.

   Apart from this, in all ante natal and post natal services, whether in a traditional setting or in new health centres, a programme of health education is being developed. These services have also assumed responsibilities in family planning, including health education of the users of the service. For these tasks a health education training programme for midwives was implemented.
3. Stimulation of interest in health and health education in associated movements, especially in consumer and parent associations and trade unions, and also in personnel working in community development.

   Apart from the international movement directed to the implication of NGOS and associations in the field of health education in Spain two health problems have strengthened this tendency.

   The first was the rape-seed oil intoxication problem which focused the interest of the people on the control and hygiene of foodstuffs and consumption in general and whose immediate consequence was the creation of the National Institute of Consumption within the

Ministry of Health and Consumer Affairs and the development all over the country of an important network of consumers' associations.

The second was AIDS which connected with the health services many movements of citizens' participation, gays associations and so forth, that had also become interested in other health and social issues such as sexually transmitted diseases, drug addiction, sexual abuse and many others, according to their area of work.

4. The need to tackle the increasing problem of drug abuse is generally recognized too. A national plan to fight drug abuse was established to unify the efforts of the administration in its search for a solution. The education programme, although mainly focused on the consumption of illegal drugs, deals also with problems linked to the use of tobacco and alcohol. Special efforts of this programme are devoted to the school population to prevent the use of these substances by young people.

5. The concern on nutrition derived from the bad situation of the Spanish population in the 1950s which was the original of the programme of 'Education in food and nutrition' established in 1961. This was an inter-ministerial health, agriculture, trade and culture initiative started as a way of teaching people ways of getting a balanced diet using mainly the country's foodstuffs. Its interest persists even after the nutritional problems have changed from deficiencies in some nutrients to a surfeit of calories and excessive consumption of fats and sugar. The new fashion of slimness and the advertising of certain products have made people, especially the young, worried about the problems related to the abuse of fats and calories. The steady increase of cardiovascular disease in recent years has also worried the health authorities and as a consequence the programme of 'Education in food and nutrition' experimented with a substantial increase in its activities in co-operation with the autonomous communities, the National Institute of Consumption, consumers' associations and CVD programmes, especially in Cataluna, Euskadi and Galicia.

6. AIDS, as a world problem, has also affected the Spanish population and alerted the health authorities. A national plan was established to unify the efforts of the country in the fight against this social and health problem. The plan, through a special sub-committee on preventative and educational actions, has developed a programme of information for the population with the use of the mass media and another of education of children and adolescents through the school system.

The work of the national plan on AIDS is connected with that of the national plan on drugs because in this country the most affected group is heroin addicts.

A very particular educational programme has been developed with the health personnel (doctors and nurses) of prisons in order to make them aware of the problem and cope with it and also to enable them to introduce health education programmes for prisoners.

With respect to health services personnel, AIDS made an important impact in education on hygienic norms about practices for the prevention of transmission of infections such as hepatitis B and many others.

7. Although immunization programmes are accepted by most of the population, educational activities are regularly carried out on this subject and some specific programmes are focused on socially or geographically marginal groups. In relation to zoonosis education, programmes are carried out by local health service personnel with the use of local mass media.

Major health problems

According to the mortality and morbidiy rates, the main health problems are those common to the developed countries.

The first one is cardio- and cerebro-vascular diseases which kill 85,000 people every year and reduce the capacity for a healthy life of many more. The educational activities focused on the reduction of this problem are those already mentioned on nutritional education, others are directed to increasing regular physical exercise, to the reduction of cigarette smoking and to the reduction of stress connected with working and social situations through mental health programmes.

The second main problem is cancer. The main educational programmes are addressed to primary prevention: reduction of sunshine exposure, reduction of cigarette smoking, nutritional education in relation to the reduction of fats and the use of vegetable fibre, and to secondary prevention mainly the self examination of breasts, the Pap test and advice of medical examination when certain signs appear.

The educational activities on cigarette smoking are directed also to a major health problem not so much for the number of deaths but rather for the incapacities and disabilities that it produces (chronic bronchitis, emphysema and asthma) which represent the causes of the highest number of hospitalization days.

Another important cause of death and incapacity is liver cirrhosis which in many cases is related to the use of alcohol as are many other health problems of the alimentary tract, the nervous system, traffic and working accidents, aggressive behaviour and social problems. Alcohol abuse is a very important problem and educational programmes on this matter have been developed over many years and form an important part of the national plan on drugs.

Accidents are another important health problem and, apart from the educational programme on traffic accidents continuously carried out by the Ministry of Transport, several programmes on the prevention of these and other accidents, especially home and school ones, have been developed by the Ministry of Health.

Diabetes is also the subject of many health education programmes both at the clinical services and community levels.

Special attention has been devoted in recent years to the education of food handlers due to the increase of food poisoning outbreaks all over the country mainly in tourist areas and big cities.

Increasingly more people eat regularly away from home in cafes and restaurants where food must be prepared some hours in advance with the corresponding increase in risk. A national education programme was established some years ago; it is implemented at local level and compulsory for all people with food handling responsiblities.

Influence of the international organizations

As in many other health activities WHO promotes health education programmes and advises and helps on their implementation. Spain participates in the 'Health for all by the year 2000' of WHO/EURO and every two years renews an agreement to participate in a collaborative programme through which it receives expert advice and information. In the concrete field of health education WHO has contributed to the development from its inception of the annual seminar providing two experts and documentation. It also sponsored the 'European conference on health education I'. The National Institute of Health 'Carlos III' participates in the core groups on health education of WHO and Spanish representatives participate in most of WHO meetings on health education. In the 'Healthy cities' programmes, Barcelona and, very recently, Madrid take part.

The International Union on Health Education has also influenced the development of health education in Spain. For many years Spain has been part of the Union, previously through a Spanish health education committee and now because the health education service of the Ministry of Health is a national constituent member of it.

Other Spanish institutions and groups are also members. This international union and the Spanish Ministry of Health and Consumer Affairs organized the 'European conference on health education I' which involved nearly 700 people from all over Europe.

The Council of Europe and the European Economic Community are also developing health education programmes that involve Spain.

In the field of health education some institutions, some autonomous communities and the central government received technical assistance as mentioned above, both in the training of personnel and in the development of programmes.

The political importance of health education is clearly mentioned in our Constitution and the General Health Law refers several times to the need for its implementation. The relative consideration given to it, measured by the number of jobs in the health services, the situation in the administrative structure of the health services and the amount of money spent on developing these activities is still very low when compared with other parts of the health system.

Nevertheless, their rate of growth, at central, regional and local levels has been increasing in recent years, even in a period of slow economic growth and with many problems in the hospital sector.

The new public health policy movement of WHO is followed very closely and will probably be taken into consideration by the authorities of the country in development of the Spanish health policy.

Future trends

Looking to the future three very important trends can already be identified. They are: the integration of health education in the general education of children until 18 years of age; the integration of health education in primary health care services; and the participation of the population in the planning, implementation and evaluation of health services.

The search for healthier lifestyles is another way to health introduced by health education services and many professional and consumers associations and many others.

The creation of the National Institute of Health 'Carlos III' as the teaching and research agency to support the Ministry of Health and the autonomous communities health services, will allow the development of research in health education which is an important part of this subject and in great need of development, both through economic and personnel dedication.

8. Programme for the eradication of the habit of smoking at the University School of Nursing in Oviedo, Spain – A CASE STUDY

M. L. Lopez Gonzalez, B. de la Torre Arrarte and J. Bobes Garcia

Summary: The attitude to the habit of smoking among health workers influences the consumption of tobacco by the public. In the University School of Nursing a programme about tobacco was carried out with three aims: to train students in the development of health education programmes; to achieve, for the first time in our country, a nursing school officially called a 'non-smoking' school; to decrease the consumption of tobacco among people – students, professors and the staff– from the nursing school. This chapter describes the method used in the development of a health education programme, which emphasized leisure activities and the positive aspects of non-smoking behaviour, and other strategies for giving up smoking, through nicotine chewing-gum, group psychotherapy and support from their peers.

Introduction

The subject of public health forms a part of the curriculum of second and third year students at the University School of Nursing in Oviedo. In the academic year of the project the students of these two year groups were invited, as a practical activity in the subject of public health, to design a programme for health education, the target population of which was to be the staff and students currently in the school. Paraphrasing the latin proverb *medicus, curate ipsum*, we said 'nurse, teach yourself'. The kernel of the programme remained to be established but it was soon agreed that the attitudes, behaviours and habits relating to tobacco use deserved priority treatment in our school.

Once the priority of the subject was established, a working party was set up whose members willingly assumed responsibility for the programme, with the support, advice and co-ordination provided by the university department of public health's staff members.

What started as a programme of health education in the field of tobacco mania, became a more ambitious 'Programme for the eradication of the habit of smoking'; this exceeded the limits of health education. In this chapter we stress the educational aspects of the programme, mentioning briefly other activities that also took place.

Aims and justification

The anti-tobacco committee consisting of teachers, administrative and service staff but mainly of students, with the typical enthusiasm of youth, formulated two ambitious aims which they considered justified. The two aims and underlying rationale were as follows:

1. That the University School of Nursing in Oviedo, in the second term (of the year), was to be proclaimed, through an agreement of its school council, the 'non smoking university school of nursing'. This would morally oblige all members, no matter what their relationship with it, not to smoke in public or in any room of the school nor in the health centres where our staff prctice nursing or medicine.
2. That at least the 60 per cent of the present smoking population *would give up the use of tobacco* in the academic year of the project.

   The overall reasoning that justifies these aims was the coherence of the new generation of nursing with the present scientific knowledge of the habit of smoking. Moreover, and starting from this coherence, other reasoning justified the already mentioned aims, according to the group. In order of priority these were:

   ☐ to set an example as nursing professionals;
   ☐ to attract the attention of the other teaching and health organizations;
   ☐ to keep and improve health.

Programme of activities

Collection of base line information at the starting point

A survey among members of the school community was carried out to discover:

1. How many smoked and the nature of their smoking habits.
2. Their attitudes towards smoking and the support which could be expected from them for our eradication programme.

A selection of behavioural results from the survey shows that:

☐ 41.22 per cent smoked daily. Among them:
   40.38 per cent smoked less than 10 cigarettes per day
   50.96 per cent smoked from 10 to 20 cigarettes per day
    8.66 per cent smoked more than 20 cigarettes per day
☐ In 50 per cent of cases cigarette smoking was mainly associated with meals.
☐ The starting age, according to the school levels, was:
   at primary school: 11.32 per cent
   at secondary school: 56.6 per cent
   at university school: 32.8 per cent. (This percentage started to smoke while studying nursing).
☐ Tobacco was bad for health according to 96.78 per cent.
☐ 90.32 per cent thought smoking should be forbidden at the University School of Nursing.
☐ 91.4 per cent supported our programme.

These figures were depicted in diagrams presented in an amusing way in order to draw attention to them and displayed on the school notice board for maximum effect.

The achievement of the aims of the programme seemed a possibility from this preliminary inquiry. The smokers were a minority and more than 90 per cent supported our idea and believed that they should not smoke in the school.

Activities to secure scientific information from the target population about the habit of smoking

We held three discussion conferences in the public health classes. All staff and students were invited to these conferences.

Cultural and artistic activities designed to sensitize the members of the community and persuade them to refuse tobacco

From the beginning we tried to show mainly the positive aspects of not smoking in an attractive and entertaining way. We started these activities with a competition of ideas that were collected in boxes placed in classrooms for this purpose. The range of contributions included slogans, subjects of posters and stickers, scripts, songs and suchlike. Requesting ideas from more than one hundred people generated an enormous quantity of material. All the ideas collected were displayed and prizes were awarded for the three best. There were however more than three useful ideas for our programme.

From the competition of ideas the following activities were selected and developed: seven drama sketches, three public demonstrations, a painting exhibition and a band of street musicians to provide backing to many of the activities.

☐ **The seven sketches**. Akin to socio-drama, their performance reduced the number of planned discussion conferences and caused a greater impact. The titles of the sketches and a brief mention of their contents to give an idea of their underlying message were as follows:
1. 'Psalmody for a blind person', in which a blind person tells of the discovery of America and of tobacco by Columbus.
2. 'The wizard Nitoko Tabako', a Japanese woman with magic powers. She takes the toxic substances from a very big cigar, in time to a tambourine roll. (In Spanish this expression has a double meaning: nitoko (I don't touch) sounds like a Japanese word.)
3. 'The lungs of Mr Alquitranio Nicotenez Chat'. Two lungs of one smoker chat about their 'smoked' life and the pathologic consequences of smoking. (Name and surname derived comically from 'tar': alquitran and 'nicotine': nicotina.)
4. 'Meeting between a healthy guy and a vicious young person', where two young people, speaking slang, defend different ways of life and attitudes related to tobacco.

5. 'Mum, damn the cigarette'. A newborn complains to her mother that she has smoked for the nine months of pregnancy and, being unhappy with her mother, the newborn elopes with the obstetrician.

6. 'Follow me if you dare, young man', where a healthy old man of 101 practising jogging overtakes a flirtatious young girl smoker. It tries to combat the myth of the false relationship between tobacco and sport in advertising.

7. 'Does smoke annoy you?'. From the rights of the non-smoker and using the mime technique, one student asks another not to smoke while studying, with different arguments.

☐ **Popular Demonstrations**. The anti-tobacco committee organized three public demonstrations in which all the members of the school were invited to participate. These demonstrations took place in the school hall and around the university campus. Statements displayed on the placards were as follows:

☐ 'Breathe health with nursing'. It was about the preservation of environment and the healthiness of the air. Many of the participants were wearing masks with ecological slogans.

☐ 'Burning of tobacco? Yes! In the bonfire'. Columbus, his sailors and the Indians, in procession, carried a pyre made of tobacco which was collected by the psalmody blind man, who asked for it from the smokers of the school. The pyre was burnt on the campus, while the characters danced around it singing a song written for the occasion.

☐ 'Come and, with your help, o cigarette – to the grave'. It consisted of an authentic burial of the cigarette coinciding with the patron saint's feast of the school. The cigarette used by the magician Nitolo Tabacko for her show, was taken within a coffin in procession around the campus, where it was buried. Over it was planted an apple tree in memorial.

☐ **Painting exhibition**. At the school hall 25 square metres of large windows were available, covered with paper, for everybody to be able to express his views against tobacco with colour, wax and finger painting. A tripod, placed strategically, advertised and invited everybody who went by to join in this activity.

☐ **Band of street musicians**. A group of vocalists and instrumentalists played the background music to many of the related activities, with music and works which condemned the consumption of tobacco.
All the artistic and cultural activities were recorded in video.

Activities to attain the primary aim of the programme

Information about the programme, at the project stage, was presented to the management team of the school. The anti-tobacco committee presented the proposed details of the project to the school director, asking for his support, which was granted at the beginning of the course.

Asking for the meeting with the school council. When we had decided on the programme of activities to achieve our stated aims we asked the director to convene the school council and to include the following item in the agenda: 'The habit of smoking in the university school of nursing: information and debate'.

It was accepted and the anti-smoking initiative was explained to the entire assembly, with obvious official backing. Then we asked for the school council to declare the University School of Nursing of Oviedo a 'health education non-smoking organization' and to inform other health education organizations so that they might follow our example.

After this council meeting everybody was morally obliged not to smoke in public when they were in the role of nurses or nursing students. The anti-tobacco committee based its request on the following facts:

☐ The results of the preliminary enquiry from which it was discovered that most people had a positive attitude towards the request made to the school council.
☐ Nowadays free countries are ruled by parliamentary democracy and as Sir George Young, Under Secretary of State for Health in the UK, said on the occasion of the Fourth World Conference on 'The use of tobacco and health', held in Stockholm in 1979: 'The solution of the medical problems at present, is found more frequently not in the laboratories of the hospital investigation but in the parliaments in the decisions taken by the local council of ministers' (1). According to these words, the 'parliament' of our school was its school council, for this reason it had to give official support to our request.
☐ The habit of smoking has been said by the WHO to be the major avoidable cause of illness and death in the world.

The school council agreed to our request with 80 per cent of its votes.

Activities to help tobacco addicts give up smoking

The programme to give up smoking was founded on the scientific contributions to this subject from the Health and Public Policy Committee of the American College of Physicians (1986), Axelsson and Brantmark (1975), Clavel and Benhamor (1984), Raw (1982, 1985), Raw and Heller (1983), Russell et al (1980) and Salvador (1986). It included:

☐ Group psychotherapy, directed by the psychiatric nursing department of the school. The group consisted of smokers and a support team made of non-smoking colleagues, whose task was to monitor the smokers who wanted to give up the habit.
☐ Chewing gum with two milligrams of nicotine in each tablet.
☐ Guide booklet presented in an amusing way to help give up smoking.
☐ Stickers to be shown publicly with the slogans (in Spanish): '**I am trying**' and '**I am succeeding**'.

Methodology

Our human resources were:

☐ The anti-tobacco committee: a group of thirty volunteer people who designed and carried out most of the programme. This committee consisted of several specialized sub-committees: sub-committee for economical subjects, theatrical committee, painting sub-committee, musical sub-committee, supply sub-committee, enquiry sub-committee, and so on.

☐ Complementary groups, such as the support group to the programme of losing the habit of smoking, in which 27 people helped as tutors to the ex-smokers and the follow up group, made up of 14 people who monitored the fulfilment of the non-smoking agreement.

The material resources were supplied by the following organizations:

☐ The Asturian Association Against Cancer, which had the necessary awareness to understand the importance of this gesture of professional coherence in new nursing promotions, and which financed most of the programme.

☐ The University School of Nursing, which provided the backup resources for the programme (photocopier, forms, and so forth).

☐ A chemical products laboratory which gave the already mentioned nicotine chewing-gum.

The Anti-tobacco committee met at least twice a week for an hour to review the progress of the programme, introduce modifications, and so on. The participation of the working team and the discussion groups were the most important methodological aspects of the programme. Prizes were given to the three students of the committee who worked the hardest, according to the votes of their companions.

The group psychotherapy was practised in sessions of an hour and a half for five days, and in follow up meetings of an hour a week, for a month. Further support was given for an hour each fortnight until the end of the course, followed by one session in each term for one academic year.

Chronological order of the programme

This is shown in Table 8.1.

Preliminary evaluation

Evaluation of the situation at the start of the project and of the level of support

This was done through **the survey** carried out at the beginning of the course; it involved 80 per cent of the people linked to the school. The most important data from it were:

☐ Daily smokers were a minority (41.22 per cent), although 54.48 of these smoked daily or from time to time.
☐ 90 per cent of the respondents supported the programme, which favoured the hope of positive results.

First term	Planning of Financing	Information Sensitization Education	Discussion-conference Sketches Demonstrations (2)
Second Term	Information Sensitization Education	Painting exhib. Demonstration Group of serenades.	Programme for losing the habit of smoking. Agreement of the school council. Preliminary Evaluation
Third term	Keeping of the sensitization	Video Group of serenades. Spirometry Sports competitions	Final evaluation

Table 8.1 *Chronological distribution of the parts of the programme*

Evaluation of the results of the development of the health education programme on its own

This was carried out through an inquiry in the second term to which 65 per cent of the community responded.
The most important results were, within the range of the *positive* influence of the programme:

☐ 10.71 per cent of the smokers gave up smoking.
☐ 27.88 per cent of the smokers smoked much less.
☐ 4.80 per cent of the smokers smoked less dangerously.

In all, 43.39 per cent of the smokers were influenced positively by the programme in their habit of smoking. Within the range of *negative* influence of the programme:

☐ 3.41 per cent of the non-smokers started to smoke.
☐ 5.76 per cent of the smokers smoked much more.

Other positive results were that:

1. 33.65 per cent of the smokers asked to participate in the programme of losing the habit of smoking.
2. 23.07 per cent of the non-smokers offered themselves to help their smoker companions who wanted to lose the habit.
3. 11.96 per cent of the non-smokers watched the fulfilment of the no-smoking agreements.

Evaluation of the results one year later

A one year follow-up programme monitoring the progress of the participants has been carried out including testing for cotinine in urine and interview work. Participants who were found to be reverting to former smoking habits received a verbal reprimand and a sticker saying: 'You have let us down'. Those who broke their agreement were more frequently the youngest students . . . and the *teachers*. Breaking the non-smoking agreement most commonly occurred at the bar, which is shared with people who are not engaged in the project and where attempts at making it a non-smoking area have not succeeded. Only 11 per cent of our smokers managed to abstain from smoking at the bar.

During this year from the starting point of 40.71 per cent ex-smokers the figure at the end was 28 per cent ex-smokers, the difference representing those who returned to smoking. However, 81 per cent of the original smokers maintained that their attitude towards tobacco had been modified in some way.

Conclusions

The margin of success of the results was perhaps less than we had hoped for but the programme has given the students a valuable experience in the field of health education. The main obstacle for the development of the programme has been the students' timetables, which allow the students very little free time, and the different timetables of different year groups made plenary sessions and any combined actions difficult to achieve.

The commitment and support from the teachers and managing staff has not been as big as the anti-tobacco committee would have wished, with the lack of appropriate places for unusual and varied activities (rehearsal of the group of serenaders, painting and drying of placards, and so on) has been a further obstacle.

The first aim has been achieved, but the problem of maintaining the numbers of those who initially agree to give up smoking remains to be solved. Our second aim however, has not been attained. The 40.71 per cent who gave up smoking after the educational programme and that for losing the habit of smoking, has decreased to 28 per cent in a year. The youthfulness and obvious vigour and health of the target population explains, perhaps, this partial failure.

References

Axelsson, A and Brantmark, B (1975) The anti-smoking effect of chewing-gum with nicotine of high and low bioavailability *Proceeding of 3rd World conference on Smoking and Health*: New York

Clavel, F and Benhamor, S (1984) Desintoxication tabagique. Comparaison de l'efficacite de differentes methodes. Resultats intermediaires d'une étude comparative *Prres. Medic* **13**, 975–977

Health and Public Policy Committee. American College of Physicians: Philadelphia (1986) Methods for stopping cigarette smoking *An. Int. Med* **105**, 281–291

Raw, M (1985) Does nicotine chewing-gum work? *Brit. Med. J* **290**, 1231–1232

Raw, M (1982) A brief guide to the smoking treatment literature. Action on Smoking and Health (ASH): London

Raw, M, Hellier, J (1983) Smokers' clinics in Britain: a descriptive survey *Proceeding of the fifth World Conference on Smoking and Health: Winnipeg*

Roemer, R (1982) *Legislative Action to Combat the World Smoking Epidemic* WHO, Geneva

Russell, M A H, Raw, M and Jarvis M J (1980) Clinical use of nicotine chewing gum *Brit. Med. J* **280**, 1599–1602

Salvador, T, Marin, D, Gonzalez, J et al (1986) Trantamiento del taboquismo: comparacion entra una terapia de soporte y una terapia utilizan do soporte, chicle de nicotina y refuerzo del comportamiento *rev. med. clin* **87**, 403–406

9. Health Education in Chile – AN OVERVIEW

Mercedes Baez Cruz

Summary: In 1952, the National Health Service was formed. Included within it was the Department of Health Education. Health education activities throughout the country were given official status in 1954 with the creation of the Health and Education Joint Commission, the structure of which is described. Health education has played an important role in improving the nation's health. Training programmes for health educators are described, as are specific health education initiatives. Future priorities centre on specific issues such as cancer and sexually transmitted diseases, training, health education in the community and evaluation of health education.

Historical background

In Chile, the goals reached in health education are the outcome of a long evolution which dates from the beginning of the Republic.

In 1822, the Board of Health (*Junta de Sanidad*) was created. Its task was: 'to establish certain norms for the purpose of making known certain useful advice for the health of the people' (Mackenna, 1933). This concern has persisted since that time, and it has been made evident by means of different laws and decrees that assign educational responsibilities and create a proper structure for an adequate organization of this work.

In 1952, the National Health Service (*Servicio Nacional de Salud*) was instituted. It included in its central structure a department of health education. At this time, health educators were given formal professional status.

In 1954, following the establishment of the Health and Education Joint Commission (*Comisión Mixta de Salud y Educación*) health education activities throughout the country were given official status. At national and regional level and in each health institution of the primary assistance level these activities took place with the purpose of producing adults who were responsible for their own health.

In 1974, the Secretary of Health (*Ministerio de Salud*) incorporated health education into the planning process as an activity to be included in other health activities. It was also made official policy that all health officials – especially physicians, nurses, midwives, dentists, dieticians, social workers, and nursing assistants – should dedicate a percentage of their time to health education and that this should be registered in the policies of the institution.

In 1979, the National Health Service was reorganized, establishing the National System of Health Services (*Sistema Nacional de Servicios de Salud*) through which it was proposed to achieve administrative decentralization, while keeping the elaboration of technical norms under central control. The role of the Department of Health Education became more one of assessing the integration of health and education.

During this same year, the document 'Policies and general norms of health education' ('*Políticas y normas generales de educación para la salud*') was written and published. It gave priority to health education at the first level of health assistance. This educational activity was to be of a general nature and would have little educational complexity. It would emphasize integral family health and community participation.

The health situation

The population of Chile is growing moderately. There has been a rapid decrease in the overall child mortality rate (1960 = 191; 1986 = 114), and the mortality rate for children under five years old has also declined (1960 = 142; 1986 = 25). Life expectancy has been extended to 71 years. There is an increase in size of the population over 65 years old.

Health education has played an important role in improving the nation's health and the people are increasingly taking preventive measures into consideration. Nonetheless, the prevalence of avoidable diseases such as hepatitis and typhoid fever would indicate that an unsatisfactory health culture still persists. Emergent health problems of particular importance are sexually transmitted diseases, alcoholism, drug addiction, and accidents.

Health education structure in the health sector

As a result of the re-structuring of the health sector, health education stopped being a section with its own administrative and functional organization, both at national and local levels.

In 1969, there were 102 health educators, and at present there are 20 professionals.

The typical health educator in Chile is a professional high school teacher, usually of biology, with a post-graduate and Master's qualification from the School of Public Health of the Faculty of Medicine of the University of Chile. This represents a total of 18.5 years of study. Of these 20 professionals, two are in the Ministry of Health (*Ministerio de Salud*), and eighteen at health services level.

To solve the problem of shortages, two strategies have been used:

a. recruiting teachers of biology into the health services;
b. the setting up of committees with a wide representation of health education professionals which have the responsibility of promoting educational activities.

Health education development

As a result of examining morbidity and mortality indicators during the last ten years, by making projections to the year 2000 and studying particular risk groups, the problems of health were prioritized. Emphasis has been placed on relevant aspects that are deemed to be susceptible to health education activities.

To plan the most appropriate strategies in education, the outcome of two national investigations into health-related behaviour that took place in 1974 and 1979 have proved extremely useful. It was concluded:

> that in some health problems – diarrhoea, bronchopneumonia and that sort of illness, mothers had the proper knowledge, but this did not mean a change of behaviour (PESMIB, 1971). The officials declared that education was important, but they did not give the necessary directions in their contact with the consultants (CONPAN, 1979).

Likewise, a significant percentage of officials were identified as not being sufficiently skilled in modern educational technologies to be able to achieve changes of behaviour. This determined the need to:

a. Begin training health personnel in the management of educational techniques that would meet the needs of the learner and encourage individual learners to take responsibility for his or her own health.
b. Establish a system that would allow the evaluation of effectiveness, and an assessment of the educational concepts acquired, especially at primary level.
c. Promote inter-sectional co-operation. There are many other state and private institutions that have the potential to solve health problems by working in co-operation with the Department of Health Education.

Training of health education personnel

The training of personnel using new methods began in 1979 when maternal breast-feeding workshops for all the regions of the country were established.

Following evaluations of these workshops it was clear that the time given to education was insufficient. This determined the need to establish a specific course for those involved in leading these workshops. This course was run for the first time in 1983 in the Health Service of Nuble. Subsequently the course was used by four health educators who trained 650 officials who had been appointed to a specific rural health plan.

In spite of these efforts, it was clear that it was necessary to establish a progressive training plan that would produce an improvement in teamwork, reflect current points of view, describe evaluated projects, and focus on ways of incorporating the community into the educational process. This task began with the training of health educators through a continual annual education programme.

Later on, the health authorities set up the 'Learning to teach project' (1984–1988). This gave training to all health personnel, particularly those working at the primary assistance level. The purpose of this project was 'to promote the expectation – through participant educational activities – that people, families and communities will take for themselves the responsibility of their health, and develop the capacity for their participation in solving the main local health problems' (Secretary of Health, 1984). To develop this project, three successive levels of training were established:

1. Interpersonal relationship improvement: humanist focusing methodo- logies centred in the person, family and community; use of communi- cation media;
2. Educational evaluation; health community work;
3. Operational investigation development.

The numbers of participants involved in this project and the number of workshops held are shown in Table 9.1.

	NUMBER OF OFFICIALS BY LEVELS			NUMBER OF WORKSHOPS		
YEARS	LEVEL 1	LEVEL 2	LEVEL 3	LEVEL 1	LEVEL 2	LEVEL 3
1984	2,850	–	–	60	–	–
1985	2,850	2,850	–	60	60	–
1986	2,850	2,850	2,850	60	60	60
1987	–	2,850	2,850	–	60	60
1988	–	–	2,850	–	–	60
	8,550	8,550	8,550	180	180	180

Table 9.1

This project considered personnel training on three consecutive levels, one per year. Participants were required to pass the previous level before starting the next. It is based in the principle of active learning. Notes are mostly not given to participants, especially at the first level. This surprises many of the professionals on the first day, especially as they are used to taking and receiving notes in other courses.

Each level consists of a multi-disciplinary workshop that lasts four or five days, followed by practical application and development during the rest of the year of what has been learned. This practice is supervised by health educators.

The workshops consist of three units. The intention of the first unit is to improve interpersonal relationships. This is achieved through:

a. exercises that help to enhance greater personal knowledge and self esteem;
b. exercises that promote interpersonal knowledge;
c. exercises that promote creative imagination.

Through this unit an atmosphere of trust is achieved which helps to overcome many blocking attitudes that participants may have.

During the second unit which is entitled 'Consideration about the educational process' factors are analysed by means of participation in exercises involving drama, role play, problem-solving, and so on.

In the third unit which has the title 'Applying what was learned', the students are left free to develop their educational ideas, educational material aids, evaluation instruments, action plans and so on. In all the workshops, special emphasis is given to the affective aspects of human behaviour. This unit varies its subject according to the level that is most appropriate.

The wide involvement of participants in this project at the first level has resulted in a significant improvement in the educational performance at primary assistance level. Through it, the prime health problem in each first aid and consulting office was defined, and educational units with appropriate material were developed.

The first level evaluation (Secretary of Health, 1985) gave the following results:

a. *Knowledge*. In the Initial test 28 per cent achieved a score between good and very good. In the final test (administered after completion of the first level) this was increased to 98 per cent.
b. *Attitude*. This was tested by means of a Lickert scale which was submitted to a factorial variation with an outcome of 0,89.
   Importance given to education. In the initial test 45.3 per cent of the responses were very good. In the final test this had increased to 87 per cent.
   Interpersonal relationship workshop impact. 75 per cent of the participants stated that the workshop had positively influenced their relationship with the others.
c. *Abilities and skills achieved*. Four hundred educational units together with mini flip-charts were developed.

At present, the development of the second level workshop is almost complete. It consists of community work, with special reference to the community groups organized by town councils in the different counties of the country. Also, the personnel throughout the country are being encouraged to evaluate their educational performance, and in particular to detect risk groups and find out the people's needs in order to achieve their active participation.

The third level is at the validating stage. This workshop has also been tried in a variety of institutions.

Educational activities in specific health problems

One of Chile's health problems has been the progressive decline of maternal breast-feeding. In 1978, an educational programme started for individuals, organized groups, and the community in general. Manuals, educational units, notebooks for mothers, flip charts, and ten television spots were produced. This education programme, which was maintained for four consecutive years, has reversed the process. In 1972, the percentage of mothers breast-feeding was 26.7 per cent. This had increased to 63 per cent in 1982 (Mardonnes, 1987). At present, educational efforts are being made at the local level and at national level in order to maintain this behaviour.

At present, education in health problems is being extended to cover areas that will be major issues towards the end of the century. These include for example, venereal diseases, other chronic transmissable diseases and cancer.

Since 1987, health education activities have been carried out with the purpose of controlling and prevening HIV infection. They have been intensified in 1988 through educational diagnosis and the training of personnel and teachers. Curricular changes for elementary school and high school have been made and educational materials have been developed.

In 1985, the 'Prevention and control of the smoking habit programme' started. Its target is elementary and high school students in an area of Santiago. Educational support materials and curricular insertions for students have been prepared, and the health personnel and teachers of the institutions included in the programme have received skilful training.

In 1987, an integrated 'Mother-child health programme' was started (UNICEF, 1988). It is intended to improve the health condition of families that live in extreme poverty in outlying districts. The objectives of this programme are to increase the use of the broadened immunization programme, decrease and prevent child malnutrition, intervene in the most frequent causes of infant mortality such as respiratory diseases, diarrhoeas, parasitosis. In order to fulfil these objectives, the personnel are being trained and educational material such as manuals, self instruction modules, brochures, slides is being developed.

Alcoholism primary prevention programme

In Chile, alcoholism has been a significant and persistent problem which has led to the implementation of strategies to lessen it. One of the most important is perhaps the 'Alcoholism primary prevention programme'. It starts by inculcating in children an awareness of alcohol abuse, in the hope that in the future they will be moderate drinkers, with the subsequent benefit that that would bring for national development. It was designed in 1974, by the Secretary of Health and the Secretary of Education. Its target was all elementary schools, and since it became official policy in 1977, its use in school has become obligatory. As a result, the programme has been incorporated into the programmed activities of the school curriculum and now 2,333,400 school students (in approximately 6000 elementary schools) are being educated about this issue. The programme respects the present curricular objectives in the school, and includes specific content about alcoholism (Secretary of Education, 1983). In this programme, the teachers act as social action leaders confronting the problem.

In 1983, this programme was officially incorporated into high schools, where it would theoretically reach 480,000 adolescents. The school prog-ramme insertions were introduced in different subjects such as Spanish, economics, history and geography, mathematics, natural science, foreign languages and art (Dobert, 1984).

An evaluation performed in 1984 pointed out that only 74 per cent of elementary school teachers use the materials and carry out activities with sufficient frequency during the school year. In general, the teachers exhibited a favourable attitude towards the programme although one of the greatest problems has been the lack of systematic training and a shortage of educational material (Figueras, 1984).

The dental health programme

Chile is classified among the countries with a high prevalence of dental problems. This programme has changed the principal dental treatment policy from extractions to repair. A high percentage of treatment time is set aside for school student assistance and 3 per cent of the whole treatment time is for health education.

An intensive dental assistance programme has been implemented. It starts with dental repair programmes for first grade elementary school children. These children are followed until they finish the last year of elementary school. It is combined with dental health education activities for teachers and parents. This is designed to promote a favourable attitude to the fulfilment of the programme, and to promote in the students a responsibility for their own health care. The preventive action is performed by teaching proper teeth brushing and fluoride rinsing.

In evaluations that took place in some health services, it has been observed that, through the educational actions and specifically through fluoride rinsing, in three years the oral hygiene index has decreased from 2.31 to 1.5 and the cavity average has declined from 6.6 to 1.08 (Melchafsky et al, 1986). Likewise, the degree of rinsing acceptance among the students was 98.2 per cent (Fernandez, 1986).

Child helps child programme

This programme is operating in elementary school educational institutions and is designed to encourage children to help each other on health issues. The programme also trains teachers to lead and assist the work of the

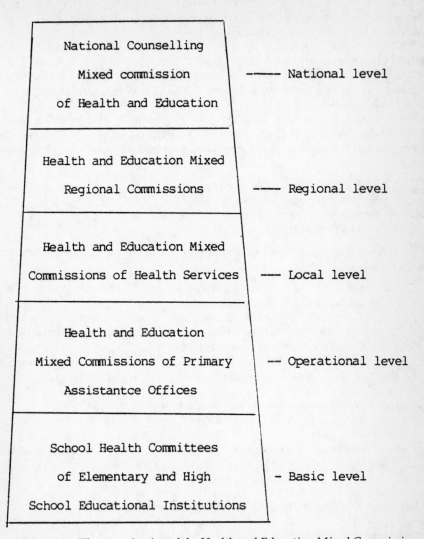

Figure 9.1 *The organization of the Health and Education Mixed Commission*

children. At present, this programme extends to all the institutions in the country.

The structure of the Health and Education Mixed Commission

Since its beginnings, the Health and Education Mixed Commission has functioned specifically at the primary assistance level. It is composed of representatives of both the Secretary of Health and the Secretary of Education. Its goals are intended to: broaden health education programmes through teacher training, incorporate health programmes into the school curriculum, consolidate the home-school ties, and disseminate health education throughout the community.

The levels of organization and functioning of the Health and Education Mixed Commission are shown in Figure 9.1.

In general, the Health and Education Mixed Commission objectives are focused on two fundamental subjects: the health of the student and school health education.

To achieve its objective, at all levels, the Health and Education Mixed Commission has a central board and sub-commissions (work groups) who have studied the most relevant school student health problems. They are as follows:

- [ ] Child and Adolescent Sub-Commission;
- [ ] Dental Health Sub-Commission;
- [ ] Environment Protection Sub-Commission;
- [ ] Mental Health Sub-Commission;

Throughout its 33 years of functioning, this Commission has contributed specifically to:

- [ ] the elaboration and development of a school health programme in a conjunctive health and education form;
- [ ] the creation of the health co-ordinator teacher function; a teacher trained to take for himself health responsibilities and act as a co-ordinator of these actions in his institution;
- [ ] the granting of training courses to the health and education personnel;
- [ ] the monitoring of the cleaning and repairing government school buildings;
- [ ] the development of a school student health manual to inform the personnel of both the Secretary of Health and the Secretary of Education;
- [ ] the monitoring of the training of those concerned with the manipulation of food.

The most demanding issues in health education

The priorities in health education are as follows:

1. to rank the most relevant and significant health priorities, with particular priority given to those that will prevent problems in adults;
2. to develop personnel in more efficient educational techniques in the management of health problems such as cancer, chronic sexually transmitted diseases, and AIDS;
3. to reinforce the personnel with community work techniques;
4. to train community agents to develop educational work;
5. to develop simple instruments which allow the evaluation of the

educational work that is performed and behaviour changes that take place in the community.

The objective of health education is to make every person responsible for his or her own health, and to ensure that everybody contributes to the achievement of healthy lifestyles for his or her family and community.

Much has been achieved but much remains to be done. Only through an effective inter-institutional co-ordination, and ensuring that the people take responsibility for their own development, shall we continue to advance.

References

Dobert, M Teresa (1984) *Prevencion Primaria del Alcoholismo en la comunidad Chilena* Asociacion Iberoamericana de Estudios de los Problemas del Alcohol

Conpan (1979) *Lactancia Materna en Chile*. Santiago, Chile

Fernandez, O, (1986) Programa de prevencion de caries escolares en un servicio de salud de santiago, *Monografia 4a Jornada de Salud Publica* Chile

Figureras, T (1984) Thesis El Programa de Prevencion Primaria del Alcohol desde la perspectiva del Profesor; un Estudio Socio-psycologico en cuatro Regiones del pais Chile

Mackenna (1933)

Mardones, S F (1987) *Breastfeeding Determinants in Chile* Santiago, Chile

Melchafsky *et al* (1986) Programa de atencion odontológica incremental, *Monografia 4a Jornada de Salud Publica* Chile

PESMIB (1974) *Conocimientos, Actitudes y Practicas de las madres en relacion con el Embarazo, Parto y Puerperio* Santiago, Chile

Secretary of Education (1983) Information: Santiago, Chile

Secretary of Health (1984) *Proyecto Aprender a Ensenar* Santiago, Chile

Secretary of Health (1985) *Monografia 3as jornadas nacionales multidisciplinarias de educacion para la salud*: Santiago, Chile

Secretary of Health (1988) *Programa Integrado de Salud Materno Infantil* Santiago, Chile

Vicuna, M B (1933) *Los Medicos de Antano en el Reino de Chile* Editorial Ercilla: Santiago, Chile

10. The organization of health education in the Nuble Health Service, Chile – A CASE STUDY

Nilda Segura Cid

Summary: Nuble is a province of Chile with a population of 400,000. Health-related activities are organized by the Nuble Health Service through various health programmes. The chapter describes the development of health education in Nuble since the 1950s. Health education was given official status in 1978. In 1982, the Health Education Committee (HEC) was created to oversee health education activities. It is particularly concerned with the training of the different health personnel who work in the health teams. Health education activities are closely monitored by the HEC through a reporting system, and evaluation has a high priority.

At present, health activities in Chile are carried out by the health services national system under the control of the Public Health Ministry, which has the task of regulating the health activities for the whole country. The health services are bodies created to carry out integrated activities in a co-ordinated way for fostering protection, recovery and rehabilitation.

Nuble Health Service

The Nuble Health Service (NHS) is in the Nuble Province, which has a population of about 400,000 inhabitants, 43.5 per cent of whom come from rural areas.

Health activities have been determined according to the needs of the people considered in the 'health programme'. These programmes are aimed at people and the environment. They are carried out by the health teams from the following establishments: seven hospitals, five urban surgeries, 13 rural surgeries, 49 rural medical offices and the 113 rural medical posts. The latter are managed by the hospitals, surgeries and medical offices. All of these institutions are dependent upon Nuble Health Service Office for specialist support.

The health programmes are developed through diverse activities, one of which is health education with individuals and groups. It has been included in all the programmes from the very beginning.

Since the 1950s, this activity has been mainly performed by social workers and health inspectors. The social workers formed educational groups and used various methods. They encouraged the other members of the health team to participate in health education. To do this, they took responsibility for the number of sessions, and the delegation of different units to professionals according to the professionals' experience and training (social workers, nurses, midwives or dieticians), supporting them in their work. This meant that the social worker was responsible for the organization of health education.

Over a period of time, the health education activities have been modified both in method and technique and in the time allocated to them by the health teams. The changes are as much a reflection of the importance given to education itself as they are a consequence of the changes which have taken place in the methods employed in its delivery.

In 1978, health education activities were given official status and became part of the activities of every employee. These activities have been evaluated in the same way as the other activities in each programme, that is on the basis of the number of programmed activities carried out as a percentage of the number of activities planned to be completed.

In 1981, an analysis of health education up to that time was made by the senior management at the NHS office. It identified a need to carry out an increasingly detailed and thorough revision of health education, and to employ a multi-disciplinary approach. Following this, in October 1982, the HEC was created, which had as its main objectives the co-ordination, assistance, supervision and evaluation of health education. The HEC comprised representatives of the different departments of the NHS Office: a health educator, social worker, nurse, hygienist and a physician from a collaborating body called: 'Programa de apoyo en extension de salud materno-infantil' (Programme to support the promotion of infant and mother healthcare).

With the objective of knowing which health institutions were carrying out health education, who gave it, and how they were carrying it out, the first step taken by the HEC was a diagnosis aimed at gathering and collating this information. For this purpose a questionnaire was distributed to the professional staff at 17 urban and rural health institutions of different levels of complexity from hospitals to health posts. To the data was added information collected during supervisory visits which are carried out regularly from the NHS office.

From the above data, it was concluded that there was a lack of knowledge and capability in educational methodologies. In addition, there was a lack of awareness about the importance of the quality of education as opposed to the quantity that was necessary to bring about the desired change in behaviour and the attainment of the proposed health goals.

Health Education Committee proposals

In the light of the above problems, the HEC proposed from 1983 the adoption of diverse strategies, which could be included in the annual programmes of activities. These have been modified according to periodic evaluations. The following are the most significant strategies.

Health co-ordinators

The awareness of the HEC amongst al

would be increased by means of 'health co-ordinators'. Such co-ordinators had to be professionals from the health team and their function would be to oversee the favourable development of health education carried out by the team members by working very closely with them and maintaining permanent contact with the HEC. At the beginning the co-ordinators were appointed by the NHS Office, without prejudice to their job functions, and for an indefinite period. After one year of work, modifications were made at the suggestion of the co-ordinators themselves; the health team itself would designate the co-ordinator, there being two at any one time and rotating every two years.

Training

It was proposed to expand, maintain and renew training in participatory educational methods and educational support materials. As part of this process they received assistance and advice direct from the Ministry of Health as well as from private organizations. The HEC is able to count on a wide variety of educational materials and audiovisual equipment at the health education office, which is at the NHS Office. The health teams from different institutions can turn to these materials as required.

Monitoring

The system of monitoring and evaluation of health education would be improved both quantitatively and qualitatively.

Advice and support

Advice and support would be given to the health teams in the programming and development of health education. This help should be as appropriate as possible to the resources available in each establishment and to the characteristics of the sectors of the population that used the facilities of the establishment.

Workshops

The organization of workshops would be aimed at analysing health education and laying emphasis on the use of health education as a fundamental tool for the improvement of the level of health of the population.

The above mentioned strategies have been included, among others, in the following activities of the HEC:

1. The advice and supervision is given by the members of the HEC to health teams by means of the 'advisory visits' that formed part of the programmed activities of each of the departments of the NHS Office, to which these people are attached. There are meetings of the HEC with the health teams and half-yearly meetings with all the co-ordinators.

2. The health education monitoring forms were created, revised and analysed. For example, the educational report was instituted. On this are included name and profession of the person carrying out the activity, the people to whom it is addressed, the techniques employed, the time spent and the content of the educational unit. This report is written immediately after the educational session has been completed and is particularly concerned with registering the characteristics of group participation, interest and motivation, as well as other elements that may seem relevant to any new activity. This document also has importance for whoever has performed the educational activity in the sense that it is used as an instrument of self evaluation. The information that is collected on these educational reports by any given health team is incorporated into the three-monthly summary, which is sent to the HEC during the course of the year. The HEC makes a consolidated report twice a year with the information received from all the institutions of the NHS which gives an overall vision about the health education situation in Nuble.
3. Communication and co-ordination with similar committees from other health services in the country was promoted for the exchange of experiences in relation to health education and the role of the HEC.
4. Periodic evaluations were carried out based on the analysis of the information sent in by the varius health teams, the data collected during the supervisory visits and above all the information given by the education co-ordinators themselves during the two annual meetings that are held. To this information was added the regular report (quantitative) made by each professional of his daily activities on the forms issued by the informatics department. This is also incorporated into a half yearly consolidated report, the information contained in which, once revised, is sent to the Ministry of Public Health.

Evaluation

From the evaluations that have been carried out to date it is important to highlight that at the beginning of 1985 it was necessary to analyse the place that health education should occupy as a strategy of great relevance for the achievement of the goals fixed by the NHS.

Thus it was felt important to consider in our work the study of the significance of the strategy of Primary Health Attention (PHA), placing education within PHA and maintaining it as a reference framework. This led us to expand upon our activities to the extent that technical meetings were organized in which the primary health emphasis of NHS was discussed. These meetings were intended to involve all the directors of health establishments in Nuble, with the objectives of getting to know and analysing the said strategy and especially health education.

As a result of the problems articulated by the health teams during these meetings, the HEC felt it appropriate to establish a project 'Policies and community participation' and to prepare and publish a 'Manual of community participation in health', to be used as a practical guide by the health teams. In addition to producing the manual they organized workshops for training staff in participative educational methods.

According to the evaluations made since 1982 there has been a progressive increase in interest and motivation of the health teams in becoming trained. This has allowed them to carry out health education in the best possible way. However, for approximately the last two years progress has been uneven and it has been possible to detect a decrease in the quantity of activities carried out and also in their quality.

Table 10.1 shows the progress of health education in the NHS in a quantitative way. In the table, the 'Health of the environment programme' does not appear because there has been a progressive increase in health education in this area during this period.

Years	Programs								
	Maternity			Dental			Total		
	Planned	Performed	%	Planned	Performed	%	Planned	Performed	%
1982	2391	2318	97	310	290	94	2701	2608	97
1983	2688	2673	94	768	945	125	3456	3620	105
1984	4516	3875	84	2047	839	52	6643	4714	71
1985	8061	6004	75	2409	790	33	10470	6794	65
1986	6933	4585	66	752	386	51	7685	4970	65
1987	6003	3950	66	201	146	73	6204	4096	66

Table 10.1 *Educational activities of the health service in Nuble from 1982–1987*

Among the factors that have influenced this evolution, we can highlight that the health teams remain motivated and interested in bringing into use the new methods while an intensive training programme was maintained. All of this coincided with the 'Year of health education' in 1985.

To the above we can also add other factors that we think are important: the lack of resources both human and material; organizational obstacles at the level of the health-teams in the areas of professionalism, motivation and willingness to reach out to the population groups to be educated; the lack of integration of the health-teams into the community to which they belong; and a lack of appreciation on the part of some professionals especially the doctors of the importance of health education. The last factor has been

Health Personel	Total Number in Public Health	Total number trained	Number trained remaining in NHS	% Trained Personel
Social workers	23	23	17	74
Dentists	58	31	27	47
Nurses	55	53	51	93
Mid-wives	41	34	31	76
Dieticians	28	28	27	96
Doctors	50	26	27	54
Health inspectors	13	13	13	100
Paramedics	69	66	46	67
Others	11	11	11	100

Table 10.2 *Training in educational methods Nuble Health Service 1983–1987*

aggravated by the fact that the doctor is typically the director of the health establishment.

Although approximately 70 per cent of the health personnel have been trained in educational methods, this is not reflected in practice. We believe that a fundamental factor influencing this phenomenon is that the efforts made so far to improve the level of knowledge of health personnel have not been sufficient to meet the educational needs of the population of Nuble. Thus we think it would be very useful if the health personnel, especially professionals, could receive these elements in pre-graduate training and/or their knowledge be updated and renewed as part of their in-service training.

The permanence of HEC as a technical/administrative body has permitted the development of a type of work that has been orientated fundamentally at the level of health-teams, to increase their awareness, and to create an awareness in those cases where it is absent, of the importance of health education in professional practice. In addition to this, an emphasis has been placed on the programming, monitoring and execution of health education to be considered as an activity equally valuable in comparison to others considered basic to other health action programmes.

Nowadays there is concern to ensure that the activities carried out by the HEC should be recognized by the heads of the different departments within the NHS Head Office as activities closely tied to each one of their programmes and, as was established from the very beginning that the HEC should completely fulfil its function of being a source of co-ordination and advice for those departments; the said co-ordination is being achieved in some measure thanks to the contributions of the members of the HEC.

Conclusions

The evolution of health education in our service, as described above, has required dedication and many hours of work which have exceeded greatly what was originally envisaged at the time of the constitution of the HEC. This has led us to propose the establishment of a more permanent work-group, which would be valuable in fulfilling the functions described above, but with more time allocated for the carrying out of these functions and having more people assigned to it. Despite having devoted six years of uninterrupted work to this project which has born some fruit we are conscious that this is a slow process which requires greater perseverance. Given the time and resources we believe that the people working in health will take on the task of health education with the dedication required to make a real contribution to the improvement of the level of health of our people.

11. Health Education in Jamacia – AN OVERVIEW

Ivy McGhie, Jean Tullock-Reid and Cathrine Lyttle

Summary: The chapter describes the history of health education, the nature of present activities, influences on health education and future trends. First initiatives were aimed at improving sanitation and the control of disease following the 'Asiatic cholera epidemic' of 1850. Health education has been recognized as important since the turn of the century and there has been increasing health knowledge since that time. In 1926, the Bureau of Health Education (BHE) was formed, initially with very limited resources. With increased resources and activities, it was responsible together with other agencies for many initiatives from 1945 to 1956. In 1956, the Jamaican Medical Department amalgamated with the Ministry of Health. The two main components of this system were medical services and public health services. During the 1960s, health educators' role shifted from being providers of information to being facilitators and enablers of other health and allied workers. The many developments since 1974 are documented and future trends are outlined.

Background information

Jamaica is the largest English-speaking island in the Caribbean with an area of approximately 4411 square miles and a population of just over 2.25 million. In 1986, 35.5 per cent of the population was between 0 and 14 years while 12.5 per cent of the population was over 65 years. A former colony of Britain with a plantation economy, Jamaica gained independence in August 1962.

To understand the development of health education in Jamaica it is helpful to review the development of organized public health in Jamaica.

The year 1850 – the year of the 'Asiatic cholera epidemic' – is a landmark in the development of public health services in Jamaica. The picture at that time was one of squalor and disease, contaminated water supplies and a total lack of sanitation. Arising out of the report of Dr Milroy who was sent out to investigate the causes of the epidemic by the Colonial Office, the following was the circular despatch from the Duke of Newcastle to Governors of the West Indies Colonies:

> To request you to exercise such authority and influence as you possess to procure the institution of such measures as may both improve the general sanitary condition of the colony under your government, and tend to avert from it such conditions as those which have recently desolated the island of Jamaica.

His Excellency, the Governor of Jamaica, Sir Charles Gray, being of the opinion that the powers vested in him under the Quarantine Act of the Island were not sufficiently explicit for the requirements of the emergency, pointed out to Chambers 'the necessity of conferring additional powers for the regulations'. Both the Council and the House of Assembly expressed the willingness to co-operate.

The legislature then passed an Act requiring the formation of a local board of health in every parish to make rules and regulations which they might consider necessary 'for the prevention and to avert the spreading of the Cholera in the parish'.

In 1851, a Bill for the establishment of a central board of health was passed. This Board expired in 1864 but was re-established by Law 6 of 1867, which gave the Governor, Sir John Peter Grant, powers to appoint a central board of health and to constitute municipal boards as local boards of health subordinated to the central board of health.

Concern about the lack of medical care was high and for many years the need for medical service in the island was impressed on the legislature. In 1868, the government medical service was started. The island was divided into 40 medical districts and 15 additional medical practitioners were appointed as district medical officers. These medical officers had to 'reside within the limits of their respective districts' and were required to:

'undertake the medical charge of paupers on the parochial rolls, and of any hospital, almshouse or prison in their districts; to attend upon the Constabulary; to exercise a general control and super-intendence over the Government Dispensaries in their districts; to vaccinate; and to advise the government and parochial authorities in questions affecting public health'.

The period between 1868 and 1919 brought increased knowledge about the cause and mode of infections and spread of disease resulting from the work of scientists such as Pasteur, Lister and Koch. It was within this period that quarantine regulations, general sanitation and control of infectious disease by isolation, came into effect in the island. But there was still no organized public health service as such, the policy being one of passing laws in an effort to control epidemics. Up to 1875, Kingston was the only parish with a commissioner of health. In other parishes officers and sub-officers of police served as 'inspectors of nuisance'.

The beginnings of co-operative health work 1919 to 1939

Organized public health really began in 1919 with the entry of the International Health Division of the Rockefeller Foundation on the invitation of the Government. The Foundation's general plan of work was to make a survey of a particular disease and to develop control measures effective in its prevention. During the survey the Foundation provided members of its staff to make a preliminary study, usually assisted by a government medical officer who later on took charge of the control programme. The team involved in these programmes generally included a medical officer, sanitary inspectors and nurses. Special attention was given to the education of the people, not only about sanitation and the improvement of water supplies but in disease prevention generally. Hook-worm was the first disease to be tackled and the campaign against this disease continued for 17 years. Campaigns against other diseases such as malaria, yaws, tuberculosis were initiated and ran concurrently.

The pioneering days

Health education has been recognized as an essential component of public health programmes in Jamaica since the early part of this century, predating even the establishment of a central health organization. At that time hookworm, tuberculosis, malaria and yaws were among the major epidemic diseases in the island. Special commissions were set up in collaboration with the International Health Division of the Rockefeller Foundation to study and control these diseases. Dr B E Washburn, the first director of the Rockefeller Foundation activities in Jamaica, founded the Bureau of Health Education (BHE) in 1926, under the auspices of the Central Board of Health, in response to the demands of teachers, sanitary inspectors and members of the public for more information about personal hygiene and the spread and prevention of prevailing diseases.

Although the objective of the BHE was to develop the health consciousness of the public, it had no full-time staff, no funds and no office of its own. It depended on the leadership of Dr B E Washburn and on whatever time could be spared by the various other members of the health team. A large part of BHE's work was mass education using film shows, distributing printed materials and giving lectures in school. In addition BHE carried out a sort of supervisory function with regard to the sanitation campaigns, receiving reports and taking general responsibility for the financing of the several health units which worked under the direction of the various commissions.

Jamaica, like the other West Indian islands, then colonies of Britain, was greatly affected by the world economic recession of the late 1920s. The poverty and distress of the people resulted in so much unrest that a Royal Commission was sent out in 1938 under the leadership of Lord Moyne to study the reasons for the uprisings and to make recommendations to the British Government. The need for improvement in sanitation, housing and medical services, for relevant education in health and hygiene and for the preparation of teachers and medical personnel in public health matters was clearly identified. Sir Rupert Briercliffe was subsequently appointed Medical Advisor to Colonial Development and Welfare (CD&W) in 1941. He emphasized the need for a more organized approach to health education with special staff appointed for that work. Full implementation of the recommendations were delayed by World War II and it was not until 1943 that plans got off the ground within the Medical Department in Jamaica and an officer was assigned to work in the field of health education.

It was recognized that the leadership needed for this special thrust in health education required a person with specialized training. Accordingly the officer was sent to the University of Michigan at Ann Arbour USA for specialist training in health education, on a Rockefeller Foundation Scholarship, prior to appointment. The appointment of Miss Gladys Morrison MA, the first Health Education Officer, in October 1945 presaged the beginning of a more organized and structured health education effort in Jamaica. The staff was increased in 1946 to include a temporary clerk/typist and a technician.

Financial support for BHE was provided initially under the Colonial Development and Welfare Act of 1940. The amount of £7010.00 was granted for the first five years with the expectation that the Government of Jamaica would assume full responsiblity at the end of that period.

The Bureau of Health Education 1945 to 1956

The first decade of BHE's life was a time of rapid and intensive expansion of programmes and increased demand for advisory and programme services from the 13 health departments in the island. However, growth in terms of staff was relatively slow and it was five years before the Health Education Officer was able to get an assistant health educator to join the then existing team of four – health education officer, typist, technician, and messenger.

The BHE carried out its work on an island-wide basis, in line with the priorities identified by the Medical Department. The main objective was to disseminate health information with a view to arousing individuals and groups to assume greater responsibility for personal and community health. In spite of the lack of personnel every effort was made to carry out a comprehensive health education programme. The projected programme included among other things working with local health and medical services in planning health educational programmes in the various parishes; stimulating, organizing and guiding in-service training programmes of personnel working in the field of health; collaborating with official and non-official agencies to promote health education, for example with the Jamaica Agricultural Society, the Jamaica Social Welfare Commission and other extension services; preparing publishing and distributing all materials for health education as required from time to time for example bulletins, pamphlets, posters and so forth; holding health exhibitions and health film shows throughout the island; planning radio broadcasts on public health matters; reviewing new health educational materials and public health literature from available sources and bringing them to the attention of medical officers, nurses, public health inspectors, teachers and others. The approach used was mainly the mass media – lectures, films and film strips, pamphlets, posters, health exhibitions and press releases on health matters. A quarterly bulletin *The Jamaica Public Health* which was published, and widely circulated especially to schools, was sometimes used as a test in classes on health and hygiene.

A special joint school health education committee was set up to promote school health education. Membership of the commiteee included representatives of the Education Department, the Medical Department, the West Indies School of Public Health, the Teachers' Association and Parent Teachers' Association. Special effort was made to have school health education included in the curriculum of teacher training colleges and in-service training in school health education was organized for teachers.

Intensive two-week courses were held with teachers drawn from rural and urban primary schools. A special feature of the programme was the follow-up by the Health Education Officer of projects designed by the teachers during the course for implementation upon return to their classes. Materials for use in school health education programmes were also produced by BHE. The BHE worked closely with the West Indies School of Public Health providing training in health education principles, methods and techniques for students doing basic training in public health and for in-service training of health staff.

The BHE was also responsible for library services in branches of the health and medical services, ordering all books and periodicals and checking on libraries in the hospitals, laboratories and suchlike. It also operated a loan library of public health books.

In addition BHE served as liaison between the Island Medical Department and all voluntary social agencies in matters relating to health. Churches, youth and other voluntary agencies were given assistance with health programmes. The Health Education Officer participated in summer schools and took advantage of every opportunity to stimulate interest in health education.

1956 to 1974

In 1956, the Medical Department amalgamated with the Ministry of Health. A Chief Medical Officer was appointed in charge of all technical aspects of the health care system in Jamaica. The two main components of this system were:

a. medical services,
b. public health services.

The BHE was included in the Public Health portfolio which was under the direction of a Principal Medical Officer (Health). But the Health Education Officer was free to work across the board with both the public health and the curative services which were under the direction of the Principal Medical Officer (Medical).

Under this new organizational arrangement BHE continued to give leadership in the planning and implementation of health education programmes and activities at national and local levels in response to the stated problems and priorities of the Ministry of Health. It also continued the programme of film shows and health exhibitions with the local health departments. Special areas of emphasis were, maternal and child health with particular attention to DPT and BCG immunization, breast-feeding, nutrition, sexually transmitted diseases, malaria and family planning. A variety of methods and approaches – surveys, staff conferences, orientation workshops, radio and subsequently television programmes were employed as well as the production and use of relevant audio-visual materials and teaching aids.

By 1956 the appointment of two additional assistant health education officers brought the staff complement to 11 persons which included one health education officer, three assistant health education officers, two stenographer typists, two drivers, one messenger. Their appointments made it possible for BHE to carry out more direct health education activities with people at the parish level. It was decided to select three parishes to receive concentrated attention. Each of the three assistant health education officers was assigned to reside and work for the greater part of each week in one of the three parishes. Using the community organization approach they worked through existing groups for example 4H Clubs, agricultural extension services, church and welfare groups, and community development officers to stimulate greater consciousness of community health problems and to encourage participation in the programmes of the local health department. The officers also worked closely with the public health staff in these parishes identifying priorities for health education and in planning and implementing appropriate programmes. This preferred way of working with one health educator to a parish was difficult to maintain with the small number of trained health educators available to service the 13 health departments, as well as carry out functions at the national level. The BHE, was now faced with the dilemma of how to deploy the slender technical resources to give effective health education service and at the same time greater island-wide coverage.

Unfortunately, in spite of having received training in health education during their basic public health preparation, many health workers felt that it was the responsibility of the designated health education officer to carry out the educational activities. This perception may well have developed as a result of the earlier emphasis on dissemination of information and with the advent of the 'specialist' it was seen to be primarily their responsibility. In 1959, the effort to shift this perspective of health education as the dissemination of information, and to enable health personnel at all levels to become more aware and accepting of their responsibility in health education, particularly at the point of the delivery of service, was intensified. The decision was taken to work on a regional basis. The island was divided into four regions with the Health Education Officer and all of the Assistant Health Education Officers each having responsibility for working with the health departments in one region.

The BHE also worked in close collaboration with other Ministries and the Government Information Service and with special interest groups in mounting programmes for 'Mental health week', 'Dental health week', 'Home and family life week', 'Child Month' and so on. It also took the initiative in developing a co-ordinated approach to family-life education and sex education in schools in collaboration with the Ministries of Education and of Youth and Community Development.

The continued increasing demands for programmes and services from the health departments, placed undue pressure on the staff and highlighted the need for technical advice in addressing the problem. In 1956, the Ministry of Health held discussions with the International Co-operation Administration (ICA) of the USA which resulted in a project agreement. The project, funded jointly by ICA and the Ministry of Health, aimed at improving BHE as a technical branch of the Ministry, preparing and training professional staff to ensure continuity of health education services for the country, and enabling BHE to select and procure basic educational equipment and materials needed for the proper functioning of the health education services. A health education consultant was made available by ICA to work with BHE for almost four years beginning February 1957. A detailed plan was developed which aimed at increasing the number of trained health educators to 10 for the island by 1966, and providing the necessary technical support staff (typists, writer, librarian, projectionist) for BHE to function efficiently.

Throughout this period considerable effort was made to recruit suitable persons with a minimum qualification of a bachelor's degree or its equivalent from a recognized institution. It was anticipated that after some practical work-experience in health education, such persons could be sent for advanced training. Unfortunately, the whole effort was hampered by the low level of emolument BHE was able to offer which made it impossible to compete with other Civil Service positions, let alone with opportunities on the open market for the calibre of persons needed. When the post of Health Education Officer was first created the salary scale was comparable to that of positions of similar responsibility in other Government Departments such as Education and Agriculture. In the major reorganization which took place at the time of the amalgamation of the Island Medical Department within the Ministry of Health this comparability was lost. The anomalies created were not adequately rectified and over the years the gap continued to widen. The BHE's ability to retain staff was also affected and there was a rapid turnover among the health educators, particularly males. None-the-less by 1964, there were six assistant health education officers on the staff. Subsequently three of these officers went on fellowships to the USA for further professional preparation, and by 1973 four of the health educators had received the MPH degree.

During the mid 1960s as a short term measure while national staff were studying overseas, Peace Corps Volunteers served as health educators in some of the parishes. In this period too, a system of recruiting graduates from the Univesity of the West Indies as health education trainees was tried as a means of building a pool of candidates suitable for appointment to assistant health education officer positions when they were created.

The BHE was still concerned about establishing closer working relationships with health personnel and community leaders at the community level on a parish basis. Experience had shown that this approach encouraged greater involvement of local health staff and other workers in the educational aspects of their daily work. Gradually perceptions of the role of the full-time health educators was shifting. From being seen only as providers of direct health education services, their role expanded to one of facilitating and enabling other health and allied workers to see health education as an integral part of their work, and to help them to carry through that responsibility effectively.

Another development in the early 1960s was the introduction of health education in the training programme for medical students at the University of the West Indies, Mona Campus. Initially students in their five-week clerkship in the Department of Social and Preventive Medicine visited the offices of BHE for orientation to the health education services and programmes in Jamaica. The Department of Social and Preventive Medicine (DSPM) saw health education as an essential component in the preparation of doctors and in the mid-1960s the Health Education Officer of BHE was invited with the approval of the Ministry of Health to serve as an honorary lecturer in health education to the DSPM. Subsequently the DSPM procured the full-time services of a health educator through the Canadian Government.

There were also developments taking place in the DSPM in relation to family planning which strengthened the need for continuing health education services within the DSPM. In 1971, as part of a special family planning project a post of lecturer in health education was created. Later the health education programme expanded to include inputs into other university programmes.

By the late 1960s links had been forged not only with the University of West Indies but with universities overseas. The BHE was serving as a place for the field training of graduate and undergraduate students majoring in health education for periods of three to eight weeks. Students originated from countries such as Pakistan, India, Ethiopia, Ghana, Libya among others.

Over the intervening years BHE's audio-visual services were strengthened to meet the demands for film shows and exhibitions from the parishes. The production and distribution of suitable health education materials and visual aids was always a priority task. In the early days the printing was done by the Government Printing Office. As the demand for materials increased it often became impossible for publication deadlines to be met due to pressures on the printing office from the various Government Departments. To meet programme needs it became increasingly necessary to use commercial printers and this put a heavy strain on BHE's budget.

In 1967, financial assistance from UNICEF made it possible for BHE to set up its own printery. During this period it had the assistance of an audio-visual consultant provided by the US Agency for International Development. Starting with one press, a printer and an audio-visual attendant the printery rapidly developed to include a second press, silk screen equipment and a silk screen printer. The audio-visual section was recognized and enlarged with the addition of a third artist. In 1968, a writer and a communication media officer were appointed.

1974 to the present

Two events significantly influenced the development of health education during this period – the integration of the family planning education officers to the National Family Planning Board with the staff of BHE and the primary health care thrust with emphasis on health education and community participation.

A background of the relationship between the National Family Planning Board, BHE and the Ministry of Health during the years preceding integration may be helpful.

A family planning programme under the auspices of a voluntary organization existed in Jamaica since the 1930s as a result of an awakening social conscience. With increasing concerns at the rapidly rising population and the social and economic problems that were resulting, the government in 1967 accelerated the 'Family planning programme' by the establishment under the Ministry of Health of a National Family Planning Board. In addition to nurses and other health personnel within the Ministry of Health and Environmental Control engaged in the provision of family planning services, the Board appointed its own staff which included Family Planning Education Officers (FPEO) who operated at the parish level. By 1974, each of the 14 parishes in Jamaica had 3 parish officers.

Through an agreement between the Ministry of Health, the Family Planning board and BHE, the latter was made responsible for the educational aspects of the 'Family planning programme' in Jamaica and for the technical guidance and supervision of the FPEOs.

The BHE also had a responsibility to train the FPEOs and assisted in the pre-service and in-service training programmes sponsored by the Board for physicians, nurses, midwives, clerks, social workers and other personnel. Educational materials in support of the 'Family planning programme' were also developed and prepared by the BHE.

As a consequence of an evaluation of the 'Family Planning programme' in relation to national needs, a decision was made to integrate the field services of the Board with the staff of BHE. The decision was implemented in April 1974 when 46 staff positions on the Board were transferred to BHE. For the first time in its history, BHE had staff available to work full-time at the parish level throughout the island. With integration, head office staff of BHE provided guidance and supervision to the field offices in the planning, implementation and evaluation of health education programmes and activities. The health educators were responsible to the Medical Officers of Health for their day-to-day operations.

An intermediate level of administration between headquarters and the parishes was also introduced in the form of Regional Health Education Officers.

As mentioned earlier, another significant influence on the development of health education in Jamaica was the 'Primary health care' strategy to which Jamaica subscribed and in which the role of health education and community participation were highlighted.

The formation of health committees at the community level became one of the main thrusts of the government. In a policy document, 'Primary health care – the Jamaican perspective', the pivotal role of health education, the educational responsibilities of full-time health educators and all members of the health team were clearly spelled out. At the field level, health educators spent a considerable amount of their time in spear-heading, strengthening and nurturing health committees through which community participation, intersectorial collaboration and the partnership role of individuals, communities and health workers in the promotion and maintenance of health were promoted. At present, there are several health committees throughout the island, and a number of community projects (most of which are income generating) were implemented through these health committees.

Over the years, in an effort to facilitate the smooth functioning of health committees and help communities gain a fuller understanding of their role in promoting and protecting their health, much health education emphasis was placed on training. Training components included the objectives of health committees, the functions of health committee members, how to conduct meetings and record minutes, interpersonal relationships and the roles and responsibilities of group leaders and group members.

Other imputs centred around prevailing health concerns. For example, committee members were taught about immunization and the importance of having infants and children fully immunized. The main problem which existed with immunizations was that there was usually a great out-pouring for the first dose and the numbers petered out when it came to the second and third doses. Through the health committees, communities helped parents and guardians to have their children completely immunized. Another example of a programme in which health committees were involved was the use of oral rehydration salts when the emphasis shifted from the use of drugs to fluids in the treatment of diarrhoea. The health educators had the main responsibility for planning, co-ordinating, implementing and evaluating the training programmes.

Much credit for the success of health committees and community projects must go to all members of the health team. In this connection the contribution of community health aids who work closely with communities on a day-to-day basis has made a significant contribution to primary health care over the past two decades.

Perceptions of health education

For a long time health education was perceived to be the responsibility of the full-time health educator. It was also perceived as a process of telling people what to do. There was a feeling that the provision of information was sufficient to bring about desired behaviour change.

These perceptions have changed, and markedly so within the past two decades. Today, it is safe to say that the majority of health workers perceive health education to be a process in which they have an important role. Increasingly, there is a desire to understand and use the principles and theories from the behavioural and communication sciences that affect the practice of health education.

Opportunities for training

Since January of 1975, in response to a request from Caribbean Governments, the Department of Social and Preventive Medicine of the University of the West Indies, commenced an 18-month programme leading to the Diploma in Community Health (Health Education). The establishment of the 'Diploma programme' opened up opportunities for nurses, public health inspectors, teachers and community workers with at least five years working experience to enter the field or receive formal training as health educators. The Diploma in Community Health (Health Education), is accepted as the basic preparation for health educators in the Caribbean. Between 1975 and 1985, 53 candidates from ten territories graduated from the programme. The programme was suspended in 1985. By request of various Ministries of Health in the region, it is to re-commence in October 1988.

Over the years staff of BHE have been intimately involved in the 'Diploma programme' through training imputs and as part of the selection committee and panel of examiners. The BHE has also served as a placement centre for health education interns from Jamaica and other countries in the region during their six months internship period.

In October 1985, the Department of Social and Preventive Medicine in collaboration with the Sparkman Center of the University of Alabama, USA, offered a 15-month programme leading to the Master of Public Health Degree. To date three health educators have been enrolled in the 'Master of public health programme'.

Career prospects

Generally, emoluments of full-time health educators are still not adequate enough to attract and retain personnel. However, a number of trained health educators have moved to related agencies and industrial firms. For example, the National Family Planning Board, the Training Division of the Ministry of Health, Carreras of Jamaica and the Drug and Substance Abuse Secretariat.

Aspects of health education currently being promoted

In keeping with a long established policy, the priorities of BHE are in accordance with the health priorities of Jamaica and the Ministry of Health. Areas of emphasis are influenced by prevailing health problems and concerns. At present, the main areas of concentration are maternal and child health including family planning, immunization and nutrition, sexually transmitted diseases including AIDS, drug and substance abuse, accident prevention, diabetes and hypertension, oral health, cancer screening and ageing.

The promotion of health education takes various forms, such as working with local health departments and schools at the parish level in planning and implementing programmes, providing training in the basic principles and practice of health education to trainee public health nurses and inspectors, trainee nurses and school teachers, holding health fairs and health exhibitions throughout the island, preparing and delivering talks through radio and television, working with scouts, guides, school children and non-government organizations on special projects, working with communities in the development of projects designed to improve their health status and carrying out operational research.

Central control in the promotion of health education

In theory, central control in the promotion of health education lies with BHE of the Ministry of Health. However, over the years there has been an increase in the number of non-government organizations and other health related agencies involved in health education programmes and projects and a number of new associations now exists. These include the Diabetic Association, The Heart Foundation, The Cancer Society, The Society for the

Control of Sexually Transmitted Diseases, A Drug and Substance Abuse Secretariat and number of insurance companies. The BHE is involved in the development of educational materials for these organizations and is often called on to participate in the planning of educational programmes. However, BHE is not usually involved during the early stages.

The Ministry of Health has the major responsibility for the health of the nation but realizes that many other agencies and Ministries are responsible for services and activities that contribute to good health. In a policy statement in 1984, the Ministry proposed a National Co-ordinating Committee to co-ordinate the implementation of inter-sectoral action for health. Such a committee could help to ensure that scarce resources are appropriately and effectively used and that programmes and activities are meeting national goals as well as individual, family and community needs.

Recognizing the benefits of a co-ordinated approach between the Ministry of Health and non-Governmental organizations and Agencies, BHE has recently received a grant from the Pan American Health organization to facilitate the development of a mechanism for co-ordinating and monitoring health education projects and activities.

Political importance of health education

Over the years, the governments of both political parties have valued health as a vital component in the thrust for development and have re-iterated that emphasis should be given to activities that promote public education, stimulate active community participation in all health programmes, and encourage people to take responsibility for the maintenance of their health and that of their community. Health education has also been promoted as the responsibility of all members of the health team and an integral part of their functioning.

Future trends

During the 1970s, the post of Director of Health Education was created. The Director is part of the management team of the Ministry of Health. The BHE now has posts for 52 health educators. Twenty-one of these are presently filled. Included in the present complement of health educators are three Peace Corps Volunteers. The Volunteers serve for two-year periods and it is envisaged that their services will be required in the future if the existing salary structures remain. Efforts are also being made to recruit the services of United Nations Volunteers to help supplement the staff of health educators.

While emphasis will change in terms of programme developments, trends indicate that from time to time priorities will be established within the following areas:

☐ health and family life education in schools,
☐ maternal and child health including family planning, sexually transmitted diseases including AIDS, drug and substance abuse, accident prevention, chronic diseases and ageing.

Individual and community responsibility for the promotion and maintenance of health will continue to be promoted and community participation encouraged.

In terms of limited resources as a developing country it is fundamental that a para-professional corps should be developed as an integral part of the strategy for implementing health programmes.

The basic training for health educators is the Diploma in Community Health (Health Education). However, there is still the need to develop specialist health educators at policy and management levels.

It is now necessary to strengthen the staff of BHE by an infusion of give specialist health educators over a five year period to develop and effectively implement the management of programmes. It is suggested that such senior professionals should be prepared up to the level of a Master's degree in Public Health.

The Department of Social and Preventive Medicine of the University of the West Indies should be involved and work closely with BHE and other agencies in carrying out research and developing training programmes in health education.

For the development and implementation of government and other health education programmes more emphasis needs to be placed on documentation, operational research and the continuing evaluation of health education projects and activities.

12. A participatory and intersectoral approach to community development — the Deeside community project St Catherine, Jamaica — A CASE STUDY

J Tulloch-Reid and M Reid

Summary: The chapter describes a health education initiative in a community in Jamaica. The project had three main components: co-operative farming, latrine construction and health education. The work of the project included collection of baseline data about the community, identification of problems, development of inter-personal skills and latrine construction. The outcomes of the project are described as are future plans. The difficulties faced by the project are outlined. Some of these were to do with perceptions and attitudes of those involved. Others were of a very practical nature. The lessons learned from the project are described.

Introduction

Globally, there has been an increasing realization that health conditions cannot be improved without the involvement of individuals and communities. The promotion of health and the alleviation of many health problems in developing countries necessitate priority attention being given to socio-economic conditions and a multi-disciplinary and educational approach as integral parts of their solution. Jamaica, along with other countries of the world, subscribes to the Alma Ata Declaration of 'Health for all by the year 2000' with community participation, health education and inter-sectoral collaboration as essential components to the achievement of this lofty goal.

It is recognized that among the underlying purposes of the educational approach to health is the development of a sense of personal responsibility for one's health and the health of the community as well as the ability to participate responsibly and constructively in programmes designed and administered for the well-being of the community.

Undoubtedly, well-organized and co-ordinated health education programmes are necessary if people are to be stimulated and prepared for participation in health programmes and to continue the developmental process. Health workers and workers in fields such as social welfare, education, community development and agriculture as well as politicians are all concerned with the quality of life of individuals, families and communities and appreciate the importance of a collaborative approach to individual and community development.

This case study shows how a rural community's capacity to address local problems and issues is strengthened by members of the health team and other departments working collaboratively. It is also an example of how the Ministry of Health and the University of the West Indies worked together in the promotion of health and development. The study highlights the basic health education principles of participative planning and community self-renewal. It also illustrates the importance of the partnership role between health workers and other professionals and the community.

Background information

Jamaica is an island in the Caribbean Sea positioned at around longitude 18 degrees north and latitude 17 degrees west with an area of 4,244 square miles. It has a population of about two and a quarter million, and is divided into 14 parishes. Jamaica became an independent country within the British Commonwealth in 1962.

Settlement and early history of Deeside (project area)

Deeside is a small rural community in the parish of St Catherine, Jamaica. It is located about 25 miles from Kingston, the capital city, and 12 miles from Spanish Town, the capital of St Catherine.

The families in Deeside live on about 40 acres of 'captured' land which was part of the property of a technical high school. The land which was idle for some time was used by the school for the rearing of animals.

At present, there are about 150 families in Deeside. The population developed gradually beginning in 1970 with four families. By 1975, there were 18 and in 1980, 33 families. When the project on which this study focuses started in 1985, there were 64 families. The original settlers had subdivided portions of land and sold lots to persons who were interested in building homes in the community. The terrain is hilly and the soil fertile. Trees such as ackee, breadfruit, coconut, bananas and citrus can be seen as well as a few vegetables.

The development of a community spirit and the evolution of self reliance

Because they occupied 'captured' land which had been idle for some time, the first inhabitants of Deeside settled as far as possible from the road so that their presence might be undetected. However, their presence was soon discovered by an alert school principal who permitted them to remain on the land because they were farming.

Conscious that they lived on 'captured' land, residents were at first hesitant to ask for outside help. Between 1975 and 1980, as the families grew, they began to meet on Sunday afternoons to discuss their problems and possible solutions. These meetings led to the formation of a Citizens' Association. The families contributed money to assist with the laying of pipes for their water supply, and, with the assistance of their local Member of Parliament, the community was provided with piped water and electricity.

Members of the health team take an interest in Deeside and a relationship is established

Sickness of a community member's daughter and her treatment at the health clinic established a link between the Deeside Community and the St Catherine Health Department which grew and flourished. An alert public health nurse and health educator decided to do follow-up home visits in Deeside as part of their treatment plan for the sick child who was apparently suffering from an allergy. During their visits to Deeside they listened to the citizens and gained their perceptions of their problems and the developments the citizens wanted to see take place. Members of the community report that many useful suggestions were made by the health team including the planting of catch crops and the rearing of animals to help meet the community's nutritional needs.

Over the years, developmental assistance was given to the community by the Social Development Commission. The officers of the Commission helped the young people in the community through their 'Youth club plan' and implemented cultural programmes and skills training. Officers of the Jamaica Movement for the Advancement of Literacy (JAMAL) also worked in the community.

The Ministry of Health's manpower development plan

The Ministry of Health in Jamaica began a 'Health manpower development plan' in October 1981 through a grant from USAID. The objective was to improve the quality of life and health status of select communities through the development of income generating projects. The guiding principle was that communities in collaboration with members of the health team and other relevant agencies and organizations would identify their problems and work towards solutions and the building of self-reliance.

The health department's knowledge of Deeside, the initiative of its citizens, and the willingness of the citizens to help themselves, led to the selection of the community for a project grant of twenty thousand Jamaican Dollars in February of 1985. The project had three components – co-operative farming, latrine construction, and health education.

Aims and objectives of the Deeside project

Through a series of workshops the aims and objectives of the Deeside project were identified by community members and members of the health team as follows:

1. the development of pig and poultry farming;
2. the training of 10 community members in pig and poultry farming, money management and co-operative farming;
3. the training of 16 community members in the building and maintenance of latrines and environmental sanitation;
4. the construction of 16 latrines;
5. training in inter-personal relationship, problem solving and leadership skills.

Preliminary Development

Development of project document

The project was conceptualized to reflect the principles of community participation and inter-sectoral collaboration.

In keeping with these principles, community members and members of the health team participated in writing up the project document. This was followed by a series of workshops with resource persons from the Ministries of Agriculture and Health. Training included:

1. how to manage piggery;
2. administering simple medications;
3. the rearing of birds;
4. the maintenance of latrines.

The sessions were both theoretical and practical and included tours of poultry and pig farms for demonstration purposes.

Selection of a management committee

The project was managed by an executive committee consisting of:

1. the Medical Officer of Health who was the project manager and principal project facilitator;
2. the president of the Deeside Citizens' Association;
3. a representative of the Ministry of Agriculture;
4. the parish Health Educator – who was the co-ordinator.

The intervention of health education interns of the University of the West Indies

In January of 1985, the co-ordinator of the project was given the opportunity of doing a three-month certificate course in community health at the University of the West Indies.

The Medical Officer of Health who was the project manager, felt that the release of the co-ordinator at that time would be disruptive to the project. Mrs J Tulloch Reid, who was both co-ordinator of the certificate course and co-ordinator of the health education aspects of the diploma programme, offered to assign two health education interns who were pursuing the diploma in community health course to co-ordinate the programme and act as project facilitators. The plan was for the interns to reside in Deeside but as no accommodation was available, they lived nearby and commuted on a daily basis.

The nature of work

The establishment of baseline data

The initial approach to the project implementation was the establishment of baseline data and gaining community acceptance. This data was collected by the interns and community members. The methods used were observation, discussions with community leaders and health personnel, participation in community activities and functions, examination of records and a question-naire. The questionnaire was designed by the interns in collaboration with community leaders and administered by the interns and community members. The community members were prepared by the interns to administer the questionnaire.

RESULTS OF SURVEY
The community profile revealed the following information:

☐ There were 64 homes, 16 of which were made of block and steel and 48 of board. Twenty-six of the homes had two rooms, 22 one room, and eight consisted of three or more rooms. None of the homes had water piped into the house. The community used 37 stand pipes and 22 of the households collected water in drums. When there was no water in the pipes, residents used the river.

☐ in 1985, the population which was estimated to be between 285 and 310 persons, was a young one with 65 per cent under 24 years of age. Most of the adults were housewives and farmers. In the community there were also teachers, a secretary, a nurse, a midwife, a mason, a carpenter, an auto-mechanic, a butcher, a painter and a dressmaker. Over 63 per cent of the community members had a primary school education and 17 per cent received a secondary education.

SOCIAL PROBLEMS IDENTIFIED BY THE COMMUNITY IN ORDER OF PRIORITY
1. Inadequate water supply. There was a need to ensure that water reached all parts of Deeside.
2. Poor access road. The road to and within Deeside needed to be repaired.
3. Lack of land ownership.
4. Unemployment and lack of skills development for the young people of the community.
5. Lack of a basic school.
6. Lack of co-operation among some villagers.
7. Poor housing and lack of money to provide for basic needs.

HEALTH STATUS AND HEALTH PROBLEMS
Health problems were identified which included: skin infections, head lice, upper respiratory tract infections and dental cavities. While the immuniza-tion coverage for polio, diphtheria, whooping cough and tetanus were good, measles coverage was 40 per cent which was considerably below the national target.

Eighteen per cent of the births were delivered by Nanas and 50 per cent of the population were not practising, nor interested in family planning. Over 60 per cent of the community utilized the maternal and child health services at the health centre.

COMMUNICATION AND UTILITIES

In 1985, there were 43 radios and 11 televisions in the community. The main source of information was the spoken word. The road to Deeside was rough and full of trenches. The residents dug mall from a pit and repaired the road which was useable by motor car. While 50 homes were wired for electricity, only 27 had electricity as 23 units were disconnected because residents could not meet the high cost of electricity bills. Kerosene lamps were widespread and wood and charcoal were the main sources of energy for cooking. Forty-one homes had latrines, 11 had latrines under construction and seven were without latrines.

The building of a community training centre

The first objective of the community was the building of a training centre. The citizens of Deeside used to meet in a church building for their monthly meetings and other functions. However, they decided that they wanted a meeting place of their own which could also be used as the training centre for their project activities. Using local lumber felled from the banks of the river adjoining the community the citizens erected a framework for a community centre in February of 1985 to coincide with the official launching of the project. Pictures were taken of the centre during all stages of the construction. A local company was so impressed with the efforts of the community that they offered the Medical Officer of Health (the project manager) sheets of zinc at a reduced rate to help roof the building.

In keeping with a Jamaican tradition, a major effort was planned for Labour Day in May of 1985. From as early as five o'clock in the morning community members started their activities. The following were accomplished:

1. the planting of trees bordering the community centre;
2. a 'Welcome to Deeside' sign by the young members of the Citizens' Association;
3. the bushing of the ground of the community centre;
4. completion of the roofing of the centre;
5. flooring of the building with cement;
6. building a latrine for the community centre.

Approximately 90 per cent of the community members participated in the Labour Day activities. The Medical Officer of Health and the interns also participated. The centre was completed and officially opened on 15 June 1985. The residents proudly invited the press to be present at their opening.

An extract from JAMPRESS, the official information service of Jamaica captured the essence of the community effort.

A fine example of self help effort has been shown at Deeside in St Catherine a small district of people with big minds who have established a community centre. It is nothing elaborate just a simple rectangular structure made out of wood, zinc, concrete and stones. But they will tell you proudly that soon, very soon, they will be involved in bigger things such as pig and poultry farming, art and craft and a basic school. There is also a latrine project in progress. (*The Daily Gleaner* June 1985)

The health education component

TRAINING

In response to the community's request, sessions were held covering the following areas:

- ☐ inter-personal relationships;
- ☐ human sexuality;
- ☐ sexually transmitted disease;
- ☐ personal hygiene;
- ☐ family planning;
- ☐ immunizations;
- ☐ leadership;
- ☐ community organization;
- ☐ problem solving.

In keeping with the educational level of the community and the participatory approach, educational strategies included role play, drama, buzz group exercises and broken squares. The following are examples of approaches that were used:

1. Aim: To identify community problems. Groups were asked what they would do to improve Deeside if they received a gift of $20,000 to help develop their community.
2. Aim: To develop leadership. The following task was set. You are the foreman in charge of the latrine construction project in Deeside. Your ten men crew are not performing the amount of work that you expect. Demonstrate through role play how you would try to deal with the situation and get more work done.
3. Aim: To develop problem-solving skills. The following task was used. You are members of the Deeside Citizens' Association and have a problem with a water shortage in the community. Demonstrate what actions you would take to deal with the problem, bearing in mind that your poultry and piggery project is at stake.

Latrine construction

Community members organized themselves in work groups and with the help of the public health inspector for the area selected sights for their latrines. Most of the digging of the pits took place at nights as the members reasoned that the nights were cooler and they could work more effectively.

This aspect of the project was facilitated by inputs from the health education interns who were former public health inspectors.

Outcomes of the programme February 1985 to June 1988

A visit to Deeside in June 1988 demonstrated community initiative and the remarkable transformation that has taken place. The specified objectives have been achieved and there have been many additional spin-offs some of which are listed below:

1. The community centre which was completed in June of 1985 is well utilized for meetings, recreation, workshops and as an immunization centre when the health staff visit the community. The centre is often rented and the money used to help defray electricity bills.
2. All homes in Deeside now have piped water.
3. A block factory has been established in the community by one of the project participants and most of the homes which are now three and four bedroom buildings with inside bathroom and kitchen, are made of block and steel.
4. The access road to Deeside is well paved.
5. Deeside has been surveyed by Government Surveyors and the machinery for granting land titles or leasing the land is in place.
6. All 17 latrines were built, are being used and are in good condition.
7. Thirteen families are now engaged in pig rearing.
8. The community won the better community competition for the Parish of St Catherine, while the football team won the parish prize for the best disciplined team.

One of the most outstanding success stories is told by Mrs Hyacinth McKenzie, one of the original settlers in Deeside who had been interviewed in 1985 at the beginning of the project. Mrs McKenzie relates how she was helped in the building of a fowl pen for her chickens. She succeeded in rearing all of the first batch of chickens received. When she sold them, she paid some of the profits into the fund. She brought a second batch of chickens but experienced difficulty in rearing them, so she switched to pig rearing. Her pigs have done very well. She is able to feed herself and her five grandchildren adequately, and has bought furniture such as a second hand refrigerator, chairs, a table and hassocks, and can find one thousand Jamaican dollars in cash at any time. She is no longer dependent on her husband, but is in a position to help him. She is extending their home which is being changed from board to block and steel. Mrs McKenzie expressed pride and gratitude at her involvement in the project. She recalls the training sessions in which sticks were used to demonstrate the difference between working alone and working co-operatively.

Another outstanding success story is that of the president of the Citizens' Association. Through proceeds from her poultry rearing, she has started a block factory. The factory provides employment for some of the residents and the blocks are sold at a cheaper rate than on the open market.

Difficulties faced by the project and how they were overcome

1. At the beginning some community members were sceptical about the project. They wondered if it had political or partisan overtones, others decided to wait and see. A detailed explanation of the funding of the project and the role of the community helped to allay their fears.

2. In learning about traditional health practices the interns collected some of the plants and herbs used by community members. The local *obea* man accused them of being involved in abortion practices. When they explained why they were collecting the plants, he assisted them and provided information about the uses of the plants.

3. Deeside community like any other is not without its problems caused, essentially, by personality conflicts. These conflicts often resulted in community efforts being dissipated. The Medical Officer of Health project manager through her involvement with the community was instrumental in helping community members solve their conflicts and in developing conflict resolution skills.

4. The citizens of Deeside are quite anxious to legally own the lands on which they reside. Late in 1987 they saw a notice in one of our daily newspapers that persons who settled on land illegally should contact the Ministry of Agriculture. The citizens led a delegation to the Ministry of Agriculture who sent a representative to Deeside to meet with the residents. The land is being surveyed and a list of names have been submitted for titles.

5. Many problems were of a very practical nature as illustrated by the examples given below:

☐ During the construction of the latrines some moulds which were imported were late in arriving. The community members decided to do without them and build the toilets in their traditional manner.

☐ On several occasions it was difficult to dig to the required depth for a latrine due to the nature of the soil. Some sites were abandoned, but drums were utilized in other instances.

☐ The community members decided that larger pipes rather than a tank would solve their water problem. The cost of laying the pipes was estimated at seven thousand Jamaican dollars. The members felt they could not afford that amount. They suggested to the water authorities that if they would provide the expertise, the community would provide the labour. The water authorities agreed, and adequate piped water was brought to their homes through this collaborative effort at a considerably reduced cost.

☐ The poultry rearing proved to be costly and difficult. This aspect of the project has been abandoned and the concentration is now on pig rearing.

Future plans

1. The community is planning to change the community centre from a wooden to a concrete building.

2. So far the community has developed haphazardly. It is hoped that it will develop in a more orderly manner with the granting of land titles.
3. The pig rearing which came later in the project is going well. It was designed as a revolving scheme. Some of the members who participated in the project have began to sell their pigs and have made returns so that others can benefit from the project.

Existing problems identified

The basic school is being held at the home of the teacher rather than at the community centre as was planned. In an interview the teacher explained that the young people in the community used the centre for recreational purposes and it is not cleaned up in time for school. He also observed that there were children of school age who were not attending school.

The president of the Citizens' Association was concerned that the adult members were reluctant to follow through with their meetings if she could not attend. However, the younger members of the community managed well, even in the absence of adults. Those involved in managing the project observed that the president had been on a number of training programmes and they felt that the opportunity to participate should be extended to other members. In this way, she could have an under-study and the kinds of knowledge and skills she possessed could be more widespread throughout the community.

Some lessons learned

☐ The motivation for continuity and self renewal which are essential for personal and community development are assured when community members experience the joy and excitement of participation and success.
☐ It is useful for facilitators to learn about and utilize the experience of others, to build upon the established traditions of the community.
☐ When communities are involved in identifying their problems, developing project proposals and setting the agenda for action, commitment, self respect, pride and confidence-building are enhanced.
☐ Resources are available in every community that can be identified, developed and channelled towards improved health and well-being.
☐ Data on community health activities often offers more positive inducements to further action including financial commitment and assistance than morbidity and mortality data.
☐ It is important to involve community members in data collection, share the results with as wide a cross section as possible and develop strategies and action plans with the community.
☐ Inter-sectoral collaboration and team work are desirable ways of working. At the operational level, however, projects often go wrong when individuals or agencies have low levels of commitment and let down the community. Someone has to be alert enough to fill the gap

otherwise the trust and credibility which are so difficult to build can be lost over-night.

☐ Communities have problems and conflicts which can divert and diffuse their energies. A facilitator who is respected and who can foster conflict resolution is a tremendous asset.

☐ Success attracts further success. All communities have problems and practices which are not conducive to health. Rather than dwelling on the problems, for example low acceptance of family planning, it is useful to find something positive about the community and to show how the community can be helped to develop further.

☐ Accurate accounting procedures are essential but often difficult to sustain. The importance of accounting for moneys spent, and keeping supporting receipts carefully is not always appreciated.

☐ Documentation of a project at every stage of its development is not only a useful evaluation tool but also a prime motivator.

☐ Field work placements have impact when interns work with a programme in which they can apply principles, concepts and skills learned in the classroom and receive support and supervision in using principles and skills.

☐ The quality of the leadership, level of commitment, inter-personal relationship skills, moral support and the integrity of facilitators are vital components in community development.

☐ Developmental rather than dependency relationships must be the goal of facilitators in helping community members and communities realize their potentials.

The leadership, level of commitment and involvement of the Medical Officer of Health makes a difference to the success or failure of community projects.

13. Health education in Canada – AN OVERVIEW

Kenneth Allison

Summary: Health education is seen as a component of health promotion. The division of health education was formed in 1978. The changes in health education – strongly influenced by Michael Palko – which took place in the context of major social and health changes, are described. In the 1970s, health education and promotion were increasingly criticized for over-emphasis on life-style problems and individual responsibility for health. Under the heading current status, the chapter describes community health education, school health education and other health education settings. There are few programmes to train health educators for either school or community work although provision of continuing education in health education is increasing. There are two major lines of research: evaluation studies and studies of factors affecting health behaviour. Research is funded from a number of sources. Important future trends: changes in health problems; the increased emphasis on health promotion; and the prospects for professionalization are discussed.

Introduction

The scope of health education activities in Canada, like the country itself, is wide and diffuse. There is neither central control over these activities nor is there, at the present time, any mechanisms of control by the Government or the profession over who practices health education. On a conceptual and organizational level, health education in Canada is considered to be one of a number of approaches under the general umbrella of health promotion. Thus, on several fronts, health education in Canada is not unlike the field in many other countries.

There are, however, some distinctive features of the field of health education in Canada which bear examination. In the following pages some of these features will be described: a brief history of Canadian health education, the current status of the field and possible trends for the future.

Although there are many excellent examples of programmes and research in the twelve Canadian provinces, the present chapter does not represent a comprehensive treatment of health education in this country. Instead, the purpose here is to provide the reader with a brief overview of some of the major characteristics of health education in Canada and to discuss some of the factors affecting future trends.

Historical development of the field

According to Dr Robin Badgley (1978), the first formally constructed
government body focusing on health education was a Division of Public
Health Education of the Ontario Provincial Board of Health in 1921, followed
by similar departments in other provinces. On a national level, a section on
Publicity and Health Education was formed in 1938. At that time, health
education was seen as being the responsibility of all public health workers
and consisted primarily of lectures and the development of news releases.
There were only a few health education specialists employed by provincial
and municipal health departments (*Health and Welfare Canada*, 1982).

The field began to gain momentum in the 1960s with the first national
symposium on health education in Saskatoon, Saskatchewan in 1961 and
the formation of a Health Education Unit in the federal Department of
Health and Welfare in the same year. The role of this unit, under the
direction of Michael Palko, was to co-ordinate educational activities and to
promote the exchange of information on educational innovations across the
provinces (Badgley, 1978).

Michael Palko was one of the founding fathers of health education in
Canada. Palko combined his academic training with a keen insight into the
problems that health educators face, based on his 'grassroots experience'
with the Saskatchewan Department of Health and the City of Vancouver. In
the 1960s, as the newly appointed Health Education Consultant or the
federal Department of Health and Welfare, he travelled throughout Canada
meeting with provincial health educators and promoting the field in general
(*Health and Welfare Canada*, 1982).

One of the greatest contributions that Palko made to the cultivation of
health education in Canada was the foundation and editorship of a
publication called *Health Education* in 1962. This began as an eight page
newsletter which served as a form of clearing house for information on
health education, such as advice on preparing visual aids (*Health and Welfare
Canada*, 1987). Funded by the Department of Health and Welfare, the
publication has evolved over time and is now entitled *Health Promotion*. It
contains feature articles, national news, a research update, regional news,
community initiatives and a review of resources.

Michael Palko was also instrumental in helping to found the Canadian
Health Education Society (CHES) in 1962. Originally, CHES was an
organization for health education specialists but it is currently open to all
individuals involved with health education as part of their work. The
organization has made some important contributions to the field, including
publication of a newsletter and a series entitled *Technical Publication*, as well
as the awarding of the S R Laycock Bursary for a student engaged in
graduate work in health education. A major accomplishment for the field of
health education in Canada was CHES hosting the IXth International
Conference on Health Education held in Ottawa in 1976.

It should be recognized that these developments in health education were
very minor in comparison with some of the larger health and social issues
affecting Canada during the 1960s. The most important health issue during

this time was the introduction of national health insurance, with its implications for health status, health care costs and health professions. Badgley (1978) points out that neither the report of the Royal Commission on Health Services (Government of Canada, 1964) nor the report of the Task Force on the Cost of Health Services in Canada (Government of Canada, 1969) dealt to any significant degree with health education.

Publication of the federal green paper, 'A new perspective on the health of Canadians' (The Lalonde Report) in 1974 represented a national interest in improving health status and curbing health-care costs through prevention and health promotion. Much of the emphasis in this report, and in its programmatic manifestations was in the area of improving 'lifestyle' through such behaviours as avoiding tobacco, eating a nutritious diet, exercising regularly and wearing seat belts.

The conceptual distinction between health education and health promotion was not clear during this time, although most agreed that health promotion was something more than health education, including such diverse approaches as the use of mass media, social marketing techniques and attempts to change social norms. One of the most successful programmes to be developed during this period was the 'Participation campaign', consisting of a series of mass-media messages encouraging Canadians to improve their levels of physical fitness.

During this 'lifestyle' period, health promotion became institutionalized, as an increasing number of departments were established under this heading, both in government and in voluntary health agencies at federal, provincial and municipal levels. Health education, as an organizational structure and as a profession appeared to be in danger of being absorbed by health promotion.

In the later 1970s in Canada (as in other parts of the world) health education and health promotion came under increasing criticism for an over-emphasis on 'lifestyle' problems and on individual responsibility for health. Writers such as Bolaria (1979) and Labonte and Penfold (1981) argued that the 'lifestyle' focus of health promotion was ideologically based and diverted attention away from the social and environmental factors over which individuals have little or no control. As a corrective, Labonte and Penfold endorsed the approach of developing 'critical consciousness' concerning health issues in communities, and for increased social responsibility on the part of government and the corporate sector.

With publication by the European Office of the WHO's document on the 'Concept and principles of health promotion' (1984), the conceptual distinction between various approaches and strategies became clearer. Health promotion was described as a generic approach that includes 'communication, education, legislation, fiscal measures, organizational change, community development and spontaneous local activities against health hazards'. Since the mid to late 1980s, this (the WHO) notion of health promotion is the one most usually espoused by government and voluntary health agencies at various levels.

In Canada, another document was important in the evolution of health promotion. In the document 'Achieving health for all', federal Minister of Health Jake Epp (Ontario Ministry of Health, 1986) emphasized such strategies as 'co-ordinating healthy public policy' and 'fostering public participation' to deal with current health problems. Within this context, health education was clearly relegated to a more minor role than it had had in the past in disease prevention and health promotion.

To summarize the history of health education in Canada, it appears to have reached its developmental apex in the 1960s and early 1970s and is now considered to be one of several strategies under the umbrella of health promotion. Canada is probably better known for its contributions in the area of health promotion than for its development of health education as a profession, or for research and programmes in this field.

Current status of the field

Community health education

In Canada health care is a provincial responsibility, with the exception of the health of native people which is a federal responsibility. Hence the extent to which health education is a component of local or regional public health services is largely dependent on decisions made on a provincial level. For example, in Ontario, the Health Protection and Promotion Act (Bill 138) (Ontario Ministry of Health, 1983), specified that health education was to be one of the mandatory services of Ontario public health units. This legislation has precipitated the hiring of at least one health educator in 29 of 44 boards of health in Ontario by 1988 (Ontario Newsletter, 1988). Similarly, there is now provincial support for the hiring of health educators in community health centres in Ontario. For the practicing health educator, Ontario appears to be providing the most employment opportunities at the present time.

The largest group of community health educators is located in the Health Promotion and Advocacy Section of the City of Toronto's Department of Public Health. This section, under the direction of Dr William J Shannon, includes six full-time health educators, as well as several health promotion consultants.

Other developments which have supported the growth of health education in Ontario include the founding of a provincial chapter of the Canadian Health Education Society in 1983, the hiring of a Health Education Consultant in the Public Health Branch of the Ministry of Health, and the formation of a professional organization, the Ontario Association of Health Promotion Specialists in Public Health, in 1986.

In 1986, the Ontario Ministry of Health commissioned a project team to develop guidelines for the new positions. Entitled, 'The role and functions of the health educator in Ontario Boards of Health', the resulting document suggested five areas of responsibility for the health educator: needs assessment for health education, programme planning for health education, resource development and co-ordination, implementation/communication, and evaluation of health education programmes. These guidelines have proven useful for Boards of Health interested in establishing health education positions both in Ontario and other provinces.

Organizationally, the community health educator in Canada normally reports to the Medical Officer of Health or his or her designate (or in a large unit, a health promotion section head), rather than to a department (nursing, inspection) head. There is wide variation in background academic training, job responsibilities and salary levels of health educators in Canada.

School health education

There is reason for optimism when assessing the status of school-based health education in Canada. On a national level, Dr Gordon Mutter, Chief, Education and Training of the Health Promotion Directorate is involved in a number of initiatives which support increases in the quantity and quality of health education activities available in the schools.

Some of the problems that school health education has been beset by in the past are duplication of effort, disparity in resources available and under-utilization of resources (Mutter, 1988a). Furthermore, there has been (and continues to be) wide variation in terms of the number of class hours devoted to health education and the relative abilities of staff to teach subject matter. Health education is normally required only through grade eight and is often taught by general classroom teachers with little or no training in health (Cameron, 1987). Many teachers who are required to offer health education in their class are not prepared for discussions of such sensitive areas as drug use or sexuality.

Although the federal government has no legislative jurisdiction in the education matters of individual provinces, Mutter and his colleagues in the Education and Training Unit have facilitated several activities throughout Canada in support of school health education. In Winnipeg, Manitoba at a national conference entitled 'Exchange '88', a network of seven major national education organizations was formalized in order to advance comprehensive school health in Canada. At the conference, the National Agencies for School Health came into being. The majority of provinces now have Agencies for School Health in place for purposes of co-ordination and co-operation between the various government and voluntary agencies involved with school health.

Two other initiatives supported on a national level are the surveys of student knowledge, attitudes and behaviour conducted by researchers at Queen's University (see Beazley and King's chapter in this volume), and a comprehensive approach to health education in the schools at Dartmouth, Nova Scotia. The Dartmouth approach, currently being tested, provides sequential health instruction from kindergarten to the end of high school, supported by inter-agency co-ordination, and family and community support (Mutter, 1988b).

In addition, to these activities, there are several examples of the development of school health education in government, university departments and voluntary health agencies on municipal and provincial levels. In Calgary, Alberta, for example, all school boards must now provide a sexuality component within their school health programme and high quality curriculum materials have been developed in order to facilitate this (Seaborn, 1988). The province of Manitoba has now implemented a core health curriculum for students in kindergarten through to grade twelve with mandatory health classes up to grade nine (Harvey, 1988). At the University of Regina, in Saskatchewan, prospective teachers can receive training in health education by taking the health sciences major of the undergraduate degree in education (Gray, 1988).

There are few employment opportunities in Canada for specialists in school health. Most teachers involved in health education on a secondary (high school) level have their training and primary appointment in the area of physical education. While many provinces have health education consultants in the ministries of education and some of the larger municipal boards of education employ consultants, there are not a large number of these positions in total.

Other settings

Thus far in this paper the focus has been on community and school health education. However, it should be noted that health education occurs in other settings as well, such as in institutions (hospitals, clinics) or in the workplace. For example health education, most usually programmes dealing with tobacco or alcohol use, has traditionally been a component of employee assistance programmes in the workplace. Shain and his colleagues at the Addiction Research Foundation (Ontario) are presently engaged in examining a more expanded role for health education as part of an integrated approach to health promotion in the workplace (Shain, Suurvali and Boutilier, 1986). This approach involves the enhancement of a sense of competence or self-efficacy among workers and attempts to deal in a constructive way with issues surrounding job satisfaction and worker participation in decision making.

There does not appear to be much activity in the area of health education in institutional settings in Canada. However, some hospitals are beginning to employ health educators to work with patients directly or to develop programmes located in hospitals for general community use (smoking cessation programmes, weight loss courses, stress reduction).

Professionalization of the field

There are currently no controls in Canada over who practices health education. While it is apparent that many existing health professionals (nurses, physicians, public health inspectors, nutritionists) engage in health education as part of their work, there is no consensus about who should have claim to the title, health educator. Thus far, neither government nor the professional organizations have attempted to regulate entry into the field. This has resulted in wide variation in both the academic qualifications and work experiences of existing health educators.

Beazley and Belzer's paper (1984) on the professionalization of health education in Canada was useful in identifying the academic background and job responsibilities of individuals engaged in health education. More importantly, the paper provided a 'report card' on the field in Canada against the criteria established by Rubinson and Alles (1984) for professionalization of an occupational category. To summarize, Beazley and Belzer believe that, while there is recognition of the need for a health education specialty, the infra-structure necessary for that to occur has not been constructed. Thus far, no professional organization has established itself as a spokesman for the terms of such issues as establishing academic training requirements or standards of practice. Furthermore, there have been no steps taken in Canada to provide accreditation of programmes or certification of practitioners. Finally, health educators in Canada have neither established that they provide a unique service nor developed a code of ethics for the profession (Beazley and Belzer, 1984).

It is clear, based on Beazley and Belzer's analysis, that the level of professionalization of health education is in its infancy. This is even more apparent when compared with developments in the United States that have recently culminated in the formation of the National Commission for Health Education Credentialing, an organization that will provide a process of certification of health education specialists.

Training programmes in health education

There are few programmes in Canada designed specifically to train full time health educators for either community or school settings. Dalhousie University in Halifax, Nova Scotia offers Bachelor and Master of Science degrees in health education through the Health Education Division of the School of Recreation, Physical, and Health Education. Bachelor's degree students can specialize in either community or school health education for potential work in the field. The Master of Science programme involves the completion of a thesis for preparation as researchers in health education.

Most other bachelor's level programmes in the field offer combined degrees in physical and health education, although the University of Waterloo (Ontario) offers both bachelor's and master's degree programmes in Health Studies. The University of Manitoba offers a master's degree in education with a specialty in community health education. A more general programme of graduate level training is the Master of Health Science degree, with a health promotion specialization, in the Department of Community Health, University of Toronto.

In addition to the bachelor's and master's level programmes in health education or related fields, there is an increasing number of academic institutions offering either continuing education in health education or one or more courses in health education for another programme (nursing, environmental health). The University of Western Ontario has prepared a certificate programme in health education for professionals already employed whose jobs include a health education component. At Ryerson Polytechnical Institute, the Department of Environmental Health offers two courses in health education for bachelor's level students training for positions as public health inspectors. Thus, there is a modest number of academic programmes in health education in Canada both for the training of full time specialists and those health and education workers whose jobs include health education.

Research

In Canada there are two major lines of research relevant to health education. First, studies evaluating the effectiveness of various interventions and materials and second, studies examining the factors influencing health behaviour. While there is not a great deal of research currently being conducted here relative to the United States, there are pockets of activity in various provinces. Probably the best known research in Canada on an international level are the studies on various aspects of smoking conducted at the University of Waterloo (Best *et al*, 1984). Also at the University of Waterloo, the Centre for Applied Health Research has been recently created to facilitate research on various aspects of health promotion and health service delivery.

A few other examples of current research activities are: an evaluation of the 'Healthstyles' programme in Ottawa (Collishaw, 1986); studies on the determinants of drug use and the effectiveness of drug education programmes (Goodstadt, 1982, 1986); studies dealing with the health knowledge, attitudes and behaviour of Canadian school children (King *et al*, 1985); a longitudinal study to be conducted in the province of Alberta to evaluate the effectiveness of the Peer Assisted Learning programme (reported by Seaborn, 1988); studies on the health beliefs and attitudes of children currently being conducted by Dr Ilze Kalnins in the Department of Behavioural Science, University of Toronto; studies of health education and health promotion in the workplace (Shain *et al*, 1986) and the ongoing work of Beazley and his colleagues at Dalhousie University. This list is not meant to be a comprehensive inventory, only a summary demonstrating the diversity of research activities in Canada.

Funding for research on health education in Canada is derived from a number of sources. The National Health Research Development Programme (NHRDP), the provincial ministries of health, and various voluntary health agencies all support research in health promotion (including health education). The Canadian Heart Foundation has a specific interest in studies in health education and behavioural science. The various funding agencies normally support research in terms of grants, student fellowships, and longer term awards to full time researchers in universities or related health institutions.

Future trends

It is difficult to project a clear path for the development of health education in Canada. As the previous pages have illustrated, there are some positive signs which bode well for the field namely, the support for positions in public health units and community health centres in Ontario, funding for research by government and voluntary health agencies, and the proliferation of Agencies for School Health. But there are also some barriers to further development of the field, including a lack of control over who practices health education and the scarcity of Canadian academic programmes to train health educators. While there are many factors that will determine health education's future, only three of these will be discussed here. First, changes in the designation of health problems, second, the current emphasis on health promotion and third, prospects for professionalization.

Changes in health problems

In Canada, as in many other countries, health priorities change as a function of both epidemiological and political factors. Changes in health priorities, of course, have implications for health care services, including health education. Two current examples of this phenomenon are concern about AIDS and drug abuse.

In the case of AIDS, although the number of cases in Canada is relatively small, departments of public health at national, provincial and municipal levels are attempting to deal with their perceptions of the public's need for education. Thus, many of these departments have established positions or even whole units (such as one within Toronto's Department of Public Health) dealing with AIDS. Over the past few years several positions as health educators have been so designated and, in Ontario, a new organization has recently been founded, the AIDS Health Education and Development Group, comprised of health educators in public health units and various community agencies dealing with this condition.

A second example of how changes in health priorities can affect the field of health education is the case of drug abuse. In Canada, there is now a National Drug Strategy (Government of Canada, 1988) to deal with alcohol and other drug abuse. Included in the National Drug Strategy are six initiatives, one of which deals with education and prevention. As a result of a concern by government and the public at large about drug abuse, health education programmes and services have been affected in departments of public health and boards of education throughout Canada.

In Toronto, for instance, one event served as a collective 'cue to action' (Becker, 1974) for local politicians to declare a 'war on drugs'. A fourteen year old student took LSD at a rock concert and was later discovered drowned near the docks at Lake Ontario's waterfront. Within a few months of this event, members of an inquest offered a series of recommendations to combat drug abuse, a mayor's task force was established to deal with the problem, and the Toronto police department declared the need for 96 new officers to deal with drug problems in the city. On a provincial level, the Ministry of Education soon announced that drug education was to be mandatory in all Ontario schools. Similarly, the Ministry of Health included drug education as a component of their revised guidelines for public health service and programmes in the province.

The examples of AIDS and drug abuse clearly demonstrate that changing health priorities have affected the field of health education in Canada. Health educators need to keep up with an increasing amount of new health information. Given this problem, it appears that health educators require process skills which they can apply to any of the several content areas of practice.

Emphasis on health promotion

Another influence on future trends in health education is the current emphasis by government on other aspects of health promotion. In Epp (1986) the document 'Achieving health for all', as a framework for health promotion is presented. Included in this framework are three strategies for implementing the various health challenges: fostering public participation, strengthening community health services and co-ordinating healthy public policy. These three implementation strategies, and indeed the entire Epp framework, have profoundly influenced the way in which health promotion activities are organized in Canada. Research funding priorities, conference themes, and public health priorities all reflect the emphasis of Epp's framework. In comparison to the more progressive rhetoric of 'Achieving health for all', health education sounds unexciting. There is now a tendency to equate health education with an older, more conservative era of public health.

Because health education is not professionalized, there is no unified voice which can re-state the importance of health education and identify its contribution to the more visionary goals to which health promotion aspires. While such strategies is healthy public policy, advocacy and community development are necessary correctives to past tendencies towards the individualization of health problems, they were not meant to replace health education. Exactly how health educators will respond to the challenge of re-establishing the importance of their work remains unclear at this time.

Prospects for professionalization

The European office of the WHO (1984) in its paper on the 'Concept and principles of health promotion' contains a warning that health promotion may become the exclusive domain of one profession. However, it is unlikely that health education will achieve this position of pre-eminence in Canada, even if it were desirable. But while health educators do not threaten to monopolize the 'territory' of health promotion, there may be several advantages to professionalization. As mentioned earlier in this paper, there are no guidelines as to who practices health education, what training should be acquired or what the basic skills and competences of the practitioner should be. This is problematic in that it results in wide variation in the quality of programmes in both community and school health education. Many health educators may be high on enthusiasm and implementation skills, but weaker in such areas as theoretical frameworks underlying health behaviour, or in planning and evaluating programmes.

While there may be strong reasons for health educators to professionalize, there does not appear to be consensus on this issue among those currently practicing. Some health educators may feel threatened by more rigorous standards of training and practice. Others do not want to be limited to being educators, and would prefer to be known as health promoters, presuming that they can be experts not only in health education, but in community development, advocacy and social marketing as well. Still others reject the idea of professionalizing on ideological grounds believing that this would necessarily imply a self servicing position, uninterested in the health of the public.

In order for health educators to professionalize in Canada the following changes would need to occur:

1. health educators themselves must recognize the advantages of professionalization,
2. a strong professional organization must emerge to provide momentum for the task,
3. health educators must agree on the core skills and competencies for various levels of practice, and
4. appropriate academic programmes must be developed to train prospective health educators.

Currently, there is not a great deal of change occurring in any of these areas. Most notable, perhaps, is the lack of activity on the part of the Canadian Health Education Society and the Canadian Association for Health, Physical Education and Recreation in providing current leadership and direction to practitioners. The extent of future professionalization of health education in Canada remains unknown.

Conclusion

Various factors have influenced the history and present status of health education in Canada. In many instances these factors were outside of the field itself, such as government positions on health promotion, legislative decisions affecting public health services or changes in health priorities as a result of public concern (AIDS, drug abuse). It is expected that future trends in health education will also be influenced by epidemiological, political and economic factors beyond the control of the field itself.

Health educators can, however, exercise some control over their fate. In order to improve the quality of practice and thereby more positively affect the health of the population, health educators may decide to professionalize. Professionalization would imply more control over such issues as the training of health educators, their roles and responsibilities and qualifications for practice. At the present time there is no consensus in the field concerning professionalization. It appears that the lack of a strong and unified professional association is hindering further development of the field.

Canada is considered to be a leader in developing and refining the concept of health promotion. But while health education is considered a component of health promotion, its importance is currently downplayed in favour of structural approaches, such as the co-ordination of healthy public policy. In order for health education to make a greater contribution to an integrated approach to health promotion, the quality of preparation and practice must improve.

References

Badgley, R F (1978) Health promotion and social change in the health of Canadians, paper presented at Conference on Evaluation of Health Education and Behaviour Modification Programmes, Canadian Health Education Society, December

Beazley, R and Belzer Jr, E G (1984) The professionalization of health education in Canada *CHES Technical Publications* Canadian Health Education Society 7, Fall

Becker, M H (1974) The health belief model and personal health behavior *Health Education Monographs* 2

Best, J A, Flay, B R, Towson, S M J, Ryan, K B, Perry, C L, Brown, K S, Kersell, M W and d'Avernas, J R (1984) Smoking prevention and the concept of risk *Journal of Applied Social Psychology* 14

Bolaria, S (1979) Self-care and lifestyles: ideological and policy implications in Fry, J (ed) *Economy, Class and Social Reality: Issues in Contemporary Canadian Society* Butterworth and Co: Toronto

Cameron, H (1987) Status and trends in school health education in Canada, paper presented to School of Physical and Health Education and Recreation, Dalhousie University, November

(Ontario Newsletter) (1988) Canadian Health Education Society Ontario, Chapter 3, 1, March

Collishaw, N (1986) Healthstyles: final results, presentation at 77th Annual Meeting of the Canadian Public Health Association, Vancouver, British Columbia, June

Epp, J (1986) Achieving health for all: a framework for health promotion, *Health and Welfare Canada* Ottawa

European Office, World Health Organization (1984) Health promotion: a discussion document on the concept and principles, Copenhagen

Goodstadt, M (1982) An evaluation of two school-based alcohol education programmes *Journal of Studies on Alcohol* 43, 3

Goodstadt, M (1986) Factors associated with cannabis non-use and cessation of use: between and within survey replications of findings *Addictive Behaviors* 11

Government of Canada (1964) Royal Commission on Health Services, Queen's Printer, Ottawa Vol 1

Government of Canada (1969) Task force on the cost of health services in Canada, Department of National Health and Welfare, Ottawa

Government of Canada (1988) Action on drug abuse: making a difference, Ottawa

Gray, G (1988) Personal communication, September

Harvey, D (1988) Personal Communication, September

Health and Welfare Canada (1982) Perspectives of the past: twenty years of health education in Canada, an inteview of Michael Palko by Frances Sgro *Health Education* 21, 1, Summer

Health and Welfare Canada (1987) Then and now: reflections on a quarter-century of change, *Health Promotion* 26, 2, Fall

King, A J, Robertson A S and Warren W K (1985) Summary report, Canada health attitudes and behaviours survey: 9, 12 and 15 year olds, Kingston, Ontario, Queen's University Social Programme Evaluation Group

Labonte, R and Penfold, S (1981) Canadian perspectives in health promotion: a critique *Health Education* 19, 3–4 April

Lalonde, M (1974) A new perspective on the health of Canadians, Department of Health and Welfare, Canada

Mutter, G (1988a) Education and training unit: school health component, mimeo

Mutter, G (1988b) Using research results as a health promotion strategy: a five year case study in Canada, unpublished paper, Health and Welfare Canada, March

Ontario Ministry of Health (1983) Health Protection and Promotion Act, Bill 138

Ontario Ministry of Health (1986) The role and functions of the health educator in Ontario Boards of Health, Public Health Branch, March

Rubinson, L and Alles, W F (1984) *Health Education: Foundations for the Future* Times Mirror/ Mosby College Publishers: Toronto

Seaborn, J (1988) Personal communication, September

Shain, M. Suurvali, H and Boutilier, M (1986) *Healthier Workers: Health Promotion and Employee Assistance Programmes* Lexington Books, D.C. Heath Co., Lexington

14. Research findings lead to improvements in health education for Canadian youth – A CASE STUDY

R P Beazley and A J C King

Summary: The chapter describes two surveys carried out to establish the health education needs of young people in Canada. The purposes of the Canada Health Knowledge Survey (King *et al*, 1983) are described. The target population were Canadians aged 9, 12 and 15 years. A two-stage cluster sampling method was used. The content of the survey was validated by an advisory body of health education specialists. The findings indicated major need of improvement in the knowledge of several health topics. The Canada Health Attitudes and Behaviours Survey (Comprehensive Healthcare Consultants Ltd, 1985) surveyed health-related attitudes and behaviours of youths aged 9, 12 and 15 years. The findings are described. They were disseminated through a series of workshops, written reports and the media. The evaluation of the dissemination was positive and although the workshops were too short, common health education strategies emerged across Canada. Policy and programme changes and health education initiatives motivated by the findings of the two surveys are described.

Introduction

A research-based initiative was undertaken recently to improve health education for Canadian youth. The Canada Health Knowledge, Attitudes, and Behaviours Surveys; 9, 12, and 15 year-olds (King *et al* 1983) were designed and conducted by a research team at Queen's University in Kingston, Ontario, with funds from the federal government; following which, both researchers and government health educators collaborated in disseminating the findings throughout Canada. Because health education for Canadian young people is improving as a result of this initiative, the authors consider it important to describe the research and dissemination processes which is the principal purpose of this chapter.

This initiative did not emerge suddenly, nor by chance. Rather, it was conceived as an integral part of a developing federal government commitment to health promotion, it was skilfully planned, and the application for funding was convincingly supported by Gordon Mutter, Chief of the Education and Training Unit of Health and Welfare Canada.

It is important to understand the Canadian context in which the initiative took place. The immensity of the country, the largely dual language composition of the small Canadian population, federal/provincial fencing over health and education, developing health promotion policies, and traditional perceptions of health education all had to be considered in designing and conducting the research, disseminating the findings, and implementing changes.

The Canadian context

PHYSICAL DIMENSIONS AND POPULATION DEMOGRAPHY
Canada is the second largest country in the world and is divided into ten provinces and two territories. Its population is small, consisting of approximately 26 million people who are distributed unevenly across provinces and territories. Although the country as a whole is sparsely populated, over three-quarters of Canadians live in urban environments.

The linguistic and ethnic composition of the Canadian population is diverse, but 88 per cent of Canadians report their ethnic origin and mother tongue as English (61 per cent) or French (27 per cent). Inuit and Indians represent only 2 per cent of the population.

JURDISDICTION OVER HEALTH AND EDUCATION
The Constitution Act of 1867 allocated to the provincial legislatures jurisdiction over the establishment, maintenance, and management of health care institutions and all health care matters generally of a local nature. The constitution gave the federal parliament the power to spend money on health matters as long as its spending did not interfere with provincial authority. This power to spend has enabled the federal government to influence the introduction of universal medical and hospital services insurance, the nature of health-related research, and the creation and distribution of health information. That is, provincial/federal co-operation is common in the health field.

The Constitution Act of 1867 placed education exclusively under the control of each province. The federal government assumes direct responsibility for the education of persons beyond the bounds of provincial jurisdiction: Indians, Inuit, armed forces personnel and their families, and inmates in federal prisons. Over the years, however, federal participation in education within the provinces, largely in the form of financial aid, has been extensive.

HEALTH POLICY
By the early 1970s Canadians enjoyed a quality of life equal to or better than that of most other countries because many of the communicable diseases of the past had virtually been eliminated, and medical and hospital services insurance had been introduced in every province. At that time, efforts to improve the health of Canadians began to focus more on the early detection and treatment of health problems, the reduction of risks to health, and the promotion of healthy lifestyles and community environments. Following publication of its health care policy statement 'A new perspective on the health of Canadians' (Health and Welfare Canada, 1974), the Government of Canada adopted a comprehensive health promotion policy aimed at motivating Canadians to adopt health-enhancing lifestyles and to refrain

from engaging in behaviours that involve a self-imposed risk to personal health.

To implement this policy, the Health Services and Promotion Branch, with its health Promotion Directorate, was created within Health and Welfare Canada in 1978. The mandate of this Branch is to conduct research and implement programmes that effectively promote personal and community responsibility for health.

HEALTH EDUCATION FOR YOUTH

Health education for Canadian youth had a low priority in the early 1980s. In schools, as a consequence, the time committed to it was inadequate, teachers were unacquainted or at best superficially acquainted with health education content and teaching techniques, the resources allocated to it were minimal, and it usually was taught in tandem with physical education or another 'parent' subject. Even though many Canadians agreed that the acquisition of health knowledge and lifeskills and the adoption of positive attitudes were the principal objectives of health education, there was considerably less agreement on what the content of a health curriculum should be. In reality, health education was viewed as crisis management.

The health knowledge, attitudes, and behaviours of young Canadians were unknown at the time. Consequently, their specific health education needs were unknown also. It was recognized that one way to identify curricular content would be to assess the needs of the intended learners through survey research. Need, in this sense, is defined as the difference between the present situation and the preferred situation where the larger the discrepancy between the two, the larger the need.

Members of the newly formed Education and Training Unit (ETU) of the federal Health Promotion Directorate, believed that the health education needs of Canadian youth could be identified by comparing their health knowledge, attitudes and behaviours with what education and health professionals believed health-wise students should know, believe and do. This belief led them to instigate a collaborative relationship with the Social Programme Evaluation Group (SPEG) at Queen's University for the purpose of assessing, first of all, the health knowledge of Canadian youth aged 9, 12, and 15. SPEG's proposal to conduct such a national study was funded by the federal government's National Health Research and Development Programme (NHRDP) in 1982.

The Canada health knowledge survey

Purposes

'The Canada knowledge survey: 9, 12, and 15 year-olds' (King *et al*, 1983) had five purposes:

1. to provide a base of reliable information about Canadian young people's health knowledge;

2. to explore a role for the ETU in the development of health education in the schools of Canada;

3. to develop a sound design by which to conduct health-related surveys of Canadian youth;

4. to develop a framework for disseminating the findings of research throughout Canada; and

5. to initiate a concept in provinces/territories for the co-ordination of various agencies' efforts toward health education for young people.

From the beginning, one political reality was viewed as having the potential to hinder seriously the accomplishment of the survey's purposes. As mentioned earlier, both education and health are primarily provincial responsibilities, and interventions into either by federal government personnel are viewed suspiciously in some provinces and with outright hostility in others. To obviate provincial/territorial antagonism, ownership of the survey was given to Queen's University, with branches of the federal government providing promotional assistance and financial support. Also provincial/territorial leaders were engaged early in the process to facilitate access to students through schools, widespread dissemination of the findings, and substantive changes in health education policies and programmes.

Methodology

The population for this survey consisted of Canadians aged 9, 12 and 15 who were in grades 4, 7 and 10 respectively. Age 9 was selected because it is the youngest age at which children can handle paper and pencil self report instruments capably and this is the most cost effective method of collecting information. Age 9 is also when health knowledge is beginning to be intellectually absorbed. Age 12 was chosen because it represents a critical stage in growth and development; most 12 year-olds are in the early changes of puberty. Age 15 was selected because it is the age when Canadian youngsters are in what is often their last year of formal health education in school. Also, age 15 represents the stage where young people encounter considerable pressure to engage in a variety of risk taking activities. At all three age levels, adequate knowledge of important health concepts is essential to prepare young people for a lifetime of healthy living.

Two important considerations helped to determine the study's methodology. First, the sample of respondents had to be drawn in such a way that reliable findings could be reported for the country as a whole and for each of the ten provinces and two territories. This necessitated using a two stage cluster sampling design. Selection of participating school boards/districts/divisions, the systematic sampling design based on a confidence level of 90 per cent. In other words, the selection was done in such a way that 90 out of 100 times, the scores obtained would be the same as if all students in a province, for example, had been surveyed. The number of respondents was 9,424 for grade 4, 10,032 for grade 7, and 9,449 for grade 10 for a total of 28,905. These numbers represented 97 per cent of the target sample.

Second it was essential to ensure that there was consensus as to the most important health concepts about which young Canadians should have knowledge. To handle this issue, a national advisory group of health and education specialists was established. The group assisted the researchers, not only in identifying and refining the health concepts to be covered in the survey, but in determining appropriate standards of 'needs for improvement' in health knowledge. Since this was a study of respondents' general rather than specific health knowledge, the decision was made to cover a large number of concepts, each with relatively few items; consequently, none of the concepts was covered in depth.

Findings

The main finding of the survey was that the percentage of correct responses given by the grades 4, 7 and 10 students were 58, 53 and 49 respectively. The advisory committee of health and education professionals judged the performances of 45 to 60 per cent of the students as inadequate, and indicated 'major needs for improvement' in the knowledge of several health topics; for example, alcohol and other drugs, human growth and development, physical fitness, nutrition, dental health, communicable diseases, and safety and first aid.

Such findings from the survey were organized and presented to create interest among health and education professionals, parents, members of the general public, and media personnel. It was felt that interested, and perhaps concerned, people would question the *status quo* in health education and seek changes to remediate the identified gaps in the health knowledge of Canadian young people. Therefore, the findings were compared to national scores and the 'highest' and 'lowest' scores achieved by other unidentified provinces/territories. As well, the scores of females and males were compared.

The Canada health attitudes and behaviours survey

'The Canada health attitudes and behaviours survey: 9, 12, and 15 year-olds' (King *et al*, 1985), like its predecessor, was conducted by SPEG with the assistance and financial support of the ETU and NHRDP. This survey complemented the earlier knowledge survey by providing additional information from which health education and promotion initiatives could be taken to promote healthy living among young Canadians.

The purpose of this Survey was to identify the attitudes and behaviours of youths aged 9, 12 and 15 with regard to selected health and safety issues. The design for conducting the research and the strategies for disseminating the first findings were identical to those used in the previous study. Because the health knowledge study had been so successful, the receptivity for this one was very high. Returns were received from 10,833 (grade 4), 11,291 (grade 7) and 10,987 (grade 10) respondents; that is, from 99 per cent of the target sample.

Findings

The main findings of the Survey were categorized as health problem areas, relationships between health-related attitudes and behaviours, and significant provincial/territorial differences. The health problem areas included nutrition, physical and leisure time activities, use of drugs, dental health, safety, and self esteem. All of them were considered to need educational attention.

The relationships found between health-related attitudes and behaviours were believed to be particularly important in the design of education interventions. Generally speaking, the attitudes held by 9 year-olds could not be linked to their behaviours, but there were many instances of strong relationships between behaviours and attitudes for 12 and 15 year-olds. Particularly relevant for future interventions were findings such as a common pattern of risk taking evident among young people, that cut across diet, safety, dental care, and the use of drugs; or the finding that when young people have positive relationships with their parents they are more likely to have more healthy lifestyles.

Significant differences exist among the provinces and territories on a number of measures. Some of the major differences showed up in connection with regular seat belt use, eating a balanced diet, use of alcohol and other drugs, and the school as a major source of information about sex.

Dissemination of results

The traditional practice of Canadian researchers in the health field has been to communicate the results of their work to colleagues by presenting papers at professional conferences and publishing in professional journals. These modes of communication have not stimulated necessary changes in the actual practice of health education because they have left those who influence change, such as the voting public, senior education and health administrators, and elected government officials, largely uninformed. More effective dissemination of the results of research is critical if ensuing changes are to occur.

Stimulating improvement in health education for Canadian youth was a goal of the 'Canada health knowledge, attitudes and behaviours' surveys. Consequently, the attempt to inform influential leaders at the national and provincial/territorial levels through a systematic and widespread dissemination process was deemed necessary. Beginning with the earliest stages of planning for these surveys, strategies for communicating the results widely and in detail were developed. The findings were communicated through workshops, written reports, and the media.

Workshops

The research findings were disseminated mainly through workshops that were held in several cities, about one year after each of the surveys was conducted. Professionals and parents who were in positions to influence changes in health education through their leadership in policy and programme planning were invited to attend these workshops at which provincial/territorial results were released in English or French. Three major objectives to be achieved at workshops were: first, to review provincial/

territorial findings in a forum where participants could speak directly with the researchers; second, to explore strategies for improving the health knowledge, attitudes and behaviours of youth; and third, to formulate recommendations for action that could improve health education at the provincial/territorial level.

A 'ripple' effect was created when many workshop participants returned to their places of work armed with photocopies of the visuals used in the researchers' presentations. They, in turn, made overhead transparencies and presented the findings to colleagues, school and health department administrators and field personnel, professional education and health association members, health education and education students, and perhaps most importantly, to school board members and parents.

Written reports

The researcher agreed at the outset to write a national report and provincial/territorial reports that would be free of statistical terminology and research jargon. These presentations of the findings were to be clear and concise, consisting mainly of precise text which would be supported by simple tables and graphic representation of the major findings. The goal of the reports was to present the findings in a manner that intended readers (parents, media representatives, elected government officials, school personnel and community health professionals) could easily comprehend. By May 1987, over 4,000 copies of the 'Canada health attitudes and behaviours survey' report and 2,100 copies of the 'Canada health knowledge survey' report had been distributed.

The media

The media were invited to participate in the dissemination of the results at the national and provincial/territorial levels. Their coverage of the national press conference where the results were first released generated public awareness within a very short time. Specifically, the initial release of the findings by Canada's Minister of Health and Welfare made front-page news across the country within 24 hours.

In the provinces/territories, media coverage focused on local results in comparison to the national results, and followed immediately the presentation of findings at workshops.

Collectively, the media's reporting of local results kept the findings in the news somewhere in Canada for several months. This reminded education and health professionals of their commitment to work for the advancement of health education for youth.

Evaluation

One purpose of the 'Canada health knowledge attitudes and behaviours' surveys: 9, 12 and 15 year-olds' (King *et al*, 1983; King *et al*, 1985) was to provide reliable information about Canadian youth. It was felt that such current, broad, and accurate information would motivate individuals and groups to reformulate health education policies and programmes. According to this strategy, believable information accruing from research would alert members of health, education, and parent organizations to the need for improved health education for young people. These organizations, in turn, would interact with provincial/territorial departments of education to bring about improvements in school education.

In May and June 1987, Comprehensive Healthcare Consultants Ltd (CHCL) evaluated both the process by which the survey's findings were disseminated and the impact of the findings. The comments that follow are very largely extracted from the CHCL report (Comprehensive Healthcare Consultants Ltd, 1987) with the addition of specific details that were provided by Cameron (1988) and Roberts (1988).

Process evaluation

The CHCL evaluation of the workshops found that the one-half day allowed for a workshop was too limited to accomplish all of the objectives, particularly the identification of strategies for improving the health knowledge, attitudes, and behaviours of children. Participants felt it would have been beneficial to extend the workshop to a full day, or to have follow-up meetings. None-the-less, in the short time given to formulating recommendations, the following ideas emerged commonly across Canada:

☐ mandate an adequate number of hours of health instruction in schools;
☐ provide quality pre-service and in-service teacher training in health education;
☐ establish within each province/territory an organization whose main purpose is the advancement of school health education;
☐ develop a profile of high-risk youth through further research and plan educational programmes that effectively intervene among their risk-taking behaviours, and consider further the nature and role of self-esteem in the lives of young people and the need for esteem-enhancing educational strategies.
☐ the consultants concluded that the combination of workshops, reports, and media coverage resulted in the findings of the Surveys being effectively disseminated to many of Canada's opinion leaders in health education.

Impact evaluation

UTILITY OF THE FINDINGS
The surveys' findings were received very positively and a number of initiatives, at least partially due to the findings, had begun. According to 87 per cent of the respondents, the findings included new information and ideas that would be useful to them. The majority (70 per cent) indicated that they were already using the findings in planning and developing health education policies and programmes in their local areas. Similarly, a high percentage of respondents said that the findings confirmed and clarified

what they already thought about the health knowledge, attitudes and behaviours of young Canadians and this reinforced their commitment to seek improvements in health education. Other respondents agreed that the findings had changed their perspective, generally believing that important gaps in school health education had been identified for them.

APPLICATION OF THE FINDINGS

As mentioned above, 70 per cent of the respondents indicated that they already were using the findings in their work. Specifically, they used the written reports as:

☐ resource documents from which to provide information to colleagues;
☐ an impetus to collaborate with professionals in the field;
☐ an impetus for policy development concerning health education; and
☐ as a basis for additional surveys of local students' health knowledge, attitudes and behaviours.

Policy and programme changes that had been motivated by the findings included the following:

☐ policy regulating milk and snacks available in schools (Newfoundland);
☐ policy making specific schools smoke-free spaces (Ontario and Nova Scotia);
☐ policy leading to the development of a family life or sex education programme (Prince Edward Island and Alberta);
☐ curriculum improvements in health education (Newfoundland, Prince Edward Island, New Brunswick, Nova Scotia, Ontario, Manitoba, Alberta, British Columbia, the North West Territories and the Yukon);
☐ new or increased emphasis on the teaching of topics such as adolescent suicide, self-esteem, oral hygiene, nutrition, drug abuse and stress;
☐ research to evaluate, over a five year period, a community approach to comprehensive health education (Dartmouth, Nova Scotia); and
☐ in-service programmes for teachers (several provinces).

A FEDERAL ROLE IN EDUCATION

By sponsoring these surveys and guiding them through dissemination of the findings, members of the ETU hoped to forge a role for themselves in advocating improvements in health education for Canadian youth. CHCL reported that many respondents were unfamiliar with the federal government's limitations relative to education; to the contrary, they expected the ETU to undertake health education enhancing activities. They suggested activities such as the following:

☐ develop and evaluate innovative health education programmes in the areas of smoking cessation and sexualtiy;
☐ document and distribute information about effective Canadian health education programmes, including ideas for involving parents, and those with resources, efficiently and purposefully;
☐ support school health education-related research, especially research that aims to assess the extent to which comprehensive health education works;

☐ spearhead provincial/teritorial and national conferences wherein health and education professionals, school trustees, and parents can come together to share and learn about specific health topics and ways to improve school health education; and

☐ support the establishment of a national organization to speak for school health education.

While some concerns were expressed, the evaluation results predominantly indicated that the initiatives taken by the ETU in disseminating the surveys' findings was positively received.

Ongoing initiatives

Initiatives begun in part as a result of the survey's findings are maturing, and, the advent of AIDS as a serious pandemic has increased the interest of adults in health education for Canadian youth, even among some of those who previously were complacent. Policy and programme changes, which are the vanguard for improved school health education, are occurring across Canada. Evidence of major changes at the national level have emerged and are emerging; they include: 'Exchange 88', the development of a national organization for the advancement of school health education, the 'Canada youth and AIDS survey' (1988), and the 'Canada health attitudes and behaviours survey' (1989).

Exchange '88

In June 1988, 275 people attended 'Exchange '88' in Winnipeg, Manitoba, collectively to confront AIDS, child sexual abuse, substance (drug) abuse, and school health education. Canadian society is faced with these three urgent issues and school systems across the country are working to develop and expand their repsonses to them, most commonly through health education/family life programmes.

Included among the five expected outcomes of 'Exchange '88' were the following:

☐ to create a better understanding among key provincial/territorial leaders of the value of school health education as a construct through which to respond to urgent health and social issues, such as AIDS, child sexual abuse, and substance abuse; and

☐ to create a national network of school health educators (that is, an organization devoted to the advancement of school health education).

This conference generated enthusiasm for placing education about youth-orientated health and social issues within the context of school health education; as a result, delegates returned home with new or renewed vigour for the task at hand.

National organization for school health education

Over the past eight years in Canada, coalitions of 'agencies for school health' have been organized in six provinces. Their primary purposes are to advance school health education through collaborative activities and to provide a networking structure for individuals, organizations, institutions and agencies within a province. This idea, which originated in Manitoba, has developed loyal supporters, not only in the six provinces where they exist, but at the national level as well.

It is not surprising that the desire for a national organization for the advancement of school health education has surfaced. Consequently, at the expense of the ETU, several of the delegates to 'Exchange '88' were invited for the purpose of considering the initiation of such a national organization. The delegates voted to support the concept in principle and selected co-chairs for a meeting to be held in the fall of 1988 to consider the concept in detail. In the meantime, representatives from the provinces/territories who have yet to form 'agencies for school health' agreed to investigate the desirability and feasibility of doing so.

The Canadian youth and AIDS survey (1988)

The 'Canadian youth and AIDS survey' was conducted to determine the knowledge, attitudes and behaviours of Canadian Youth (aged 12, 14, 16 and 18 to 21) with respect to acquired immuno-deficiency syndrome (AIDS) and other sexually transmitted diseases (STDs). The relationship of these findings to other aspects of young peoples's lives such as self-esteem, mental health, relationships with parents and peers, peer pressure, homophobia, tolerance for people with AIDS, use of drugs, and socio-economic indicators was examined in order to identify the characteristics of those most at risk of contracting AIDS or other STDs.

The ultimate purpose of the survey was to provide reliable information that would be used to develop further AIDS-related health education initiatives directed at young Canadians both provincially/territorially and nationally. Like the past national surveys this survey was funded by the National Health Research and Development Programme and was conducted by the Social Programme Evaluation Group at Queen's University in Kingston, Ontario.

Its protocol and design and the thorough dissemination of its findings throughout Canada by way of workshops, reports, and media coverage was a replication of those methods that proved successful with the 'Canada health knowledge, attitudes and behaviours surveys'. The final report of the 'Canada youth and AIDS survey' will be released in October 1988. It is awaited by Canadian health and education professionals and its impact on the further development of AIDS education as part of school health education is expected to be felt within a short time.

Canada health attitudes and behaviours survey

The 'Canada health knowledge, attitudes and behaviours surveys' provided Canadian researchers and government health educators with a sound design for conducting national survey and a framework for effectively disseminating the findings of research across the country. These could be utilized by researchers and government personnel in other countries as well as by those in Canada.

In recognition of this, the European Regional Office of the WHO invited Canada to associate with eleven member countries in surveying the health attitudes and behaviours of youth aged 9, 12, and 15 in 1989. Core health areas will be included by all 12 countries, with the addition of other areas at each country's discretion. Participating in this international study fits into the planned five-year sequence of surveys in Canada in 1984, 1989 and 1994.

Conclusion

There is excitement among Canadian health educators today. After years of trying to convince people of the importance of school health education, without much success, momentum for the idea is now building. The advent of AIDS, along with the persistence of health and social issues such as child sexual abuse and drug abuse, has hastened the realization that crisis management health education is ineffective; and, that something more thoroughly planned and implemented is necessary. The 'Canada health knowledge, attitudes and behaviours survey: 9, 12 and 15 year-olds' (King et al, 1983) pointed out specifically the need for better health education for Canadian Youth. They put young people's lack of knowledge and risk-taking behaviours before Canadian adults in a form that could not be ignored. These surveys jolted many professional and parents out of their apathy about the preparedness of young people to prevent illness and injury. They helped create a climate for change and actually motivated change. The health education that Canadian youth is receiving now can be traced, at least in part, to these two landmark surveys.

References

Comprehensive Healthcare Consultants Ltd (1987) *Impact Evaluation of the Canada Health Knowledge Attitudes, and Behaviours Surveys* Health and Welfare Canada, Ottowa
Cameron, H (1988) Personal communication
Education and Training Unit (1988) Exchange '88: *A National Exchange on Health and Social Issues in Education* Health and Welfare Canada, Ottawa
Health and Welfare Canada (1974) *A Perspective on the Health of Canadians* Ottawa
King, A J C, Robertson, A S, Warren, W K and Fuller, K A (1983) *Summary Report Canada Health Knowledge Survey 9, 12, and 15 Year-Olds* Queens's University, Social Programme Evaluation Group, Kingston, Ontario
King, A J C, Robertson, A S and Warren, W K (1985) *Summary Report Canada Health AH and Behaviour Survey 9, 12 and 15 Year-Olds* Queens University, Social Programme Evaluation Group, Kingston, Ontario
Roberts, G A (1988) Personal communication

15. Health education in Australia: seven queens — AN OVERVIEW

V A Brown

Summary: Australia is a country with an Asian climate, a British legal and parliamentary system, and an American style of State and Federal organization. Despite this borrowing, Australia, 200 years after British settlement, is also very much itself. Health education in Australia, as with health education everywhere, tends to reflect the values of the country, forged from this historical background. Later local influences include forty years of steady immigration from all European, and a few South East Asian countries. The population is now sixteen million; about that of Greater London, in area larger than all Europe, concentrated in five large and about twenty smaller cities. Thus the overall health profile is that of a modern, urban industrialized country with a generally European lifestyle.

Introduction

What is health education?

Also like health education everywhere, there is considerable confusion about the use of the term itself. Taking the continuum from maintaining good health, to minimizing need for treatment of disease, to successful rehabilitation, health education supplies the knowledge needed for each of the three stages.

This knowledge takes a different form for children, parents, medical practitioners, hospital administrators, politicians and health educators themselves. Australians tend to confine use of the words health education to school health education and the instruction on lifestyle risks delivered by the family doctor. Other activities that promote the country's health, such as mass media campaigns, courses which extend lifestyle choices and policy and management initiatives tend to be labelled health promotion, health management and health advancement respectively.

Just how idiosyncratic this labelling is, is reflected in the fact that in New Zealand, Australia's nearest neighbour in cultural terms, the order is reversed and health education covers media health campaigns, and health promotion describes school programmes. To reflect current trends in Australia, and also to match the leadership provided by 'World Health Organization', I will use health promotion throughout this chapter as the umbrella term for improving the health of the population, and assume that it is synonymous with health education wherever there is learning involved.

The most characteristic aspect of health education in Australia is not a matter of names, but a reflection of the state/commonwealth division of responsibility for health matters. Although the Commonwealth Government, meeting in the national capital, Canberra, collects the taxes, and makes national policies, the taxes are given to the states to spend, and in the area of health at least, state policy rules.

States and queens

This sense of individuality in the different states is so strong that each has its own representative of the Queen of England, in addition to the commonwealth representative, who is known as the governor-general. So firmly do the states guard their autonomy that diplomatic representatives of other countries must present their credentials to the governor of each state, as well as the commonwealth. No wonder a new, and confused Belgian ambassador was heard to say, after travelling 20,000 kilometres on this errand, 'In this crazy country, you have seven queens'.

National health

Workers in health education share his frustration. There are, in fact, six states and two territories, as well as the Commonwealth Government; and all nine administrations have to agree, before a national nutrition, AIDS education or drug policy can be formulated. As we shall see, different values about sexuality, drug use, and even education itself dominate in different areas. Thus Australia has neither a national health education policy, nor a curriculum. It does have a national AIDS policy, a women's health policy, national dietary guidelines, a national drug campaign and a 'National health promotion programme'. In April, 1988 a national health targets and goals strategy was launched, developed by a nationwide 'Health targets and goals implementation committee'. Thus there is now a national health promotion (or health education) strategy for the first time; five years after the first state, South Australia, announced its own such strategy.

Australia's health for all

Australia's national policy proposes three areas in which targets can be set: population groups, major causes of ill health and health risk factors. The finer details are as follows.

POPULATION GROUPS
The socioeconomically disadvantaged, aborigines, migrants, women, men, older people, children and adolescents.

MAJOR CAUSES OF ILLNESS AND DEATH
Heart disease and stroke, cancers (including lung, breast, cervical and skin cancer), injury, communicable diseases, musculoskeletal diseases, diabetes, disability, dental disease, mental illness, asthma.

RISK FACTORS

Drugs (including tobacco smoking, alcohol misuse, pharmaceutical misuse, illicit drugs, and substance abuse), nutrition, physical activity, high blood pressure, high blood cholesterol, occupational health hazards, unprotected sexual activity, environmental health hazards.

Not so healthy

The items in the list reflect the national style. While sharing the international health risks of heart disease, cancers and injury as the primary causes of early death, they also reflect a seriously disadvantaged indigenous population (25 years less life expectancy than their colonizers), sharp differences in the successes of health education with different client groups, the high national level of prescribed drug use, and a lack of health services designed for women. Kane and Ruzicka (1987) have calculated that cardiovascular disease has been reduced by one-third in the higher educated, higher income groups, and not at all in the lower. This can be taken as a sharp message to health educators, about the literacy and cultural levels at which they are targeting their messages.

Australian epidemiologists, Broadhead, (1985), McMichael (1985) and McMichael and Hetzel (1987) have provided detailed figures which identify early deaths, under 65, at one and a half times greater for lower than upper socio-economic males, for cancers; and three times greater for respiratory diseases and injury. Different risk figures show up for different ethnic groups, depending on their changes of diet and lifestyle. Australia now has zero natural population growth, but has for decades absorbed an increase by migration. One in three Australian children have parents not born in Australia. This has clear implications for the direction of school and community health education.

National health development programme

Returning to the topic of the 'National health promotion programme' (NHPP) this funds, yearly, about two million dollars worth of programmes, and influences about another ten million dollars worth, not a large budget compared with the 74 million dollars available for medical research. The effectiveness of these programmes far outreach the funding levels. At present NHPP grants include the following:

- ☐ major national education campaigns on diabetes, hearing impairment and schizophrenia;
- ☐ Australian Council for Health, physical education and recreation curriculum materials for schools; the 'Health education and lifestyle project' (HELP);
- ☐ a set of resources and community self-help materials for community development in health;
- ☐ a national database of health education materials and resources, accessed through Medline and entitled 'Health education and promotion system' (HEAPS);

- ☐ 'Workplace health education programmes', monitored by the National Heart Foundation, to evaluate their use for reaching blue-collar workers;
- ☐ 'The Family Medicine Programme', a training scheme for general medical practitioners in family and preventive medicine;
- ☐ The 'Healthy cities Australia project', in which three cities have offered to host a pilot programme introducing the so-called 'New public health' to their city administrations and to Australia, and to assist other cities with the same process.

As well as these model programmes, the national campaigns on AIDS and drug abuse have a very strong educational tone, and inject considerable extra resources into state community development and health promotion programmes. These funds provide considerable social impact, since they are often spent in very conservative areas. For instance, in the State of Queensland, homosexuality is illegal and carries heavy penalties. The state has not been able to take advantage of the excellent public education programmes run by the gay community in the other states. Commonwealth money is able to go directly to Queensland gay groups for this purpose.

The 'National campaign against drug abuse', now in its fourth year, has had a similar effect in educating a fairly hard-drinking community about the risks of heavy alcohol use, and reaching the hard drug using community, who technically don't exist.

The most ambitious national health programme is just commencing. The 'Health for all Australians' project is being set up in every state, with the support of the health departments and teaching institutions, for a three year trial period.

An important organization with a responsibility to inform and protect the Australian public on health matters is the National Health and Medical Research Council. Traditionally medically and research oriented, the council is slowly accepting the responsibility of informing the Australian public on social health issues.

Within the past three years, recognition of the broad social role of modern public health has led to the development of university programmes in this area in five states. A review of medical education in Australia made the point that these, and all other health-care training institutions should include strong strands on health education and on community health. Implementation of these recommendations remains to be seen.

The health lobbyists

Four lobbying organizations play a very influential part in Australian health education. The Public Health Association of Australia (PHA) (it has just separated from including New Zealand as well) has a strong research reputation, and is supporting epidemiology and evaluation techniques which make a firm foundation for health education strategies. It produces a research journal, *Community Health Studies*, which this year is bringing out special editions on community development and new public health legislation. The Australian Community Health Association takes up different issues from PHA, mainly those of community workers, and of recognition of the need for community development in policy and resource decisions. The Australian Council of Social Services enters the health education area in its interest in the welfare of lower socio-economic groups.

The fourth lobby group is the most unusual. Established due to the protests of national consumer and welfare organizations that the Department of Health was too medically and provider oriented, the Consumers' Health Forum is an umbrella organization for over thirty consumer bodies, such as Aged Pensioners, the Arthritis Foundation and the Australian Consumers Association, and produces major reports on drug policy, health-care funding, and health consumer rights.

A strong influence on the development of health promotion in Australia has been the 'Second national conference on health promotion' sponsored by the WHO in Adelaide, South Australia in April, 1988. Two hundred overseas invited delegates, and fifty Australians attended. The conference built on the five principles of health promotion developed at the 'First international conference' in Ottawa in 1986, namely, building healthy public policy, creating supportive environments, strengthening community action, developing personal skills, and reorienting health services. This charter has come to be known as the new public health. The theme of the conference was 'Healthy public policy' and the final resolutions were first, that public policy should be directed towards equity of health outcomes, in order to remedy the social differentials in health status, and second, that all health and social services should be accountable in terms of health outcomes from their services.

Australian states and territories

Australian states are much harder to summarize, either individually or collectively, than is the commonwealth contribution to health education. This is partly due to the widely varying commitment of resources, and partly to the different political orientations. We will try to understand the overall picture by taking them state by state.

West Australia

A state bigger than Europe with the population of Sheffield, income from mining and agriculture, and a severely unhealthy indigenous population presents a challenge to health education services. The state has a highly regarded epidemiological unit, which helps focus health planning, regional health educators in the far-flung districts, heavy emphasis on radio and television, and a commitment to health education curriculum in the schools. The HELP curriculum mentioned above was developed in West Australia, because of the local expertise.

West Australia was the first state to convince its politicians of the serious health cost of smoking. The health promotion service received a two million dollar budget to develop media campaigns and anti-smoking material, which were used throughout the country.

South Australia

South Australia has the reputation of being the most socially responsible state; and it is certainly the capital of community health services. The first state to have women's refuges, domestic violence and child abuse clinics; it was the first state to publish state health targets and goals. It has seen the publication of a social health policy, a social justice paper, and a review paper on primary health care, from the Health Commission's Social Health Office in 1988. Adelaide has a model hospital health education service in the Flinders Medical Centre, and a range of specialized health centres. Noarlunga, a satellite town to Adelaide, is one of the 'Healthy cities' pilot cities, and is in the process of building a primary health care hospital.

The Health Development Foundation, also in Adelaide, is a private enterprise consultant group which designs health education programmes and curricula. It grew out of a successful joint diet and exercise programme trialled in South Australian schools in the early 1980s in conjunction with a comic book, the *Body Owners' Manual*. Evaluation of the programme showed children more alert, more interested in their schoolwork, and fitter than those without the programme.

Victoria

The Victorian Health Promotion Foundation was established this year to distribute the twenty three million dollars collected as a tobacco tax from Victorian smokers. One-third is to replace advertising for sports and cultural events which are prepared to forgo tobacco sponsorship, one third to research, and one third to sponsor programmes and projects in health promotion. One major project being sponsored is a 'Healthy Localities' project, in which local councils will bid for ten programmes of one hundred thousand dollars to implement health promotion strategies in their areas.

Health district councils are a Victorian community development strategy, where citizen's advisory councils supervise health districts, and receive some funds for health education strategies. It is from this project that the nationally funded 'Community development in health' programme arose. The Health Issues Centre is yet another Victorian innovation, where Government funds a research and policy unit in the community, to prepare independent advice from a community perspective. The Brotherhood of St Lawrence is a church organization, funded from donations, which works on social development programmes with the most needy groups in the city. Each programme is evaluated and the Brotherhood produces a series of occasional papers 'Policy in practice'.

Victoria has a range of educational initiatives in health promotion, with a Master's programme planned in 'Healthy public policy' at Latrobe University; health education diplomas at Monash University, and Burwood campus of the Victorian State College, and the first Australian degree in health promotion and information on the Rusden campus. Melbourne also has the Social Biology Resources Centre, a professional training centre for difficult social issues, such as sexuality and the disabled, and AIDS education.

New South Wales

Sydney is by far Australia's largest and most commercial city. Here is the highest incidence of AIDS, heroin use, and fringe suburb violence. Health promotion and health education are delivered through organized school curricula, or through regional health services based in hospitals. This does not give the field a high profile, and it is difficult to evaluate the impact of services. Australia's main project on evaluation of health promotion is based in Sydney, however, at Westmead Hospital, the Department of Community Medicine of the University of Sydney. In this same Department is a model hospital health education service, for staff, patients and relatives, called 'Health link'.

Sydney also has the School of Public Health which trains the epidemiologists for health promotion. The University of New South Wales trains preventively oriented general practitioners, and has just launched a Master's programme in health promotion. Health regions such as Illawarra, part of the 'Healthy cities Australia project'. Lismore with an innovative social marketing programme to lower heart disease, and Liverpool with high unemployment make New South Wales a widely varied state as far as health education is concerned.

Queensland

Queensland, as we have already commented, is the conservative state. Sex education is not permitted in schools, condom vending machines have only just been licensed, and there is serious discussion of the need to teach the creation myth in schools. Not surprisingly, there are very few community health centres. The health promotion unit of the state health department has recently been abolished, with a view to redesigning a more effective unit. The epidemiological section of the health department gives national leadership in the fields of cancer and heart disease. Alcohol and drug education are dealt with separately, through professional alcohol and drug services.

Tasmania, Northern Territory, and Australian Capital Territory (ACT)

Smaller in population than the other areas, these last three are even more different from each other. Tasmania is rural, conservative, and community oriented. Health education is in schools, and is education for living. Northern Territory has the worst health problems in Australia, with the largest aboriginal population, alcohol abuse and petrol sniffing rife, high unemployment, and very little hope of change. Nevertheless, the territory, apart from producing Crocodile Dundee, trains aboriginal community health workers, and uses high technology satellite communication to get health messages across.

ACT has the national capital and the highest level of income and education in the country. This does not mean there are no health risks, however, but only that the proportion is somewhat less, and resources are available to trial some community services, to contribute to the 'Healthy cities project', and to provide a full health advancement service, with a health education resource centre, health management courses in work-places and community centres, and volunteer training for self-help groups.

Conclusion

Australian health education services a country, small in population and large in area, with the standard health risks and lifestyle of a modern industrialized country.

Two factors distinguish Australia's approach to disease prevention and health promotion. First, there is a history of independence of the six states and two territories from the central Commonwealth Government. This has been overcome for successful national AIDS and drug education campaigns, and a newly formulated national 'Health targets and goals' strategy. Otherwise, states vary widely in their commitment to health education, from a token presence in schools, to a central role in state health policy.

The second factor reflects Australia's reliance on British and Canadian models of health care. The goal of free health care for all has led to highly expensive hospitals and renewed enthsuiasm for preventive programmes. Here the WHO models of a new public health have been influential in encouraging Australia's own preference for community self-reliance and community development strategies.

Bibliography and References

Ashton, J et al (1986) Healthy cities – World Health Organization's new public health initiative Health Promotion 1, 3, 319–321

Baum, F and Brown, V A (1988) Healthy cities (Australia) project: from vision to reality Proceedings 2nd International Conference on Health Promotion, Adelaide: World Health Organization, Geneva, 31–38

Broadhead, P (1985) Social status and morbidity in Australia Community Health Studies 14, 2, 87–97

Brown, V A (1981) From sickness to health: an altered focus for health care research Social Science and Medicine 15A, 195–201

Brown, V A (1985) Social health in a small city: Proceedings, 3rd International Conference on Health Education: Dublin

Hancock, T (1986) Promoting health in the urban context Working Paper for Healthy Cities Symposium, Lisbon: World Health Organization

Hetzel, B (1980) Health in Australian Society Penguin, Harmondsworth

Kane, P and Ruzicka, L (1987) Australian Population Trends and Their Social Consequences, Melbourne, Commission for the Future

Kickbusch, I (1986) Health promotion: A global perspective, Canadian Journal of Public Health Autumn

Marmot, M G et al (1984) Inequalities in death – specific explanations of a general pattern? The Lancet i, 1003–1006

McMichael, A (1985) Social class and mortality in Australian males in the 1970s Community Health Studies 9, 3, 220–230

McMichael, A and Hetzel, B (1987) The L/S Factor Penguin, Harmondsworth

Milio, N (1988) Making healthy public policy: developing the science by observing the art: an ecological framework for policy studies Health Promotion 2, 3

Social Health Office (1988) *Social Health Strategy for South Australia* South Australian Health
   Commission
Whitehead, M (1987) *The Health Divide: Inequalities in Health in the 1980s* The Health Education
   Council, London
World Health Organization (1986) *A charter for health promotion report of First International
   Conference on Health Promotion, Ottawa* WHO Euro, Copenhagen
World Health Organization (1988) *Australian day, papers and workshops, proceedings 2nd
   International Conference on Health Promotion, Adelaide* WHO Euro, Copenhagen
World Health Organization *Strategies for healthy public policy, report of 2nd International Conference
   on Health Promotion, Adelaide* WHO Euro, Copenhagen

16. Course development in health education and promotion – A CASE STUDY

R F Wellard and B R Walker

Summary: This paper discusses the development of a post graduate course in health education designed for health workers and conducted within a School of Health Sciences. In Australia, Colleges of Advanced Education and Universities offer a wide range of courses which are nationally registered as 'graduate diploma' courses. These courses are generally run on a part time basis and are equivalent to a year of full time study at a postgraduate level. The normal entry requirement for such courses is an undergraduate degree or equivalent and some years of work experience in relevant fields. In most states of Australia there are graduate diploma courses in health education, some of which have more of a focus on health education curricula in primary and secondary schools, whilst others have more of a community health focus. A good example of the latter is the Graduate Diploma in Health Education offered by the Lincoln School of Health Sciences, La Trobe University. The course attracts participants from most health disciplines and who work in a range of health and community agencies.

The aim of this chapter is to discuss the evolution of this course from the time it was originally proposed, over ten years ago, to the present time. The evolution of the course is examined against a background of the institutional factors and changes in the field of health education which have had an impact upon the course. The changes to the aims, content and structure of the course, described in this chapter, is a case study of the way in which changes results from a complex interplay of specific political and structural factors within organizations, broad developments within a field of knowledge (in this case health education), and the perception of staff as to how this change ought to be implemented.

Introduction

The context of course development

Lincoln Institute of Health Sciences was established in 1973 by a voluntary merger of independent schools of physiotherapy, occupational therapy, and speech therapy. At the time of this merger the institute enrolled approximately 600 undergraduate students. The original academic aims and objectives of Lincoln Institute included those of promoting and developing teaching and research 'for the practice of disciplines, sciences, professions and services concerned with health'. One specific aim focused on the facilitation of inter-professional collaboration and the promotion of better health care through the provision of academic expertise in 'such areas as health education, health promotion and health policy'. Since 1973 student numbers have increased to approximately 2,500. There are now eight undergraduate degree or diploma courses which, in addition to the three original courses mentioned above, cover areas such as nursing, podiatry, orthoptics, medical record administration, prosthetics and orthotics. In addition, there is a number of graduate diploma courses some of which are profession specific in content while others are interdisciplinary or generic in nature. The health education course is one of the latter.

Interdisciplinary emphasis

Since its inception the Institute has included programmes based on philosophies of interdisciplinary co-operation and collaboration. While the undergraduate courses remained strongly discipline specific, in the post graduate area there developed a number of generic courses that clearly ran across disciplinary boundaries. These included courses in rehabilitation studies, community health, ergonomics and health administration, all of which were established by 1980. Because these programmes did not readily fit within an organizational structure designed around profession-specific undergraduate programmes a special unit, the Academic Committee for Inter-disciplinary Studies (ACIDS), was established to 'house' these courses and promote interdisciplinary education. In attempting to fulfil this role (which it did with varying degrees of success) ACIDS administered the inter-disciplinary graduate diplomas, developed a variety of short courses, conducted staff seminars on inter-disciplinary education, proposed different models for enhancing inter-disciplinary education in undergraduate and post graduate courses. ACIDS existed, as an organizational entity within the Institute, for approximately five years. The profession-specific schools of the Institute viewed it with deep suspicion. They were concerned that ACIDS might be a device to reduce profession specific course content and replace it with inter-disciplinary content and coursework common to a group of professional courses. In the face of this opposition it was finally concluded that ACIDS would not be effective in achieving its goals. In late 1981 it was disbanded and the courses for which it was responsible were allocated to other academic units of the Institute. It was within the context of these organizational structures and internal political debates that the graduate diploma course in health education was first proposed in 1978. It was not approved until 1983 and accredited in early 1984.

Changes to the institutional context after 1983

The administrative structure of the Lincoln Institute of Health Sciences required each accredited course to have a course advisory committee responsible for advising departments on policy issues in regard to those courses. The health education course advisory committee was established with the commencement of the course in early 1984. Through these advisory committees, which were required to draw a considerable proportion of their membership from outside the institute, links were established and maintained with major organizations concerned with the field of health education. These included the health department of Victoria's Health Promotion Unit, community health centres, the Anti-Cancer Council, health promotion units of major public hospitals, the Public Health Association, Community Health Association and independent organizations such as the Social Biology Resources Centre. These connections with organizations concerned with the conduct of health education maintained a focus on education for effective practice in the field and linked the programme with major policy reviews and initiatives. For example, as the World Health Organization 'Health for all by the year 2000' initiative began to impact on the direction taken by policy reviews at state and national levels it simultaneously was being developed in the philosophy of the course.

During 1986, at the beginning of a period of major change in the Australian higher education sector, the Lincoln Institute of Health Sciences, a college of advanced education, commenced the negotiation of a merger with La Trobe University which was completed in January 1988. The change in status from College of Advanced Education to University enhanced previously limited opportunities to develop postgraduate programmes at master's, by coursework and research, and at doctor of philosophy levels. The changes took place in a climate of limited public sector resources and emphasis on education for workforce development. Both of these considerations were important in shaping master's level developments described towards the end of this chapter.

The developing field of health education

Changing frameworks of health education and promotion

Development of the graduate diploma in health education, despite the impact of institutional issues described below, reflects significant theoretical development in the field of health education and promotion. Much of this development can be understood within the framework of attempts to clarify relationships between patterns of health outcomes categorized variously by social group, disease states, risk factors, for example; individual behaviours; social and physical environments; and the mediating social structures and processes. The rationale for health education lies in its capacity to facilitate identifiable advances in health status. There are of course many issues around how those advances may and ought to be identified which will not be addressed here. Of more concern are the issues of whether the advances sought are for individuals or groups, the identification of the connections between the two and by what means they are to be brought about.

The term education is imbued with the ethos of individual development which in some general way has powerful, but difficult to specify, outcomes for the social collectivity. Health education has frequently assumed this mantle, but at the same time health educators have recognized that the outcomes sought are often quite specific, for example, reduced lung cancer rates through reduced smoking, and that many of the determinants of those outcomes are beyond the control of individual actors. Health educators have recognized that the process of advancing health is complex and involves action at different levels of social organization while still focusing their activities on individuals. The following definition of health education developed by Fisher *et al* (1986) illustrates the point:

> [Health education is] the communication of *knowledge* and the provision of *experiences* to help individuals develop their attitudes and skills, which will assist their adopting *behaviour* to improve and maintain health for themselves and their fellows. Health education aims to assist individuals, groups and communities to make informed decisions about their health. In addition health education aims to enable individuals and groups to influence and change *social policy*.

The link between individual learning and collective change via social policy is, in this definition, unclear.

The term health promotion suffers from similar problems of definition. Under some definitions might be included all attempts to advance health while under others the focus is on individual change, social marketing or other particular strategies (Fisher *et al* 1986, Tannahill 1986, Tones 1986). Nevertheless, the various definitions of health education and health promotion relate the two closely to each other. In some definitional schema health education was conceived as being an aspect of health promotion, in others the two terms are used more or less synonomously. In this chapter the term health education is used to refer to the field of activities addressed in the definitions of health education and promotion. On top of the distinctions between health education and health promotion were added others such as health advocacy, community development and legislative change. Health educators undertook activities that might fall within any of these definitions.

Practical reasons for the apparently obsessive concern with definition were very real problems of incoherence in the addressing of health issues and of anxiety on the behalf of many health personnel about the legitimacy of some approaches to health education. Of particular concern was a debate between advocates of individual change, a model easily understood by clinicians, and those who advocated social change which, for many clinically trained health workers, took health education beyond the legitimate boundaries of health practice. For health workers trained initially in the largely apolitical traditions of individual learning and individual curative techniques the political nature of some of these approaches, for example community development and health advocacy, was alien and discomforting.

When it was accepted that there had emerged a number of approaches to positively advancing the health of communities by working with social processes, both individual and collective, there was a problem of conceptualizing their relationships. How ought work on individual behaviour change relate to community development, health marketing strategies and legislative change, for example? The issue of legitimacy was associated with this lack of clarity. Practitioners required a clear and integrated framework describing how health advancement might be achieved in order to legitimate the range of activities it was understood needed to be undertaken to systematically improve the health of communities.

A number of writers developed integrated frameworks for health education/health promotion (Fry 1982, Labonte 1985, Tones 1986, World Health Organization 1986). The most widely recognized of these is the Ottawa

Charter for Health Promotion (Ottawa Charter) a statement developed and adopted at the First International Conference on Health Promotion held in Ottawa November, 1986, which was jointly sponsored by the WHO, Health and Welfare Canada and the Canadian Public Health Association. Health promotion is defined, in the Ottawa Charter, as 'the process of enabling people to increase control over, and to improve, their health' (World Health Organization 1986). The Ottawa Charter is often described as a framework developed within a social, as opposed to bio-medical, model of health. The Ottawa Charter outlines strategies in health promotion which integrate action at different levels of social complexity, on the factors influencing health. These include levels of individual and social action in economic and environmental arenas (World Health Organization 1987). The Ottawa Charter identifies five areas of action within the context of public policies for health. These are:

☐ strengthen community action for health;
☐ develop personal skills in exercising control over health;
☐ enable, mediate and advocate for health;
☐ create supportive natural and social environments;
☐ reorient health services towards health objectives (World Health Organization 1986).

As a framework for action in health education the Ottawa Charter is, it is argued here, the most coherent available and the one most likely to be understood as a source of legitimation for the range of activities involved in health education. In this context the term health refers to the WHO definition of health being a positive state of social, emotional and physical wellbeing.

In the late 1970s and early 1980s Victorians engaged in health education were, generally speaking, coming from the traditions of education that were essentially individualistic but recognized the social context of health issues and the necessity for some forms of social action. How it all fitted together was not clear. Early work on developing the Graduate Diploma in Health Education reflects this dilemma. In the mid 1980s this began to change. In 1986 the state 'Ministerial review of health education and promotion' issued its report. In this report health promotion was still defined as 'any combination of education and related organizational, economic and political interventions designed to promote behavioural and environmental changes conducive to health' (Victorian Government 1986), but this was seen as operating within the framework of the WHO 'Health for all by the year 2000' (HFA) initiative. The themes of the report were largely those of HFA-positive health, equity, multi-sectoral co-operation, action at many levels of social complexity and community participation. During 1986 to 1987 the ideas embodied in HFA and the Ottawa Charter gained a much wider currency in the health community providing the framework for some national reviews in the health field and a series of conferences. By 1987 the perspectives of HFA and the 'Ottawa Charter' were having a significant influence on the 'Graduate diploma in health education' programme.

Early development of the health education course

An initial 'concept' proposal for a course in health education was first put forward by a sub-committee of ACIDS early in 1978. In order to obtain approval to conduct courses, colleges of advanced education were, at that time, required to submit an initial proposal to the relevant state educational authority in order to obtain planning approval. This approval gave permission to the submitting college to develop a detailed course submission for educational accreditation by the state educational authority. The process was often lengthy, taking up to a year or more for completion.

Not surprisingly, the concept proposal for health education emphasized how the course would have strong affiliations with other inter-disciplinary courses including rehabilitation studies, community health and health administration. In the proposal it was contended that: 'Such courses are designed to build on the expertise of the various disciplines through an emphasis on teamwork, health maintenance in the community rather than emphasizing traditional approaches leading to increasing isolation and fragmentation of health professionals'. It was argued that the course would greatly assist health professionals by improving their ability to educate 'patients, peers and community groups about health and disease'. The educational objectives of the proposed course placed major emphasis on developing understanding of the social conditions affecting health, alternative models and underlying assumptions of health service systems, and the development of health education skills. In some respects this proposal echoed concerns that would, in the mid 1980s, be systematized in theoretical models of health education, for example, the Ottawa Charter. However, the established interests within the Institute were uneasy about developing inter-disciplinary activities and not yet prepared to recognize health education as a legitimate field of health work. When the proposal was submitted to the Institute's board of studies 'it was suggested that it duplicated some curriculum material (in other courses) and that perhaps the community's needs for training in health education could be met more effectively by continuing education programmes'. Continuing education programmes were short, non-award courses or even single events such as a one day workshop. The proposal was prevented from being forwarded to the state educational authority for reasons of the politics of inter-disciplinary education prevailing within the institute at the time. Thus, the initiative to develop a formal programme in health education was kept off the formal institute academic agenda until 1981.

Although health education developments were temporarily blocked, ACIDS proceeded to develop activities in inter-disciplinary education. These included undergraduate programmes in community health and health teamwork, public health seminars and the restructuring of graduate diploma courses in order to increase inter-disciplinary coursework and create a common structure. Towards the end of 1981 it was decided to disband ACIDS and relocate the courses it administered to other academic units. The School of Nursing unsuccessfully sought control of the health education proposal. Responsibility for the proposed course in health education and the existing course in health administration were transferred to the forerunner of their present home, the Department of Health Administration and Education. The courses in rehabilitation studies and community health were transferred to the precursor of their present home in the Department of Behavioural Health Sciences.

The original structure of the courses was maintained after this reorganization but their subsequent development was framed by more specialized departmental concerns. In this reorganization health education and health administration retained their link but the connection with rehabilitation and community health was weakened. Although in subsequent years the courses in health education and administration were overseen by separate and specialized course advisory committees, administratively they were closely connected. This became a major influence on subsequent developments in the field of health policy which ultimately involved all four of the original courses.

As part of the decision to disband ACIDS it was agreed that the institute would establish a health education course development committee. This decision turned out to be fortuitous. The Institute, as part of its annual reporting process to the state education authority, had continued to list health education as a possible future development. Around the time the course development committee was agreed to notification was received from the education authority that the course had been approved for commencement in 1984, notwithstanding the fact that there was no course and no formally approved course proposal. The course development committee was established forthwith with a membership including Institute staff and a cross section of external people involved in community health and health education. A combination of persistence on behalf of the course proponents, the decision to lower the profile of inter-disciplinary education and sheer accident cleared the way for development of a formal programme in health education.

Exploration of assumptions in the initial course development

The first meeting of the Health Education Course Development Committee was held in July 1982. It was presented with a statement of rationale and objectives for the proposed course which bore little relationship to the proposal developed some five years earlier. This first draft of the course rationale did not mention inter-disciplinarity and placed nowhere near the same emphasis on a social health perspective. Instead, it emphasized an individualistic, more 'clinical', philosophy focusing on the individuals' responsibility for their own health, lifestyle factors affecting health, and the need for health professionals to develop educative skills to assist people change their behaviour. However, the draft objectives retained some elements of the original perspective. They stated that students were to develop knowledge of political processes, of the way the health system operates and sets priorities, knowledge of alternative models and philosophies of health services and educative skills. The influence of the connection with health administration can be seen in these objectives.

By the end of 1982 the course development committee had succeeded in broadening the rationale. It was finally based on the following principles:

- [ ] an appropriate concept of 'health' ought to include physiological fitness and emotional wellbeing;
- [ ] the health status of people is strongly affected by behavioural and environmental factors;
- [ ] the medical, 'curative', perspective of many health professionals ought to be changed to a more 'positive' view of health;
- [ ] the responsibility for developing more positive health attitudes and behaviour in the community rests with individuals, families, community groups, health professionals, and governments;
- [ ] health professionals can contribute through role modelling, education, social action and political activity;
- [ ] governments have responsibility to develop health policies and provide resources to ensure that an appropriate health service infrastructure is available to members of the community.

The rationale proposed that health education was relevant for the promotion of health, prevention of illness, and coping with illness. It was thus multi-faceted and applicable in hospital settings for patients as well as community agencies. The course objectives that followed from this rationale emphasized:

- [ ] understanding patterns, processes and structures in relation to individual health behaviour, community life, and health service provision;
- [ ] developing skills in design, implementation and evaluation of educational activities.

The content of the course proposed was designed to closely reflect these objectives while at the same time fit with the Institute's common course structure for graduate diploma courses.

The course proposal underwent the rigorous external review process required for accreditation during 1983. In 1984 it was accredited, the year of the first student intake.

Course developments since 1983

The original, 1983, rationale for the Graduate Diploma in Health Education emphasized, as was considered appropriate at the time, behaviour change (health, at risk and illness behaviour) although recognizing that individual behaviours cannot be separated from the social relations in which they are learned and performed. Despite acknowledgement of the importance of social arrangements in the creation of health the course rationale argued that 'applications of education in health are relevant for people who':

1. value health and wish to maintain and promote their health and prevent the occurrence of illness;
2. perceive the threat of illness and wish to obtain a remedy and prevent its onset;
3. regard themselves as sick and wish to cope with their illness and improve their health;

4. perceive themselves to be well but adopt behaviours which are risks to health. Educational programmes directed at these four groups will be multi-faceted encompassing activities variously described as patient education, individal health counselling, health education, health promotion, community health education, public health education etc. (Course Accreditation Proposal: PG1 Health Education, 1983)

In 1983 the social nature of health was understood but a philosophy of individualism legitimated health education activity proposed in the course. By 1987, when the rationale was revised, social action had become sufficiently respectable for it to be considered a legitimate goal of education in health education. Health education and promotion operate at three levels each of which are linked to the others (French and Adams 1986):

1. behavioural change – improving people's health by changing behaviour, for example through self-management, media campaigns and legislation;
2. self-empowerment – improving health by increasing people's capacity to exercise control over their health status within constraints of their environment, for example counselling, promotion of self-esteem and self help groups;
3. collective action – improving health through change in political, social, scientific and economic arenas which create the environments within which people are constrained, for example through advocacy, community action and pressure groups.

A comprehensive approach to health education and promotion would usually involve activities and action at each level. Generally, health workers are most comfortable working at level 1 and least comfortable at level 3. On the completion of this course people should be prepared to work at all three. (Course Information Booklet: PG1 Health Education, 1988)

This discussion of levels was then located within the framework of the Ottawa Charter.

In those areas of the course dealing specifically with health education strategies there has been a significant shift in the focus of content away from education as the reference tradition towards social studies in health. This has been most apparent in the area of community health education. In that section of the course the change has been from locating specific strategies in the context of generalized problem solving skills towards studies of social relationships around themes of power and social change and the location of particular strategies within that framework. In the conduct of the strategies section of the course a theme of critical reflection has developed. In each area students are engaged in a series of activities in which they are required to act, reflect, and act again out of new insights. Paulo Freire's (1972) concept of dialogue provided the conceptual rationale for the emphasis on reflection in the process of teaching health educators. For Freire dialogue 'is the encounter between men, mediated by the world, in order to name the world'. It is a group process in which action is reflected upon in order to arrive at insights which might be shared and which serve to reframe future action. For the clinically trained health workers the exercises in critical reflection have been powerful sources of learning and personal satisfaction as they have grappled with new forms of theory and practice encountered in health education.

During 1988 the graduate diploma in health education underwent a significant reorganization as part of a process of linking five graduate diplomas into a common course structure upon which was built a master's degree by coursework. The earliest negotiations in the development of this initiative were between the courses in health education and health administration. In these discussions it was concluded that health policy constituted a common core of interest and that HFA provided a framework to link policy studies in health education and administration. Subsequently, the courses in rehabilitation studies, community health and behavioural health psychology were represented in the negotiation of a common structure. In the new framework the subjects shared by all the courses deal with the distribution of health and ill health in the Australian community, their explanations and the implications of these explanations for the construction of action at different levels of social complexity; with research and evaluation issues and techniques; with the origins, development and operation of the health system and with policy processes and strategies for health advancement. The specialist health education part of the revised programme examines the range of strategies involved in the work of health promotion systematized in the Ottawa Charter. These include strategies for working with individuals and groups on learning tasks; on group processes; on negotiation, participation, advocacy and lobbying; on social marketing and community development; on programme development, implementation and evaluation.

Conclusion

It has been argued in this chapter, that developments in the Graduate Diploma in Health Education have been shaped by internal institutional forces and by developments in the field of health education. In any final analysis both of these can be located in the context of much wider debates around the roles of health workers, appropriate activities for health services and the values and understandings prominent on the health agenda at particular points in time. In the late 1970s progressive forces in the then Lincoln Institute of Health Sciences were rallying around the issue of interdisciplinary practice. A special unit had been established to promote the idea, initiate curriculum changes and co-ordinate interdisciplinary postgraduate courses. Opposition to these developments on behalf of profession specific interests within the institute were effective in dismantling the institutional structures which had been established and in establishing an agenda for health education which was more individualistic and compatible with a clinical orientation to health services. Recent changes in the programme towards a more social perspective on health and health education have been linked to major policy debates within the health sector which extend well beyond the boundaries of the School of Health Sciences. These debates have focused on the inability of the community to afford an entirely clinical health system, on the desirability of prevention and health advancement and the recognition that many health outcomes are the consequence of activities outside the health sector. These debates have stimulated the articulation of more comprehensive perspectives and theoretical frameworks for health education which not only make sense to health workers but which also legitimate the activities which have been recognized as essential for health advancement. The most widely recognized of these frameworks is the Ottawa Charter which is a framework for health education based on the principles of the WHO HFA initiative. As the HFA initiative has gained currency in debates in the wider health policy community the Graduate Diploma in Health Education has been able to develop away from a clinical orientation towards a social perspective on health and health education.

References

Course accreditation proposal: PG1 Health Education (1983) Lincoln Institute of Health Sciences, Melbourne

Course information booklet: PG1 Health Education (1988) Lincoln School of Health Sciences, Melbourne

Fisher, K F, Howat, P A, Binns C W and Liveris M (1986) 'Health education and health promotion – an Australian perspective' *Health Education Journal* **45**, 95–98

Freire, P (1972) *Pedagogy of the Oppressed* Penguin, Middlesex

French, J and Adams, L (1986) 'From analysis to synthesis: theories of health education' *Health Education Journal* **45**, 71–74

Fry, D (1982) 'Frameworks in health education', *a paper presented at the 11th International Conference on Health Education, Hobart*

Labonte, R (1985) 'Social inequality and healthy public policy', *a paper presented at the 12th World Conference on Health Education, Dublin*

Tannahill, A (1986) 'What is health promotion?' *Health Education Journal* **44**, 167–168

Tones, B K (1986) 'Health education and the ideology of health promotion: a review of alternative approaches' *Health Education Research* **1**, 3–12

Victoria Government (1986) 'Ministerial review of health education and health promotion: report to the Minister for Health' Victorian Government Publishing Service, Melbourne

World Health Organization (1986) Ottawa charter for health promotion, Ottawa

World Health Organization (1987) Health promotion: a discussion document on the concept and principles, World Health Organization, Geneva

17. Health education in Kenya – AN OVERVIEW

N O Bwibo and J M Acham

Summary: The Health Education Division in the Ministry of Health was established in 1953 to administer health education activities. Government policy in health education places emphasis on the individual and the community. There are ten major health promotion programmes currently in operation. These cover a number of issues including family planning, environmental sanitation, provision of safe water and mental health. Family planning and the control of communicable diseases are important issues. The chapter describes the range of personnel involved in the delivery of health education. Of the various health education strategies employed, those focusing on school children are considered especially important. It is considered essential that health education strategies in local communities take into account the level of education and the culture of the people. New emphases include the development of resources, drug education, sex education, and AIDS education.

Introduction

The important role that health education plays in the utilization and delivery of health service was realized a long time ago. This realization was instrumental in the establishment of the Health Education Division in the Ministry of Health in 1953 specifically to administer and to be in charge of the functions of health education then and subsequently. The Division has been strengthened after independence and given a mandate as follows: 'to develop and conduct intensive, systematic and sustained education, informational and promotional activities against the causes of disease and their contributing factors'. The Division is a functional service like the nursing division and is directly linked to the Ministry of Health through the Chief Health Education Officer who is responsible to the Director of Medical Services through the Director of the Health Education Division.

Background

Health education is perceived in this country as an important strategy for helping the individual and the community to realize completely the value of the health services provided by the Government. It is seen as an essential component of the curative, preventive and promotive health delivery system of this country. There can be no better emphasis of this perception than the assertions and statements made by the Government in the Five Year Plan, 1973 to 1978, for the Health Education Division (Ministry of Health, 1972). This states that the primary goal of health education is 'to improve health and the general family standards of living among young people of Kenya'. It goes further to state that:

> the aim of providing health and family life education is to make it possible educationally, for the people of Kenya, to strengthen their desires, capacities and competencies so as to assist themselves and the nation in managing their own health and family planning affairs. This means that the individual and groups of individuals will go through a process of growth in health matters based on knowledge which is applicable to their ways of life . . . resulting in wholesome health practice for healthier and happier living.

This perception and policy puts emphasis on the individual and the community while bearing in mind the 'ways of life' of individuals and communities and ensuring that health education is 'based on knowledge which is applicable'. The emphasis on the community is not only logical but desirable since 85 per cent of the present estimated 21 million population of the Republic of Kenya live in rural areas. This emphasis on the individual and community also calls for ability of the individual to comprehend the principles of health education most of which are understood better with improved basic education. To make this possible, an adult education programme was established in the early 1970s, to run concurrently with basic primary and secondary education, for the purpose of improving literacy among adults.

Health education programmes

The major public health problems in Kenya are preventable. It is on this argument that the health education programme lays its weight. These major health problems are related to climatic factors, poor sanitation, poor housing, poor nutrition, inadequate and poor water supply, frequent births, and lack of knowledge about disease causation. These factors lead to infections, parasitic diseases, communicable diseases, diarrhoeal disease which the health workers cannot prevent without the people's understanding and participation.

The Government through the Ministry of Health and other relevant ministries puts emphasis on the following programmes to promote health:

1. Family Planning;
2. Extended Programme on Immunization;
3. Curative services;
4. Diarrhoeal disease control;
5. Environmental Sanitation;
6. Communicable disease control;
7. Provision of safe water;
8. Food and Nutrition Programme;

9. Mental Health;
10. Dental Health.

The activities of the health education programmes provide health educational and audio-visual aid services in support of formal training of health personnel. This is to effect the implementation of the above programmes or to train personnel in other sectors who are concerned with community development such as the various extension workers.

In carrying out the above programmes, the purpose of health education is to inform and educate Kenya's population on matters related to their health so that the people can:

a. protect themselves against communicable diseases;
b. use appropriate methods of family planning;
c. feed their children better so they will be able to learn better and grow up to be healthy and productive citizens;
d. promote their own health by adopting good health practices;
e. practise environmental sanitation;
f. practise good health habits and promote their own health through community effort.

It also attempts to:

a. ensure that as many families as possible know that the health services and staff exist to assist them in family planning matters;
b. increase support in the community and among family members for husbands and wives to practise family planning;
c. encourage parents to utilize fully, and on a continuing basis, the services provided by clinics for themselves and their children.

A high infant mortality rate in some rural areas and urban slums, together with a high fertility rate and a high population rise of 4 per cent per annum makes family planning an important but complex issue. The confusion in the minds of the people about the value of family planning in the face of high infant mortality rate can be a real problem. The role of carefully thought out and consistent health education on this issue is considered essential in implementing Government policy of family planning and birth spacing.

In all these activities, the 'Health education' programme endeavours to collaborate with, and to assist, the health workers and all those who can bring health education to the public. In other words, the activities and functions of the 'Health education' programme amplify the various strategies of the Ministry of Health, and those of other Government ministries to promote health and health practices.

Personnel involved in health education

Various cadres in the discipline of health education exist in Kenya. Although the Health Education Division was one of the earliest to be established, it still lacks staff particularly at the higher level of the profession and those with degree qualifications. There are four groups involved in the delivery of health education.

Firstly, there are the health education officers. This group forms the basis of the health education organizational structure. Typically, health education officers hold diplomas in health education. In the strategies to be followed for the 'Health education' programme it is stressed that the personnel development activities should be focused on health education officers since they are the specialist health education personnel.

The next category of personnel involved in the delivery of health education is the health workers who, while not wholly engaged in health education work, do undertake health education activities alongside their own duties. This group comprises several groups of health workers, such as doctors, nurses, midwives, public health officers, nutritionists, medical social workers and health technicians.

The third category of personnel engaged in health education activities are those workers from other sectors and disciplines of Government Ministries and non-governmental organizations (NGOs) whose duties and activities are directly or indirectly promoting positive health practices. These include teachers, agricultural extension workers, youth groups, women's groups and administration personnel.

The fourth category includes community leaders and others respected within the community. This is a very important group as the success of the community participation depends upon them.

The organization and administrative structure of the personnel in the Health Education Division is as follows. At the head of the Division is the Director under whom is the Chief Public Health Education Officer assisted by two Senior Health Education Officers and five Health Officers all stationed at the headquarters. There is a Provincial Health Education Officer in each province and a District Health Education officer at District level while at the community (village level) are the Family Health Field Educators. Other Family Health Field Educators are based at the hospitals, health centres and dispensaries. This last group carries out a patient's education programme and may do some 'outreach' work around the hospitals. The functional layout of the Health Education Division is shown below:

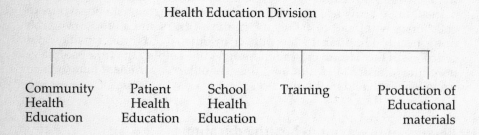

Health Education Division

| Community Health Education | Patient Health Education | School Health Education | Training | Production of Educational materials |

It should be noted that in their day to day interaction with patients, the nurses and doctors deliver a considerable amount of health education but may lack the correct communication skills to do so. There is a need for those professionals to be trained or guided by the professional health education specialists so as to enable them to operate efficiently.

Health education information is given to the patients in the clinic as they wait to be seen by the doctor, or while they are in-patients. It is questionable whether this is the most appropriate time since the patients, in pain or anxious about their conditions, might not be motivated to listen and follow what is being said even if it is relevant to their illness. No evaluation has been done to assess the effectiveness of this strategy.

Currently, there is no scheme of service for the core group of health education officers. This is being vigorously pursued with the relevant authorities. When it is achieved, it will be important in motivating and encouraging these professionals.

The Government attaches much importance to health education and hence provides the required recurrent costs and provides all the supporting and related staff in the Health Education Division. Such related staff include printing staff, audiovisual staff and photographers. The relevant supporting staff include technical staff and drivers.

Health education strategies

The health education aspects being promoted include changing people's behaviour and habits so as to improve and promote their health. This is done for groups of people for example in hospitals or health centre clinics, family planning clinics or ante-natal clinics. In such situations the health education professionals take the opportunity of helping the people who happen to be there and providing them with information on health related to their immediate conditions. The alternative strategy is employed in the community where the health education personnel organize people and provide campaigns for specific health problems which may be current in the area such as an outbreak of cholera. In both situations, whether these strategies are successful depends very much on what form of communication is to be used. Because of literacy problems, approaches that do not involve the use of written materials such as motion pictures, drawings, role play and food item demonstrations have been tried. Health education news is relayed on the national radio as transistor radios are very popular and are available in every corner of the Republic. In urban areas, the use of television for health education is common.

One strategy which appears to be very successful is the health education of school children at both primary and secondary schools.

Placing the emphasis on the health education of school children is of value because their minds are in a formative stage. They are more likely to change their habits or form good health habits when given health education so early in life. It has also been found that the school children are agents of change in their own homes as they take health messages and information to their parents and siblings. Because they can read, the school children are able to explain any health information in the news media and in pamphlets to their illiterate parents.

It is also realized that the school children are in a position to carry out some of the health education activities such as hand washing before eating and after using latrines, washing their clothes and generally keeping their bodies clean through the care of their finger nails, feet, hair and teeth. There is a very successful dental health programme on television which is geared towards school children where they convey, by means of role-play, the important message of cleaning their teeth with a toothpaste. Exercise, rest and nutrition through school lunches are prominent aspects of health education for school children.

The school health education programme also takes other forms that are important. Apart from directly providing health information to the school children, the teachers involve the children in keeping the school compounds clean by collecting rubbish and cutting grass. Inspection of the children for body hygiene is also regularly carried out.

For this programme to succeed, the teachers have to be willing to participate. Availability of visual aid material and books on health education promotes the teachers interest. Biology lessons offer a useful opportunity for teaching health education. In the neighbouring country of Tanzania, there are health education books printed in Swahili, such as the one quoted in the references *Maarifa Mapya ya Kuelimisha Afya* (Manuya) which translates *New Techniques for the Teaching of Health*. Such books can help teachers to refresh their minds and teach health education.

Health education strategies in the community have taken into account the level of education and the culture of the people. It aims to involve the various groups in the community in learning health-related information or participating in an active way to improve health status. There are usually many extension workers in the community. These together with the Family Field Educators provide health education to the people in the community.

The extension workers and the Family Field Educators are knowledgeable about the culture and beliefs of the people. They can take this knowledge into account in their work, as any activities which violate the beliefs of the people in the community are not taken to kindly. Several examples exist where cultural patterns and beliefs have to be taken seriously. These include food taboos and food preference, eating habits, food distribution within the family, pregnancy and childbirth, child rearing, use of toilets for the family members, disease causation and the care of the sick, death and funerals.

There are many NGOs that provide health care at various levels to the people in the community. It is very important that for their programmes to succeed, they seriously consider the correct approach to health care. Their success, like that of the extension workers and the Family Health Field Educators, owes much to their understanding of the culture and beliefs of the people. These correct attitudes to health education are commendable.

We shall touch briefly on the role of the African Medical Research Foundation (AMREF). This is a non-government organization which provides much health education through the news media and radio in conjunction with the Ministry of Health. Among their employees in the past was a cultural anthropologist whose role in the understanding of the people's beliefs in food and eating habits helped a great deal in dealing with people both in rural areas and urban slums of Nairobi. Those ideas he gained in working with the people are described in his book (Scotney 1976). This is one of AMREF's many printed manuals for health workers.

The AMREF participates in providing health information on the Kenya radio, on selected topics which are well presented and hence eagerly listened to. Like other NGOs, AMREF runs a 'Primary health programme' in a semi-arid area in Kebwesi in Machakos district.

The utilization of an opportunity to provide health education in Kenya has been the annual agricultural shows at provincial and district levels. At each of the shows, the Division of Health Education has a stand where health education programmes are discussed and displayed. These stands are very popular which strongly suggests that people find them informative and educative.

Youth groups, women's groups such as *Maendeleo Ya Wanawake* of Kenya and various church groups participate in health education related to their needs. Youth groups deal with the health problems affecting young people including teenage pregnancy, sexually transmitted diseases and drugs and alcohol. *Maendeleo Ya Wanawake* and the church groups deal specifically with nutrition, adolescent pregnancies, sex education and the utilization of health services.

As the majority of the childbirths occur at home and are conducted by tradition birth attendants (TBAs), the Government has taken the training of TBAs as an important health education issue. The TBAs are trained in groups, district by district. They receive instruction in methods of detecting pregnancies that are at risk, hygienic delivery, care of the newborn and care of the mother. The TBAs are respected local individuals and are therefore a powerful tool for change in childbirth procedures. They are in a position to transmit correct information on childbirth and family planning to their clients.

New Emphases

New emphasis should be placed on health education in relation to mental health. This area has so far been neglected. The establishment of the Division of Mental Health, should facilitate the setting-up of useful programmes on mental health.

The increasing availability and use of drugs also calls for greater emphasis in health education about drug use so as to avoid the problems of drug abuse, an issue that is a major concern in western countries.

As indicated above, the success of health education is influenced by the ability of those being educated to read and follow written information. As more and more children go to school, the literacy rate will greatly increase. As a result, there is a need to print more readable information such as pamphlets and health manuals for the people. The printing of such booklets should be possible since the Health Education Division has printing facilities which are not yet being utilized to maximum.

There is also new emphasis on reproductive health particularly adolescent pregnancies. The question of sex education for young people carries many emotional feelings and parents are bewildered and often uncertain as to what to do. Suggestions of family planning methods for young people in this group meets with outcry from all walks of life. Overcoming this response needs to be addressed.

We cannot finish the area of new emphasis without mentioning the efforts being made to spread the correct information on the global problem of AIDS. Various approaches are being used to educate the mass about prevention of this disease and also the care and support of victims wtihin the family.

External influences

Kenya gets assistance and support in its 'Health education programme'. Most of the international assistance comes from WHO, UNICEF and USAID. In all these, the assistance provided is to support the implementation of Government efforts rather than duplicating them. The WHO provides fellowships for training and also assists in the Postgraduate Community Health Programme at the Faculty of Medicine, University of Nairobi. The WHO also provides assistance through the programme of printing health education materials. It also sponsors regional WHO seminars like the one that took place in Harare for Community Health Education (World Health Organization 1987).

USAID has provided training facilities, teachers, printing equipment and other health education resources to the Health Education Division. It also provided teachers from the US Peace Corps. UNICEF has been instrumental in promoting health education through training, through seminars and in the provision of vehicles for transport in the field.

Future trends

The strategies and future trends of health education were carefully charted by a committee of experts in a workshop held in 1985 (World Health Organization 1987) where it was emphasized that there was a great need to have a blueprint of strategies for Kenya covering the main areas of health education activities. Since the Health Education Division is a functional arm of the Ministry of Health, the projected activities and trends have to reflect the main health strategies of the Ministry. In line with the global commitment of 'Health for all by the year 2000' through primary health care, health education has to play its role in making Kenya realize this social obligation. The Health Education Division is translating its activities within primary health care and community-based health care. It is replanning and implementing programmes and evaluating their effectiveness. In this way, it is in a position to revise the projects in the light of the evaluation.

Realizing the need to train health education manpower, the Government of the Republic of Kenya has put a great deal of effort into training. In the 1970s the Government of Kenya with the assistance of USAID sent three Health Education Officers to the USA to pursue degree courses in health education. At the same time, the Government sent three Health Education

Officers to the West African University to take the Advanced Diploma in Health Education course. In addition, a small number of Health Education Officers were first trained locally at the Division of Health Education. The Division also trained 817 Family Health Field Educators. Currently Health Education officers are trained at Medical Training College (MTC) in Nairobi. The Health Education Officers from the Health Education Division participate in the teaching of these trainee health education officers.

Health education forms an important component of the teaching syllabi for most health personnel particularly for public health nurses in the 'Advanced nursing diploma' programme and the 'Enrolled community nursing programme'. The postgraduate doctors doing the Masters of Public Health Degree programmes have a big health education component in their course. The University of Nairobi has sponsored one of the teaching staff of the public health course for a degree programme in health education in the USA. All of the above indicate that training is taken seriously. In the future this training will undoubtedly have an effect on the quality of health education in Kenya.

In order for health education to have a greater impact on the many health problems, the Ministry of Health has established a National Committee on Health Education within the Ministry of Health with adequate representation from appropriate Government officials so as to provide an adequate policy-making body. This will be important in strengthening health education efforts in the country.

References

Guilbert, J J (1976) *Educational Handbook*, World Health Organization

Koeune, E (1957) *How to Teach Hygiene, Home Nursing and First Aid: A Book for Primary School and Welfare Centres in East Africa* East African Literature Bureau

Lutwama, J S and Bennett, F J (1969) *Health Education in East Africa: A Challenge to the Schools* Longmans: Nairobi

Manuya, S J *Maarifa Mapya ya Kuelimisha Afya* East African Literature Bureau

Ministry of Health (1972) *The Health Education Division Five Year Plan 1973 to 1978* Ministry of Health, Kenya

Ministry of Health (1985) *Health Education Strategy in Kenya* Ministry of Health, Republic of Kenya

Norman-Taylor, W (1956) *A Textbook of Hygiene for Teachers in Africa* Longmans, Nairobi

Scotney, N (1976) *Health Education: A Manual for Medical Assistants and Rural health Workers* African Medical Research foundation

World Health Organization (1987) *Report of Regional Workshop on Strengthening the Training of Communication/Education for Health in Health Personnel Training Institutions* Harare, Zimbabwe 6–10 October 1986: WHO Regional Office for Africa, Brazzaville

18. Insights on health education: experience of the African Medical Research Foundation (AMREF) – A CASE STUDY

D Nyamwaya, E Oduol and C Wood

Summary: Health education has only recently become fully accepted as a special activity requiring specific professional training. As a service it has not received the serious attention it deserves in terms of budgetry and staff allocations. Until the 1970s a western model of health education relying mainly on print media was being applied in a context where the majority of the people was illiterate.

A variety of programmes have since been developed involving alternative ways of communicating health information which focus on health behaviour and which pay particular attention to the cultural background of the population. A wide range of strategies and their evaluations are described.

General background information

Although western biomedicine has existed in East Africa since the beginning of this century, it was only recently that health education became fully accepted as a special activity requiring specific professional training. Before this acceptance, medical personnel made various attempts to 'educate' their patients regarding the prevention of ill-health.

Even after health education became accepted as a special activity, this aspect of health development has in many cases been affected by a number of obstacles which have hindered effective implementation of health education campaigns and programmes. Firstly, health education as a service, has not received the serious attention it deserves in terms of budgetary and staff allocations. Health education departments, where these exist, are usually understaffed, with very small budgets. In both Uganda and Tanzania, for example, the respective health education departments have each less than a dozen professional health education staff.

Secondly, conventional health education is usually regarded as a public information service *per se*. The basic assumption underlying this view is that people do not practise appropriate health behaviour because of ignorance. However, it is clear that something more than knowledge is required to bring about health behaviour change. This understanding is brought home vividly when it is realized that most smokers are well aware of the health hazards of their habit.

Thirdly, conventional health education approaches and activities have rarely been evaluated. It has been difficult therefore to establish linkages between such approaches and activities and specific, demonstrable effect.

During the last two decades and especially after Alma Ata the conventional approach to health education has come under increasing attack from both health and non-health specialists. Various attempts have been and are being made to develop more effective approaches to health education. The African Medical and Research Foundation (AMREF), has played a role in the search for effective approaches to health education. The organization's experiences are discussed below.

AMREF's experience in health education

Based in Nairobi, Kenya, AMREF has been at the forefront of promoting a new approach to health education. The development of this new approach started in the mid-1970s and still continues. Having identified many flaws in conventional health education programmes, AMREF (1977) launched a more comprehensive programme known as 'Health behaviour and education'. The programme regards health education as a multi-stage process, which embraces the exchange of information between health professionals and the public, translating the information into knowledge and behaviour change and integrating health education with other aspects of health and other development.

This programme, which consists of several projects, is co-ordinated by the Health Behaviour and Education Department.

Establishment of the need for the programme

A survey of health education activities undertaken during the early 1970s by AMREF indicated that in spite of many attempts to disseminate health information, there were few tangible effects of the attempts. It was realized further that the approaches used lacked relevance and the programmes in existence reached only a few, especially those who could read and write. This was so because a western model of health education, relying mainly on print media, was being applied in a context where the majority of the people were illiterate. The health education programmes did not take adequate consideration of the fact that communication of messages and their translation into health behaviour are influenced heavily by the target population's culture.

Aims and purposes of the AMREF health education initiative

In order to optimize the effects of health education programmes, AMREF emphasizes the use of concepts and skills developed in the social and behavioural sciences. This is done in three ways.

Firstly, the programme encourages the undertaking of operations research on the socio-cultural aspects of specific diseases and health problems so as to improve the development and implementation of programmes designed to modify health behaviour. Such studies cover people's beliefs, customs and behaviour, attitude change processes, appropriate communication methods and strategies in so far as these relate to health improvement.

Secondly, the programme seeks to promote the development of systematic procedures for monitoring and evaluating health education activities and approaches and their impact.

Thirdly, the programme provides professional short and long-term training of health and other development workers on effective health education methods, approaches and media.

In order to realize the broad goal and purposes listed above, AMREF is involved in a number of specific health education programmes, both directly and indirectly, the latter through Ministries of Health or other non-governmental organizations.

The nature of work

Health education projects undertaken or supported by AMREF fall under three broad categories: training of health workers for effective health education, community education for behaviour change and development, and production and dissemination of health education media and materials.

Training community health workers for health development – regional programme for East Africa

The success of community-based health development programmes depends largely on community participation. Community participation remains the backbone of rural health development programmes. Training of local extension agents – animators or motivators – for health promotion/ disease prevention facilitates much needed community participation.

Among the rural poor the need for training such people is much greater. Illiteracy is common, even radios and other sources of health information are relatively few. Most information is therefore communicated verbally. People therefore have little access to health information. The goal is education of the people by the people through utilization of available human resources, hence the need for training Community Health Workers (CHW) as the link between the institutionalized health system and the community.

Training of community health workers by AMREF generally takes place in their local community and does not necessitate their leaving their home area. In-service training activities continue thereafter. These in-service training programmes are tailored to meet local needs.

The training curriculum normally emerges from the community health needs and CHWs' own personal experiences. The curriculum therefore varies from locality to locality. The teaching method has always been the learner-centred problem-posing method popularized by Paulo Freire. This provides the CHWs with inter-personal communication skills that enable them to stimulate villagers to participate in health development programmes. The training puts much emphasis on health education as a crucial component of community health services. A good example of such training is to be found in the 'Kibwezi rural health programme'. Community based health workers have been trained to teach their communities regarding child survival, water and sanitation and family planning.

Evaluations carried out show that community health workers who receive training in the methods of comprehensive health education perform better than those who have not.

Education for Community Health Action Project (ECHAP) Kenya

This programme is a milestone in Kenya's health education programmes' history. It started as 'innovative activities for the promotion of health through health education' in 1985. The rationale for ECHAP was threefold. Firstly, throughout the 30 years of health education in Kenya, it had not been possible to determine the association between health education and change in health behaviour. Secondly, health education was taken for granted and inadequate attention was given to message and media strategies and their respective recipients. Thirdly, health educators seldom instituted or built-in any mechanisms for monitoring and evaluating of health education programmes to determine programme achievements. In addition there did not exist a sufficiently defined conceptual framework or implementation strategy for facilitating active community participation in health education. The ECHAP, therefore, is envisaged as a tool for developing a prototype conceptual model for health education. The project aims at assisting health education officers to utilize low-cost forms of communicating health information so as to stimulate community action in health development programmes.

The programme is a joint venture between the Division of Health Education (DHE) Ministry of Health, Kenya and AMREF. Staff from these two institutions guide health education officers with project development, implementation and evaluation. There are now sixteen such projects in various parts of the country. Participating staff are drawn from Government and NGOs. Small grants are provided where necessary. The grants serve as 'seed money' with the community providing the bulk of the other resources needed for project implementation. With the assistance of a health educator, a community comes up with a defined health problem to be addressed through health education. A baseline survey is carried out using participatory action research methodology. The baseline survey indicates the main causes of the problem which are then addressed through the ECHAP project. Monitoring and evaluation strategies and indicators are built into the project.

The objectives of this project are:

☐ to help develop a *modus operandi* in which active community participation in health education and development can be maximized;

☐ to provide training opportunities to health education planners and workers, both in government and NGOs by involving them in design, implementation and evaluation of small-scale health education projects;

☐ to promote inter-agency collaboration in health promotion through community involvement.

At the moment, there are sixteen ECHAP projects in Kenya. Five such projects have already been completed but the activities stimulated are still continuing.

Diarrhoea control project in Mukurweini Nyeri, Kenya: an example of the ECHAP approach to health education

The overall goal of this project is to reduce the incidence of diarrhoea in the community. Other objectives are:

- ☐ to create awareness of the existing diarrhoea problems;
- ☐ to increase knowledge on the causes and factors contributing to the spread of diarrhoea;
- ☐ to provide skills on prevention and control of diarrhoea;
- ☐ to promote community participation in diarrhoea control;
- ☐ to encourage utilization of oral rehydration therapy as a means of managing diarrhoea.

To achieve these objectives comprehensive intervention strategies included, among others, baseline surveys, training community health workers and extension workers; field demonstrations and distribution of educational materials written in the local language. These had to be designed and developed.

The DHE and AMREF assisted with project design, monitoring and evaluation, and financing. Project implementation was carried out by a health educator and a team of village health workers. The health educator received the appropriate orientation in a workshop organized by the DHE and AMREF. Funds provided by AMREF were used for construction of demonstration structures and training of village health workers.

Results of monitoring and evaluation exercises indicate that there has been a marked decline in diarrhoea morbidity (43.17 per cent for 1986 to 1987). According to health centre reports, before 1986 the demand for oral rehydration salts (ORS) provided at the centre exceeded their supply. The 1987 records indicate a decline in ORS consumption because of a decline in diarrhoea cases. The health centre currently sends the remaining ORS sachets to two neighbouring hospitals! Another reason for the reduced demand for ORS sachets provided at the health centre arises from the home preparation of ORS, which is yet another result of the project.

Success of this project is also indicated by the new skills acquired by the target population. Members of the community can now make concrete latrine slabs, improved water tanks and ORS. There is more and early use of existing health (especially family planning) services, which is another indicator of project success.

The knowledge of the community regarding the causation of disease has also increased. People now understand better the connection between the physical environment and the causation of diseases such as diarrhoea and worms.

The community has formed health action groups for collecting funds, purchasing materials and sharing labour. These groups make bricks, protect springs, build water tanks and suchlike. Most of these activities are carried out using local materials and labour.

Health education media development
folk media project, Turkana District, Kenya

In developing countries where the rate of literacy is low, folk media play an important role in non-formal education. In primary health care programmes this role is consistent with the principle of using appropriate technology to enhance health development.

AMREF seeks to promote development and use of indigenous media in communicaton for health development in the community and produce a booklet on health songs, riddles, poems and drama which can be utilized by community groups and schools. A good example of a folk media project is to be found in an AMREF (1985) sponsored project in Turkana, Kenya.

The folk media in Turkana District is aimed at assisting various communities in the district to:

☐ articulate concerns, needs and demands to clarify the nature of existing health problems for example immunization, child care, diarrhoea, malnutrition, ante-natal care, personal hygiene, hydatid disease and other communicable diseases;

☐ mobilize people for participation in their own health care;

☐ assist people to take up more responsibility for their health problems and demonstrate their capacity to change and improve their health through collective efforts;

☐ inculcate positive health values among schoolchildren;

☐ develop a booklet on health songs, riddles, poems and drama in the Turkana language which can later be used by extension workers, church leaders, adult teachers in the whole of Turkana District.

The project activities during the last two years have included workshops and seminars organized for extension workers and school teachers to compose the required riddles, poems and drama as means of communicating health messages. Extension workers currently are using these forms of communication when educating community groups to stimulate discussions, raise and analyse issues, challenge values/beliefs related to diarrhoea, immunization, nutrition/malnutrition, hygiene, eye problems, and hydatid disease among the Turkana. A health song-and-drama festival is being planned in order to provide additional motivation for health actions.

Folk media have proved to be an effective technology for stimulating health action. Though no formal evaluation of the project has been undertaken yet, there are pointers that substantial health behaviour change has been achieved through these media. It is also important to stress that folk media are fairly low cost in terms of development and use. The media serve a dual purpose – they entertain, as well as inform and motivate people to change behaviour.

With time, folk media are likely to prove their effectiveness in enhancing rural health development.

Defender, a health education magazine for laypeople

The health behaviour of people, and youth in particular, begins with the values, beliefs and attitudes of their social and cultural environment and the economic realities of their families and communities. Health cannot be separated from the development of a person or society. Its presence makes fuller development possible. Its absence imposes heavy restrictions on what is attainable. But relatively few children and youth in today's world absorb from their social environment the concept that health is an asset of high priority or that they themselves can be instrumental in affecting it.

Schools do little to prepare youths for living a healthy life and for tackling the health problems and risks they will encounter. Reading materials on health are rarely available, and where they are, they are usually too technical and expensive.

Our contribution to health learning for youth, in and out of school, and adults in less developed countries, requires making available a health magazine written in simple language. The *Defender* magazine is AMREF's response to the need for health information for lay youth and young adults. The Department of Health Behaviour and Education of AMREF publishes and distributes a quarterly health magazine whose title may be taken to reflect the eventuality that d-disease, e-endanger, f-families, e- eliminate, n-nations, d-destroy, e-every, r-resource.

Twenty thousand copies of *Defender* are produced every quarter and sent to individual readers, institutions and vocational training centres in Eastern Africa and beyond. These readers include youth, in and out of school, and young and middle-aged adults in both rural and urban areas.

The overall goal of *Defender*, which has evolved since its first issue in 1968, is to assist people in Eastern Africa to be more knowledgeable about health and therefore help them to be their own primary source of health care and further stimulate and empower them to manage their health destiny and enhance the quality of their lives. *Defender* therefore aims at:

☐ empowering and encouraging people to assume a greater degree of responsibility for their own health based on more comprehensive and accurate health knowledge for better healthful living;
☐ providing a forum for people with health problems affecting their families and communities to write and ask questions about these problems;
☐ providing a health information source additional to those available through local health services, hence an opportunity for acquiring information that can immediately be used to improve living standards;
☐ encouraging a more meaningful discussion within communities on current health problems and needs so that the services of the local health facilities become better utilized;
☐ assisting in early recognition of the symptoms of diseases and helping individuals and communities respond more quickly to the need to seek treatment.

To ensure that *Defender* reaches an interested target audience assessments have been carried out in 1977, 1982 and 1985 supplemented by annual computerized updating of the mailing list. The findings have shown *Defender* meets target readers' health learning needs.

In 1977 a questionnaire was developed and included in the October issue. Readers were required to complete and return the questionnaire if they wished to receive further issues. A total of 38 per cent of readers responded. Respondents indicated that the magazine was well targeted in terms of topics covered. There was also an indication that the magazine had stimulated discussion and led to action in response to health problems.

In 1979 an increasing proportion of the material printed consisted of replies to readers' letters. By the end of that year almost all articles were based on readers' questions. The volume of correspondence continued to increase, and during the year individual copies dispatched increased from 8,000 to 9,000. Since then the increase in demand has continued. At the current circulation figure of 20,000 and an estimated readership of 100,000 in East Africa alone, the demand for readers to be included in the mailing list is estimated at 30,000 by 1990.

Defender has addressed most health problems through answers to readers' questions and topical issue. Very positive feedback has been received regarding the use of advise in *Defender* for effecting health behaviour changes and especially the enhancement of self-care.

Problems relating to the production and distribution of magazines in general have been noted in the case of *Defender*. These problems relate to change of readers' addresses and failure to respond to all questions raised by readers. Occasionally it has become necessary to write letters to readers in response to questions asked.

Production and distribution of *Defender* will continue with special attention being paid to matters relating to the health of teenagers and young adults and each issue is to focus on a particular health aspect instead of several.

Conclusions

The health education programme known in AMREF as 'Health behaviour and education' has been in existence now for over ten years (since 1976). A major evaluation of the overall programme is scheduled to take place from mid-1989, but a number of conclusions can be drawn from experiences already recorded.

The comprehensive approach to health education, that is emphasizing behaviour change rather than mere dissemination of information and the application of behavioural sciences, has proved to be quite effective in promoting and/or changing behaviours relating to health. It has been shown that a proper understanding of people's beliefs, attitudes and practices before embarking on health education activities leads to more effective health education programmes.

A number of NGOs and Government departments have been assisted to recognize the need for studies of peoples' cultures before or alongside the launching of health programmes. The inclusion of behavioural scientists in health programmes is becoming increasingly common in East Africa.

The programme has also confirmed that health education can be undertaken by non-health professionals. Teachers, community health workers and community leaders, most of whom have no health training, have been shown to be capable of contributing to health behaviour change.

The 'Health behaviour and education programme' at AMREF has faced one major problem: lack of trained manpower. There are few well trained behavioural scientists with an orientation towards health. Similarly there are few medical specialists with proper grounding in behavioural sciences. Much time and money have therefore had to be used in the training of staff wanting to be specialists in health behaviour and education.

The programme is being consolidated. AMREF is increasingly involved in advocacy for the promotion of behavioural science in health programmes. Training of staff to man the behavioural components of such programmes will continue with emphasis on district health management teams and communities.

Finally, we must stress that though AMREF considers health education as a special activity requiring specific skills, it also views it as an integral aspect of other health development activities. Health education initiatives have been shown to yield better results when they are fully incorporated into broader health programmes including curative services.

References

African Medical and Research Foundation (1977) *Health Behaviour and Education Project Proposal* AMREF

African Medical and Research Foundation (1985) *Folk Media: Communicating for Health Promotion*, Kenya communicatons support project in Turkana District in Kenya: a concept paper

Alanen, L (1985) What can be learned from progress in socialisation research?: *12th World Conference on Health Education Proceedings, Dublin* Ireland

Anderson, M G and Child, R C (1985) Systems and behaviour change: health promotion objectives in Southern Illinois *12th World Conference on Health Education Proceedings, Dublin* Ireland

Bandura, A (1971) *Social Learning Theory* General Learning Press, New York

Morley, D, Rhode, J and Williams, G (1983) *Practising Health for All* Oxford University Press

Oduol, E (1988) Health education for diarrhoea control in children under five years: a challenge for health workers *Paper presented at the Kenya Paediatric Association Annual Scientific Conference* March 1988

Oduol, E (1985) *Training Community Health Workers in Southern Sudan: A field report*: AMREF

Read, M (1957) Social and cultural background for planning public health programmes in Africa *paper presented at WHO Seminar on Health Education in Africa*: Dakar

Scotney, N (1979) Development of health education programmes. Paper presented to the Royal college of Obstetricians and Gynaecologists Study Group on Maternity Services in the Developing World: What the Community Needs: London

Shaffer, R (1984) *Beyond the Dispensary: On giving community balance to primary health care* AMREF

Ssenyonga, J Oduol, E and Nzioka, N (1986) Evaluation of innovative projects for strengthening community health action through health education. AMREF

19. Ibadan comfort stations: an experiment in environmental sanitation health education – A CASE STUDY

Z A Ademuwagun

Summary: The development of 500 Stations was the target for the programme in 1969. The building of the first station to provide toilet and laundry facilities for a community of families began in 1970. To date, 42 have been built but many problems exist in maintaining them. Greater attention needs to be paid to this very important and potentially very successful community health project.

In its conception and planning great attention has been paid to the social structure of communities and to the values held by the people. It is noted that people value privacy and cleanliness highly yet many do not understand the connection between excrement, flies and disease. Researchers and educators from outside Nigeria often misunderstand the level of organization within African communities and fail to harness this natural resource. This project does not make this mistake. Promotion of the project also relies on the cultural values rather than poorly understood health knowledge.

Introduction

The problem of liquid wastes disposal in the unplanned, crowded and congested parts which characterize most of the cities of Nigeria is a perennial one. Uncontrolled disposal of liquid wastes and human excreta contaminates rivers and streams and even leaking water pipes, thus affecting the potability of water supplies. The resultant effect is the presence of the common water-borne diseases such as ascariasis, dysenteries, diarrhoea, cholera, typhoid and hookworm infection. Ibadan is a typical city in point.

Ibadan is the largest city in Black Africa, with a population of about two million. Most of Ibadan city is plagued by problems of inadequate or absent basic social infra-structure. This problem is complicated by the unplanned nature of the inner core of the city. Slum and squatter settlements continue to present serious challenges to the engineers responsible for planning environmental sanitation improvement programmes. Environmental sanitation problems are particularly acute in the slum and congested inner core of the city with its open drains and insanitary disposal of human wastes both liquid and solid. The lack of easy accessibility to the streets, roads and alleys still precludes the construction of conventional sewage disposal systems and the routing of refuse tracks into the crowded areas of the city.

Behavioural and non-behavioural factors

Problems have been identified as follows:

1. For individuals and families:
   a. indiscriminate disposal of human wastes, liquid and solid;
   b. ignorance of health implications of (a); and
   c. poverty which prevents the construction and use of conventional human wastes disposal facilities.
2. For the administrators:
   a. Town planning defects:
      i unplanned and congested inner core of the city;
      ii open drains;
      iii lack of basic sanitary infra-structures – public toilets, public refuse bins, potable public water supply;
   b. Ineffective enforcement and management of environmental sanitation policy implementation by government functionaries, for example ineffective public health superintendents;
   c. Inadequate funding of environmental sanitation projects by the government, resulting in ineffective collection and disposal of human wastes, solid (refuse) and liquid (excreta and household waste waters) – defective environmental sanitation engineering; and
   d. Inadequate public health education – environmental sanitation health education.

The comfort station

A comfort station is a building with three compartments designed to provide toilet, bathing, and facilities for washing clothes, respectively for an extended family compound of about 300–600 persons. An 'aqua privy' (a tank filled with water), about six feet deep, built at the bottom of the building, provides a satisfactorily hygienic method of disposing of the waste waters and human excreta generated by the inhabitants of the compound. Dunghills and areas of land used for salgas in the backyards are suitable for comfort stations.

The comfort station is not a public facility but the *bona fide* property of the family who participates in its construction. Only members of the family compound who are also responsible for the cost of operation and maintenance are entitled to use the station. While the family provides land and labour, the former Western State Government with its collaborators provides a grant of about four thousand Nigerian pounds for the purchase of building materials and other equipment. Proper operation of the comfort station is essential and daily maintenance of the station is the responsibility of the owner who must ensure that toilets, showers and laundry rooms are kept clean and that repairs are made before they become a major problem.

As an intervention in environmental sanitation, the comfort stations are intended to serve as a self-help experiment in community development through active community participation efforts. Hence, to all intents and purposes, the project is an experiment in environmental sanitation health education (Ademuwagun, 1975). The founding fathers intended the experiment at Ibadan to be replicated in other towns and cities with similar environmental sanitation problems in the then Western State and in Nigeria as a whole.

Four standard designs are utilized at present to cater for most situations. One laundry and one urinal with washbasin are provided for each type.

Type	Toilets	Showers	Actual population served (maximum)	Recommended population to be served (maximum)
I	28	16	1,012	700
II	20	12	880	500
III	16	10	400	400
IV	10	6	230	250

Table 19.1 *Design for comfort stations*

An analysis of Table 19.1 shows that, on the basis of the actual population served, there is a variation in usage from 23 to 24 persons per toilet and 38 to 73 persons per shower. In most cases, this variation is attributable to site restrictions. On present indications, an optimum of 25 persons per toilet, and 40 persons per shower, could be adopted and the corresponding design population are also shown as IV.

In 1969, the former Western State Government of Nigeria (now consisting of Oyo, Ondo and Ogun States) decided to embark upon a modern sewage and drainage project for the ever-growing city of Ibadan. It delegated the Ministry of Works and Transport as the participating Government Agency and the Ibadan Wastes Disposal and Drainage Board with the requisite expertise to work on the project with international assistance for the improvement of environmental sanitation in Ibadan. The WHO and the UNDP came to the assistance of the State Government.

Plan of operation

The plan of operation consisted of two phases:

Phase one

The purpose of phase one was to assist the Western State Government in undertaking engineering and feasibility studies necessary to the preparation of master plans and construction programmes for sewage, drainage and solid wastes as well as inter-related legal, managerial and financial matters to the City of Ibadan, Western State of Nigeria.

The project agreement was signed between the Government and the WHO/UNDP on 7 January 1969 while the programme was expected to start on 15 FEbruary 1969. A sub-contract agreement between the WHO and Maclaran Limited of Toronto, Canada, was signed in Geneva on 28 February 1969, and the sub-contractor began work on 5 March 1969.

Phase two

The purpose of the project was to assist the Government in undertaking a programme of health education and construction of sanitary facilities to alleviate the urgent environmental health problems in the old city, and to complete the economic, organizational and engineering studies on the city-wide sewage system which was then being planned with UNDP assistance.

Agreement on phase two of the project was signed in 1971: by the Western State of Nigeria on 12 October 1971; by the WHO on 12 October 1971; by the Federal Government of Nigeria on 10 November 1971; and by the UNDP in 1971.

In 1972, additional man-months of expert service was provided in respect of the WHO in order to further assist the development of self-help demonstration projects and local health education programmes in support of environmental sanitation education. Specifically, the involvement of the WHO focused on the health education component of the comfort station. As stated in one of the objectives of the 'Comfort station programme' in phase two of the plan of operation by the WHO/UNDP:

> a health education programme in the field of environmental health will be developed in collaboration with national, state and local agencies, institutions and organizations with the principal efforts being directed towards the enlightenment of the inhabitants of the densely populated areas on the advantages, ways and means of improving environmental health conditions.

It is in this context that Ademuwagun (1975) described the Ibadan comfort station as an 'experiment in environmental sanitation health education'.

The inception of the comfort stations

As a result of the feasibility study mentioned above, the 'Comfort station experiment' was launched in 1970. The Government envisaged the construction of 500 comfort stations by 1980, and 25 of which were to serve as a pilot project. Apart from technical support and guidance from the Government through its collaborating agents, the first 25 were expected to be financed, built and administered through self-help by the concerned families/communities. The Government, on its part, also planned to finance some pilot stations in other parts of the state in order to introduce and popularize the experiment among the people in the state beyond the city of Ibadan. The last of the pilot comfort stations was ready towards the end of 1975. Since 1975, only seventeen additional comfort stations have been constructed through community efforts bringing the total to 42 within a time-frame of 1970 to 1988 instead of the envisaged 500 comfort stations. In summary, 25 comfort stations were built between 1970 and 1975 while 17 were constructed between 1976 and 1988.

The first nine family compounds to embrace the experiment were: Adebolu, Apena, Bara, Egbodi, Foko, Saku, Adepo, Kagunmolu, and Oyewo/Lawoye. Table 19.2 shows data on the actual environmental sanitation facilities in the family compounds with the comfort stations before the project, while Table 19.3 contains the sanitary facilities at the nine comfort stations together with other relevant information, such as when the stations were started and completed.

	Family/ Compound	Population	No. of Compounds	No. of Public Toilets	No. of Public Refuse Depots	No. of Public Water Taps	No. of Private Wells
1.	Adepolu	250	1	Nil	Nil	Nil	1
2.	Adepo	400	1	1	Nil	Nil	Nil
3.	Apena	345	1	Nil	Nil	Nil	1
4.	Bara/jaiye ade	217	2	Nil	Nil	1	1
5.	Egbodi	215	1	Nil	Nil	1	1
6.	Foko	735	1	Nil	1	Nil	Nil
7.	Kagunmalo	170	1	Nil	Nil	Nil	Nil
8.	Oyewo/ Lawoye	237	1	Nil	Nil	Nil	Nil
9.	Saku	256	1	Nil	Nil	Nil	Nil

Table 19.2 *Some data on the target communities: pre-comfort station experiment*

Comment

Since the research report of Ademuwagun on the comfort stations in 1975 an additional 17 comfort stations have been constructed bringing the total to 42 out of the envisaged 500 comfort stations by 1980. Forty-one comfort stations are now either being fully used or partially used owing to one problem or another. Some are locked-up and one at Age-Egbeomo has just been rehabilitated by the family compound, the rest need one kind of repair or another. For example, Olunloyo comfort station is locked up because the donor of the piece of land on which the comfort station was build is unable to agree with the other households on the modality of use and maintenance. Akilapa comfort station is sealed up because of an engineering defect – the soakaway pits are full and overflowing with faeces. Obisesan comfort station is also locked up because of maintenance problems and inability or failure of the people to pay the accumulated water and light bills.

It is necessary to add that formal technical health education support of the 'Comfort station project' stopped in 1975. This might have led to the substantial growth of the project.

Health education intervention

Introduction

The comfort station idea was initiated by the Government and not by the

SERIAL NO.	WARDS	FAMILY COMPOUND	LOCATION	POPULATION	CONSTRUCTION PERIOD	TOTAL ROOMS	TOILETS	BATH	WASH	HOUSE HOLDS	REMARKS
1.	NW. 3	Egbodi	Oke Seni	255	January – Oct. 1970	19	10	8	1	11	
2.	SW. 4	Foko	Foko	840	Nov. 1970 – Dec. 1971	19	10	8	1	56	
3.	SW. 5	Apena	Gege–Foko	390	Sept. 1971 – July 1972	25	15	9	1	20	
4.	NW. 3	Bara	Abebi	270	July 1972 – Feb. 1973	22	12	9	1	11	
5.	S. 4	Adebolu	Elekuro	300	March 1972–March 1973	21	12	8		14	
6.	E. 6	Oyewo–Lawoye	Ojagbo	300	March 1972 – Nov 1973	21	10	10		16	
7.	SW. 4	Saku	Foko	300	March 1972–March 1973	15	8	6		15	
8.	E. 2	Adepo	Oranyan	440	June 1972 – Sept 1973	25	16	8		21	
9.	NW. 3	Kagunmalo	Abebi	240	July 1972 – Oct. 1974	17	12	4		10	
10.	SW. 1	Osundina	Isaleosi	620	Jan. 1972 – Oct. 1972	34	21	12		30	
11.	E. 4	Ogo	Gbelekale Aperin	210	April 1972– Nov 1974	15	8	6		10	
12.	E. 4	Aperin	Aperin	1250	Nov. 1972– Dec.1974	28	8	9		59	Just Rehabilitated
13.	SW. 2	Areegbeomo	Idiarere	400	Nov. 1972 – Jan.1975	25	18	9		21	
14.	SW. 4	Olega	Foko	250	Oct. 1972 – Oct.1975	17	10	6		13	
15.	SW. 4	Babasale	Foko	380	Nov. 1972 – Jan.1975	16	10	6		18	
16.	SW. 4	Oluode	Oke–Foko	280	Oct. 1972 – Nov.1975	17	10	6		17	
17.	S. 6	Olunloyo	Agbongbon	400	March 1972 – 1975	27	16	10		23	Never used
18.	NW. 3	Abebi	Abebi	900	Oct. 1972 – 1975	33	20	12		55	
19.	"	Alaka	"	1030	Oct. 1972 – 1976	31	18	16		60	
20.	"	Epo	Idikan	908	Oct. 1972 – 1975	45	28	16		55	
21.	SW. 4	Alagbede	Foko	385	Oct. 1972 – 1975	17	12	4		20	
22.	"	Akako	Ita–maya	810	Oct. 1972 – 1975	45	28	16		51	
23.	"	Omo	Foko	155	"	17	10	6		10	
24.	"	Agiri	"	160		17	10	6		9	
25.	E. 4	Obisesan	Aperin	640	Oct. 1972 – 1977	41	28	12		31	Sealed-up due to accumulated W/Bill
26.	NW. 1	Agbeni	Agbeni	400	1972 – 1978	17	8	8		20	
27.	SW. 4	Ojojakan	Inalende	675	1972 – 1976	34	21	12		29	
28.	E. 4	Isaro	Arena	190	1972 – 1979	13	8	4		8	
29.	SW. 6	Elesude	Foko	600	1972 – 1988	40	24	16		32	Being Completed
30.	NW. 3	Ajigbai	Opo Yeosa	300	1972 – 1983	17	10	6		16	
31.	NW. 2	Akilapa	Idikan	780	1973 – 1975	34	21	12		41	Sealed-up because needs evacuation.
32.	SW. 5	Akinninganin	Foko	250	1973 – 1979	17	10	6		14	
33.	NW. 4	Atowoda	Inalende	800	1973 –1979	45	28	16		50	
34.	NW. 3	Ogodu/Olukudu	Abebi	280	1973 – 1987	12	10	2		14	
35.	"	Ladapo	Abebi	670	1974 – 1978	45	28	16		21	
36.	"	Ogala	Falaiye/Abebi	450	1974 – 1979	11	6	4		21	
37.	SW. 5	Parakoyi	Itamaya	1090	1974 – 1981	41	28	12		62	
38.	"	Oto	Foko	920	1974 – 1981	37	24	12		56	
39.	"	Oteseku	Foko	420	1974 – 1981	17	10	6		22	
40.	SW. 6	Siba	Gege–Foko	245	1974 – 1980	17	10	6		12	
41.	NW. 3	Olude	Abebi	310	1975 – 1980	16	10	6		16	
42.	"	Ololu	"	-	1975 – Date	-	-	-	-	-	Abandoned

Table 19.3 *Statistics on the Ibadan comfort stations*

people. Therefore, the idea had to be sold to the people for various reasons if the experiment was to succeed, because of the vital roles of the communities. Each community was to provide space or a plot of land for the construction of the comfort station; each community had to provide labour through self-help; and each community had to utilize, supervise, and maintain the comfort station through effective management. However, a pre-condition for all these activities was that the people should accept and buy the idea through appreciating the value and its advantages over their customary bathing, clothes washing and toilet habits.

This, in short, was the *raison d'etre* for the formal introduction of the health education component of the project in 1972, and for which a WHO health education specialists, Mr Erol Williams, was attached to the project (1971 to 1972). With the exit of the WHO health educator, the Department of Preventive and Social Medicine, College of Medicine, University of Ibadan became involved in the project: first, through a study of the health education component of the project by Ademuwagun (1974–1975) and, second, through the involvement of ARHEC staff and students in their concurrent field work in community health education activities all over Ibadan city.

Specific health education interventions

1. Educational behavioural needs assessment

The people's behavioural needs assessment in relation to environmental sanitation problems was carried out through operational researches – community surveys, study of people's knowledge, attitudes and practices (KAP), and so on in order to gather relevant baseline data for education purposes.

Community surveys on the people's toilet, bathing and laundry habits and general personal hygiene and environmental sanitation revealed the following:

a. Toilet habit: Most of the households in the inner core of the city had (have) neither water closets nor pit latrines. Consequently, the generality of the people took to defecating in hidden corners, dung-hills, open areas, streams and rivers. As much as possible the adults defecated under some cover, at least to cover their face for a token privacy.

b. Bathing habit: Most households had (have) no conventional bathrooms. In effect some provided bamboo sheds where they took their bath in privacy. While the majority of the adults bathed in secluded corners in their backyards the children took their bath at any open space around the house. The used water flowed into the open drains around the household.

c. Washing of Clothes: These were washed near open drains, channels, wells and streams or rivers. Drawing water from the few public water taps for clothes washing in the absence of wells which characterized most of the households was very cumbersome. Therefore clothes were usually washed wherever water was available such as by the wells, streams and even ponds, thus adding to the indiscriminate disposal of human wastes (liquid and solid) all over the place to constitute health hazards.

d. Personal hygiene and environmental sanitation: The people were (are) quite conscious of the need for personal hygiene and environmental/ compound cleanliness for aesthetic reasons rather than for the health implication. Thus they bathe regularly, usually twice a day in the morning and evening notwithstanding the water supply problems in most households. They also clean their houses and the surroundings regularly, indeed this is the first task in the morning before the people go about their daily rounds of duties.

As to how they dispose of the refuse gathered, the gutters or drains, roadsides or the base of the refuse bins are the usual sites. In this regard, it is necessary to observe that most of the people at the inner core of the city are a victim of an urban phenomenon. Lack of adequate and easily accessible public refuse bins contributed immensely to the indiscriminate disposal of some refuse.

Some refuse bins were inconvenient because of their height, people having to climb a series of steps before they can deposit refuse. And this is in a culture where children and women do the clearing and removal of household refuse.

The people loathe the murky waters and the offensive odours from the open drains, and associate the presence of flies and rodents with dirt and odours.

e. Value of privacy: The adults value privacy during bathing and when defecating. However, lack of conventional bathrooms and toilets in many households as well as lack of public toilets in the communities of the inner core of the city leave the masses with no option than to manage with situational realities when urinating, defecating, or bathing if only to cover their faces or private parts with an olive branch.

f. Health knowledge: A study of the people's knowledge of the health implications of indiscriminate disposal of solid and liquid human wastes showed that the majority of the people except the few educated ones did not associate these poor environmental conditions with the common water-borne diseases such as ascariasis, diarrhoea, dysenteries, hookworm infections and cholera.

EDUCATION STRATEGY/IMPLICATION

The value of personal hygiene and environmental sanitation which was (is) dearly held by the people for aesthetic reasons and the people's concern for privacy in toilet and bathing practices were isolated as the vehicle for relevant health education messages on the value of the comfort stations. In other words, we focused on what was of intrinsic value to the people. While education of the relationship between unhygienic personal habits or insanitary disposal of human wastes and ill-health (for example cholera and diarrhoea) was stressed, more emphasis for the less educated masses was on cleanliness as a value premium which must be cultivated always. So also was the need for privacy in bathing and toilet stressed as a very important value that should be translated into living realities. The comfort stations were presented as a device for the realization of the people's intrinsic values associated with cleanliness and privacy in addition to the device to stem the common water-borne diseases.

For example, the advantages of the comfort stations over the other known local environmental sanitation facilities were thus summed up:

a. safer in terms of the solid nature of the walls and floor;
b. more private for individuals bathing or using the toilet;
c. a source of more regular and convenient water supply for bathing and washing clothes;
d. more convenient with regard to the number of people per toilet; and
e. reduce environmental pollution hazards due to uncontrolled disposal of liquid wastes.

2. Community involvement, mobilization and participation

Since the comfort stations are for the people and by the people through self-help, the need for community involvement, mobilization and participation was a foregone conclusion. Community surveys with the active participation of the local people were used as strategies for collecting baseline information on leadership and power structures in the various communities, traditional ways of community education and mobilization, channels and methods of communication, and how people get things done for or in the communities for example bell rings to summon people to meetings, story telling and singing, and role playing or drama.

Our findings were very instructive. For example, one concept often branded by external researchers in Africa is 'community organization', the need to get the community organized in support of specific Government or agency projects and for socio-economic developmental purposes. This attitude implies the assumption that the communities are traditionally unorganized/or disorganized and that they never engage in socio-economic development efforts on a communal basis. This attitude was faulted by the revelation that each of the communities was well organized for socio-economic development and for the security of life and property. In this regard it dawned on us that it was nothing short of professional arrogance and ignorance for orthodox health professionals and social and behavioural scientists who are overly obsessed about the need to carry out 'community organization' activities among the African peoples in both urban and rural settings, because community organization and community development are as old as the history of each community. The concept of self-help was also as old as the history of each group.

Various local resources such as people, institutions, organizations and associations, which could be utilized (and were indeed utilized) to promote the comfort stations idea were identified. Thus, instead of creating new resources, the existing ones such as respected leaders and associations were fully tapped and utilized as partners in progress as exemplified below.

The people are used to community mobilization for the implementation of agreed community projects. Evidence also abounds of various mechanisms used by the people for community mobilization in support of various government projects in modern times through self-help. Thus, again, the concept of 'community mobilization' for community development purposes is as old as the history of the people in their natural habitats. What is then needed is the ability of the project staff to sell the comfort station idea to the people, such as by tying it to what is of intrinsic value to the people for example, value attached to cleanliness and privacy.

Group identity and communal spirit, *esprit de corps* was very strong among the people as symbolized in sharing in times of pain and joy, and this was further dramatized in the attitude and practice of 'I am my brother's keeper'.

Another dimension of this group solidarity in the traditional communities before the arrival of modern civilization was 'communal discipline' of wayward community members to enforce compliance with group will.

In the light of the findings, what the project staff did from an educational perspective was to build on the existing community structures and resources for the promotion of the comfort station idea in the various communities.

Examples of the use of local resources in support of the comfort station project

1. *The Oke-Seni/Oke Padre Community Development Society*

Through a process of a community survey, the project staff identified the 'Oke-Seni/Oke Padre Community Development Society' as one of the existing and dynamic organizations in the inner core of the city. The society became the obvious choice of the project staff for the sale of the comfort station idea and as a gateway for entering into the heart of the community and winning support for the idea.

The society, often referred to as 'Oke-Seni Community Development Society', was founded in 1966 by the local people.

In the Oke-Seni community there were 21 compounds or families with a population of over 6,000 people. The people live in large extended family compounds without modern health and related social amenities. Oke-Seni was not planned; before 1966 the area was never served by any motorable roads and communication was difficult.

In 1966, in the traditional way of the local people, the heads of the 21 family-compounds with some educated elites, civil servants, religious leaders, teachers, traders and women leaders met at a community meeting.

The meeting carefully reviewed the needs, interests and problems of Oke-Seni community and took decisions to improve it through community self-help projects. It was in this way that the Oke-Seni Community Development Society was born in 1966.

MAJOR CONTRIBUTIONS OF OKE-SENI DEVELOPMENT SOCIETY

a. In March of 1966, a programme of adult literacy was begun with the enrolment of adult pupils. By May of the same year, the pupils were able to read and write Yoruba, while market women were able to do simple arithmetic.

b. In October of 1966, the society began a one thousand four hundred Nigerian pound road project within its area which, when it was completed, made it possible to open additional shops and trading centres in that community.

c. In June of 1966, more adult pupils were registered for adult classes in English and functional literacy.

d. In 1969, the society began a one thousand Nigerian pound bridge and road drainage scheme, with financial assistance from its members and from local as well as international organizations.

OKE-SENI AND THE FIRST COMFORT STATION AT IBADAN

In 1969, the project staff, working with and through the local influentials, introduced the comfort station idea as a means of improving the environmental conditions in the community through self-help and with financial and technical assistance from the State Government. The objectives and mode of operation of the comfort stations were explained and fully discussed. The idea was embraced by the local influentials who, in turn, discussed the idea with the Oke-Seni Development Society. Because the idea was congruent with the society's self-help frame of reference, and served as a continuation of the series of local development projects, it was embraced and supported without much difficulty.

Oke-Seni community was surveyed in 1969 to identify suitable sites for the building of comfort stations as well as to explore possible land donation by the local people for the building. As a result of the survey, the Egbodi family compound of Oke-Seni Community was the first to embrace and support the idea. The building of the first comfort station in Ibadan, and first of its kind in Black Africa, was thus started at the Egbodi Compound NW3/899, Oke-Seni Community in January 1970. In October 1970, it was declared open with great fanfare to serve as a source of further motivation of exercise in 'self-help' to the Oke-Seni Community people and to other communities in the inner core of Ibadan City.

THE EDUCATIONAL IMPLICATIONS AND SIGNIFICANCE OF THE EGBODI COMPOUND COMFORT STATION

The building of the Egbodi comfort station served as a medium for demonstrating and propagating the idea. The 1971 cholera epidemic was further exploited to sell the comfort station idea in that no single death was recorded in Egbodi family, while in Apena Community in the same SW4 Ward, cholera took the toll of 10 lives. Poor sanitary conditions were capitalized upon by the project staff, through working with the local leaders, to explain the causes of the cholera attack in Apena. Particular reference was made to the isolation of Egbodi compound from the attack because of the comfort station already in use. Consequently, Apena embraced the idea and built the third comfort station in Ibadan. Foko Community being the second of the first nine communities to build their comfort station.

Thus, the demonstrated possibility and success of an existing comfort station in one community served as a major motivation to the other communities.

2. *The NW3 Ward Health Council as a local resource*

As the work of the Ibadan Wastes and Disposal Project (IWDP) became more and more involved, it was necessary that the local people should be more involved in order to face the reality of the environmental sanitation situation through the people's co-operation and active participation. The IWDP personnel had to come out of their academic shells to communicate with the ordinary citizen to discover his likes and dislikes, his beliefs and values, his total behaviours as these affect the sanitation programmes. It was during this search for the best method of involving and educating the public about the sanitation project in general and the comfort station in particular that the idea of the ward health council came into being.

Ibadan City is divided into 46 administrative wards, each consisting of several family compounds with a distinct family head still wielding some measure of authority over his own kith and kin. The family head, 'Mogaji' (traditional chief), derives this authority from the Olubadam and his chiefs. Since each family compound was broken down into a number of habitable dwelling houses which were to be provided with adequate modern sanitary facilities, it was thought that the most reasonable sizeable unit with which the project staff could hold dialogue and get favourable results was a ward council. To this council the family compounds would send their representatives who would come together to discuss and decide on what they wanted in their community. This could be done either through their usual traditional 'self help' activities or through external assistance.

INITIATING THE WARD HEALTH COUNCIL IDEA

The project staff, particularly through the technical assistance of Mr Erol Williams, a WHO health educator attached to the project, decided to make use of the existing structure and available resources of the ward system to facilitate the overall sanitation project. With the co-operation of project staff, national counterparts and the Department of Preventative Social Medicine of the Faculty of Medicine, University of Ibadan, effort was directed toward securing ward-wide acceptance and support for the project idea and making a success of it. Project staff had briefed the local leaders on the objectives of the project and the potential contributions of a ward health council; the leaders accepted and supported the idea as an intergral part of the ongoing self-help projects for community development as far as environmental sanitation was concerned. The IWDP gave the health council free technical advice in the planning, design and construction of comfort stations, public toilets, refuse depots, and other facilities essential for the improvement of environmental sanitation on the Ward.

It was in this way that the project staff, working with and through the local leaders, that the NW3 Ward Health Council was established on 9 May 1972 and formally launched on 2 June 1973.

THE NW3 WARD HEALTH COUNCIL CONTRIBUTIONS TO COMMUNITY DEVELOPMENT INCLUDING ENVIRONMENTAL SANITATION

Since its inception, the NW3 Ward Health Council has accomplished the following:

a. Supplied the addresses of approximately 80 per cent of the 133 compounds in the ward.
b. Met with Government to negotiate for the construction of:
  i. Three modern elevated refuse depots.
  ii. Two privy toilets.
  iii. Four additional comfort stations.
c. Convinced a resident to donate private land for the construction of a public toilet facility for the ward.
d. Imposed a tax of 50 kobo per month on each compound in the ward.
e. Succeeded in getting Government to evict squatters so that public conveniences can be built.
f. Produced their own stationery and writing supplies.
g. Begun to identify additional health problems in the ward.
h. The council had, in the recent past, settled quarrels between the community leaders or chiefs on the one hand, and the community at large on the other.
i. The Health Council has also (since 1973) been meeting with the Institute of Child Health, University College Hospital, to see to the possibility of the institute including child health welfare in its areas of operation.

A survey is now in progress in the area which will lead to the establishment of a clinic in the ward.

The NW3 Ward Health Council has begun to function as a very cohesive group, so much so that it is possible to exert pressure on its members and community. For example, it has organized several families to team up to build comfort stations instead of individual families building their own. Currently, the families involved include:

1. Bara/Jaiyeade
2. Idi-Igba/Eleko/Olosun/Oloya/Opadere
3. Olude/Modiyanju, and
4. Alfa/Seni/Apooyin

EDUCATIONAL POTENTIAL AND INPUTS OF THE NW3 WARD HEALTH COUNCIL

The NW3 Health Council was a pilot council with great community developmental and educational potential in the area of environmental sanitation improvement. It represented the local people's interests and goodwill for community action and dedication to overcoming sanitation problems and solving other related social problems through their own efforts and freewill. The acceptance and support was won by the project staff through the special educational input, particularly through community mobilization processes, and the active involvement and participation of the local people in planning to help themselves.

From the experience of the present council, one could predict that the success thus far demonstrated in the area of environmental sanitation would motivate other communities to form their own ward health councils. With the continuing technical support by the Government, ward health councils may in no distant future become a city-wide public forum for local involvement and active participation in planning, construction and operation of essential facilities for the entire Ibadan city, other towns and cities in Nigeria as a whole.

Monitoring and evaluation of the project

Monitoring and evaluation of the comfort stations were built into the implementation planning process jointly by the project staff and the community people working as an implementation committee. The concepts of 'effective utilization' and 'effective maintenance' of the comfort stations were defined for the purpose of monitoring and evaluation. Monitoring indicators for effective utilization and supervision as well as evaluation instruments were developed to assess quality of performance and problems encountered in overall utilization and maintenance process.

The indicators used for monitoring effective utilization of the comfort stations were that the people always:

   i.   defecated only in the aqua privy while in the community
  ii.   took their bath only in the bathrooms; and
 iii.   washed their clothes only in the laundry rooms during the day and night.

Effective maintenance involved the following checklist:

    i.   clean surroundings of the comfort stations through regular cutting of weeds and sweeping, and sanitary disposal of the refuse collected;
   ii.   clean toilet rooms, bathrooms and laundry rooms through regular washing and sweeping of the floors, and leaving the floors dry always;
  iii.   provision of covers for the latrine holes and ensuring that the holes were always covered after toilet use;
  iv.   use of water or toilet roll tissues only to clean up after using the toilet;
   v.   turning off the water taps immediately after use to prevent wet floors as well as wastage of water;
  vi.   absence of flies and bad smells at the comfort stations;
 vii.   provision of light at the comfort stations at night to facilitate nocturnal use of the station;
viii.   provision of locks to the doors at the stations for safe keeping and to prevent intruders from using them;
  ix.   prevention of damages at the comfort station, and timely repairs once damages occurred;
   x.   regular payment of both light and water bills to prevent the disruption of light and water supplies.

Inspection, supervision and evaluation formats

The need for regular performance evaluative inspection and supervision of the comfort stations in the context of the criteria developed was stressed. The general community meeting, with the technical guidance of the project staff, came up with the following general operational model:

a. Inspection of the comfort stations jointly by the project staff with at least one of the representatives of each household/family which owned the station. Inspection days were to be pre-arranged.
b. Inspection by project staff alone without heralding the day of inspection. This was to encourage constant use and maintenance of the stations by the people.
c. Documentation of both encouraging and defective aspects.
d. General discussion of the results of inspection at the individual local comfort station community or family meeting as well as at the general community meetings; and consideration of strategies for improvement.

A specific scoring format or inspection, supervision and evaluation checklist was also jointly developed. See Appendix 19.1.

Each community or family compound devised its own mode of operation for the effective supervision and maintenance of the comfort station. For example: Foko, Saku and Bara family compounds each decided to employ paid caretakers whose job was to ensure general sanitation of the inside and surroundings of comfort stations. A fee of 50 Kobo per household was made mandatory as each family compound's contribution toward the wages of the caretaker per month and for other miscellaneous running costs of the stations. All other family compounds decided on household unit labour on a rota basis. The mechanics for supervision and reports on progress and problems were also established. Fortnightly meetings on progress and problem reports were also planned.

Problems identified with the comfort stations

The problems identified with the comfort stations are of three categories viz: pre-construction, during-construction, and post-construction problems.

Pre-construction problems

INITIAL RESISTANCE PROBLEM

There was an initial resistance to the comfort stations idea when it was first introduced. The resistance was a result of an existing tax agitation among the people at the time when they were aggrieved over a flat rate of six Nigerian dollars per head. This agitation for a reduction in the tax rate was aggravated by the people's concern for lack of basic social infra-structural facilities in their communities. The police and the tax collectors who were also perceived as agents of the government and politicians became objects of hate and targets of attack and abuse from the local people. This was the origin of the 1969 tax riot in Ibadan and at the eve of the comfort stations experiment.

Thus local events at the time of the introduction of the comfort station idea were a major contributory factor in the initial resistance problem because, as events later proved, the initial resistance was to the Government of the day and its agencies rather than to the comfort station idea *per se.*

LOCAL PREJUDICE AGAINST PUBLIC HEALTH INSPECTORS/ SUPERINTENDENTS

Many of the local leaders were, at the time of launching the comfort station idea, at loggerheads with the public health inspectors otherwise called health superintendents. This was because of the prejudice which the local people had against the health inspectors over alleged corruption, exhorbitant fines, victimization, extortion and other ills since about 1963. The health inspectors were regarded as agents of the politicians and the Government in power. It was alleged that most of the charges which the inspectors levelled against them over poor environmental sanitation were calculated attempts to punish the people by 'the agents of the political party which we did not support.' Thus, any mention of the idea of environmental sanitation was calculated to be the making of the public health inspectors acting in the guise of agents of the Government in power to punish people in the opposition parties. Hence the idea was taken with extreme suspicion and caution.

Like the problems of initial resistance, the crisis with the public health inspectors could be seen as the people's indirect confrontation with the Government of the day and its political agents as well as with the inspectors for their alleged corruption.

PEOPLE'S CONCERN OVER FAMILY LAND

The people expressed grave concern over the family piece of land which they had to donate for the construction of the comfort stations. There was the fear that the government might turn round in later years to appropriate the land and take over the comfort stations. Like all over Yorubaland, the families treasured their land as a main source of security to their posterity and, as such, they hesitated to give it away *gratis.* There were some people whose concern was not with the need to get adequate compensation or with Government appropriation of their family land, but with the fact that they had to give up that treasured land for the construction of 'mere latrines and laundry facilities'. 'How on earth can we be expected to donate our land for the construction of public latrines of all the valuable uses our land can be put today?' re-echoed in most of the communities affected.

The attitude of the people can be appreciated because at that point in the history of Nigeria there were many cases involving governments' appropriation of family lands and estates in other parts of the country. Even the Land Use Decree today has not significantly changed this attitude.

During-construction problems

SHORTAGE OF FREE LABOUR

By virtue of their jobs, mainly as farmers and traders, the local people were not particularly ready for voluntary labour for the self-help aspect of the construction of the comfort stations. Rather, they preferred to hire paid labourers to do their own aspect of the work, but many of them did not pay their own levies for paying the labourers.

ACUTE SHORTAGE OF BUILDING MATERIAL

The people complained of acute shortage of building materials at different stages of the comfort stations' construction. Acute shortage of building materials at the time the experiment was undertaken had even led to the suspension of so many government and individual or personal building projects in all parts of Nigeria. This problem was aggravated by the general universal inflationary trends and, particularly, the heavy port congestion in Nigeria at the time.

Post-construction problems

Problems in this phase were those connected with the use and maintenance of the Comfort Stations.

HIGH ELECTRICITY AND WATER BILLS

Many families complained of 'high water bills' which, as they alleged, they could not afford to pay. The inability of a family compound to pay always led the water corporation to disconnect the water supplies serving the comfort stations. Without regular water supply, the comfort stations experiment would be virtually rendered useless. Similarly, because of the people's failure to pay the electricity bills, the Nigerian Electric Power Authority (NEPA) often had to disconnect the light serving the comfort stations thereby rendering maximum use and care of the stations difficult, if not impossible, at night.

INTERMITTENT DISRUPTION OF LIGHT

The comfort stations shared with other parts of Ibadan and the country at large the common experience of regular light failure which rendered the comfort stations unusable at night to most people. On the other hand, the light was often switched off at night by the community leaders to prevent meter wastage and the attendant 'high' bill. Also to make sure that the light was not used when the meter was not switched off, the doors of some comfort stations were locked from about seven in the evening to six the following morning. Another reason given for locking the comfort stations at night by the owners was to prevent 'outsiders' from making use of the stations. However, apart from NEPA failure, the main reason for the control of power-light supply appeared to be the need to keep the light bill down.

DERELICT INDIVIDUALS AND GROUPS

Some family compounds opted for direct labour to ensure the maintenance of the comfort stations instead of employing paid caretakers. One method was for each household to be responsible for the general sanitary condition of the comfort station for a specific period of time through a rotational system. Another method was that each household was allocated a number of aqua privies and bathrooms, and the household concerned was made responsible for the sanitary maintenance. The problem with this kind of arrangement was that in certain instances the work was either never done or perfunctorily performed by unreliable individuals.

COST OF REPAIR OF DAMAGES

Damages to some of the facilities, such as broken doors, taps and laundry slabs were often never repaired by the people, and lack of repairs to damaged structures often led to disuse or improper use of the comfort stations. A general complaint was either lack of money, unavailable materials, or both.

ENGINEERING DEFECTS

Some comfort stations were out of order too soon after construction due to blockage of the aqua privies. The resultant odour was offensive to the users who then gave up using the stations. The problems lingered on because a blockage was either never evacuated or irregularly evacuated by the wastes disposal board.

In summary, the problems fell under two categories: the behavioural and the non-behavioural. The first category was of those which directly stemmed from the behaviours of the target population as individuals and as a group because of lack of internalization of the value of the comfort stations; the second was of those that stemmed from situational events, engineering defect, and inadequate technical support.

The success of the comfort stations experiment in environmental sanitation health education will, therefore, depend largely on the strategies evolved to remove or reduce the identified negative behavioural and non-behavioural factors such as through improved and continuing health education efforts as well as Governmental technical and administrative supports. Strategies for resolution of the problems are currently being reconsidered both by the communities and the Ibadan Municipal Council.

A graduate student is currently (1988) carrying out his master of public health (health education) degree research under the title: *An Educational Evaluative Study of the Pattern and Degree of Utilization and Maintenance of the Ibadan Comfort Stations*. His findings will no doubt strengthen the health education component of the comfort stations. (Obadiah K Edamaku, the candidate, is a graduate student in the African Regional Health Education Centre, Department of Preventive and Social Medicine, College of Medicine, University of Ibadan. He started the evaluative study during 1987/88 session.)

Conclusion

The Ibadan comfort stations are, to all intents and purposes, an experiment in environmental sanitation health education; and the experiment is first of its kind in Nigeria and Africa as a whole. The comfort stations idea has been accepted and adopted by the target communities at the inner core of Ibadan City. However, notwithstanding the acceptance and adoption of the experiment, it was a matter for concern that only 42 comfort stations have been constructed to-date (1988) out of the envisaged 500 (out of which 25 were to serve as a pilot project) by 1980.

Evaluative study of the comfort stations from an educational perspective shows records of better utilization than of maintenance, and that formal technical health education input was prematurely terminated in 1975. The behavioural and non-behavioural problems identified, pre-construction, during-construction and post-construction, show that the target communities have not completely internalized the value of the comfort stations and the technical engineering support of the Government falls short of the people's expectation.

Therefore, given the needed political, technical, administrative and continuing education supports by the government, the experiment will be a huge success of simple practical technology in environmental sanitation health education, particularly as a means of effectively coping with the perennial problem of human wastes disposal in the inner core of the city of Ibadan.

References and Bibliography

Ademuwagun, Z A (1970) Some educational planning principles in public health programme *Journal of Society of Health, Nigeria* **V**, 1

Ademuwagun, Z A (1972) Major impediments to effective use of health services *The Journal of Health Education* **31**, 2

Ademuwagun, Z A (1972) Information and motivation in health education *The Journal of Health Education* **31**, 3

Ademuwagun, Z A (1974) The challenge of health education methods and techniques in developing countries *Health Education Journal* **33**, 1

Ademuwagun, Z A (1975) *The Ibadan comfort stations: an experiment in environmental sanitation health education*, an unpublished WHO-Sponsored research report, University of Ibadan

Bennis, W G, Benne, K D and Chin, R (1961) *The Planning of Change* Holt, Rinehart and Winston, New York

Brazzaville, (1975) AFR/HE/69 Health education in environmental health programmes WHO Regional Office for Africa

Knutson, A L (1965) *The Individual, Society and Health Behaviour* Russell Sage Foundation, New York

Paul, B D (1955) *Health Culture and Community* Russell Sage Foundation, New York

Sridhar, M K C and Omishakin, M A (1975) An evaluation of water supply and sanitation problems in Nigeria *Journal of Royal Society of Health*, UK **105**

The Health Education Project Advisory Committee: (1975) Making health education work, *Americal Journal of Public Health* **65** (October supplement)

Williams, Erol (1972) Community organization as a health education process, *Paper presented at the seminar on environmental sanitation, UCH, Ibadan*, August 15–18

1. Name of Comfort Station ....

   Is the surrounding of the Comfort Staions clean?

       (a) Very clean................1
       (b) Fairly clean.............2   1
       (c) Dirty....................3

2. Are the Latrines with covers?

       (a) Yes......................1   2
       (b) No.......................2   ----
                                   ----

3. Is the floor of the Latrine Clean?

       (a) Very clean...............1
       (b) Fairly clean.............2   3
       (c) Dirty....................3   ----
                                   ----

4. Is the floor of the Bathroom clean?

       (a) Very clean...............1
       (b) Fairly clean.............2   4
       (c) Dirty....................3   ----

5. Is the Washroom clean?

       (a) Very clean...............1
       (b) Fairly clean.............2   5
       (c) Dirty....................3   ----

6. Is the water flowing during your visit in the

       (a) Latrine?   (i) Yes...............1   6
                      (ii) No................2   ----

       (b) Bathroom?   (i) Yes...............1   7
                      (ii) No................2   ----

       (c) Washroom?   (i) Yes...............1   8
                      (ii) No................2   ----

Appendix 19.1 *Comfort stations inspection and supervision format*

7. Are there bowls for washing hands using the latrine?

    (a) Yes........................1   9
    (b) No.........................2   ----
                                           ----

8. Are there keys to the

    (a) Latrine?

                (i) Yes...............1   10
                (ii) No................2   ----

  (b) Bathrooms?

                (i) Yes...............1   11
                (ii) No................2   ----
                                        ----

9. What damages do you observe at the Comfort Stations?

    ----

10. What general remarks do you have about

    (a) Use of the Comfort Stations?

    (b) Care of the Comfort Stations?

Inspection by:--

Date: -----------------------------

20. Health education: instrument for a health oriented culture? an ITALIAN experience – A CASE STUDY

A Mongelli

Summary: This chapter describes a health education initiative which took place in schools near Verona between 1978 and 1981. The geographical, social, economic and cultural contexts are described. A model was devised through which the school medical service could bring about health education. The intervention had four stages: increasing the sensitivity of those responsible for the schools medical service; creating sensitivity to health care problems in pupils, teachers, non-teaching staff and parents; inter-systemic planning and verification of the outcomes.

Introduction

What follows is an outline of an experiment in health education that was carried out in various nursery, elementary and intermediate schools in a district on the outskirts of Verona between March 1978 and January 1981. Pupils, teachers, non teaching school staff, parents and the author – a public health nurse were all involved. [In the Italian school system the 'scuola media' is an entity in itself and provides for children from 12 to 14 year's old, after which they may or may not go on to the secondary school after obtaining the 'Licenza media'. The expression 'intermediate school' has been used for convenience.]

Methodology

A problem solving approach was used combining both inductive and deductive methods.

The theory of systems was applied and this allowed the various groups and the available human resources of the scholastic and health care systems to work together as a unit.

An integral teaching plan was worked out for parallel classes which rendered a process of on-going health education possible during these years and became a link between the various subjects and between the pupils of parallel classes and the teachers in the different areas.

The teaching model which results from the analysis of the experiment should provide an answer to the question posed in the above title.

This chapter, will take the following steps in problem solving:

1. describe the geographical, social, cultural and economic background to the experiment and the school medical service;
2. define the problems;
3. describe the instruments used in collecting the data which permitted an analysis of the traditional service which while exposing its contradictions led to a definition of the needs and problems to be faced and the formulation of a hypothesis for their solution;
4. suggest a hypothesis for a solution;
5. show how the project was planned and carried out;
6. give an evaluation of the results obtained.

The geographical, social, economic and cultural background to the experiment and the school medical service

The territory

The experiment which was begun in March 1978 and ended in January 1981 took place in a new housing area on the outskirts of Verona which up until 1956 had consisted of a small village with a history of almost 1000 years. In 1956, public sector housing increased and by 1970 practically the whole area was built up without any precise urban planning.

Some essential support structures were lacking. For instance there was a system of sewerage which did not cover the total needs of the growing population and had to be supplemented by septic tanks. In one area these frequently overflowed spilling their contents into the street near a primary school. There was a shortage of sports facilities which the local authorities tried to overcome by opening the school gymnasia to the public in the afternoons and evenings. The lack of playground, public gardens and cultural centres meant that the only meeting places for young people were the streets, the village square and the cafés. There were few schools and the whole area which had a population of 80,000 was policed by only eight officers. This area included the district where the experiment was carried out.

The social and health services

At the beginning of the experiment the social and health services in the area were: a vaccination clinic; an obstetric and paediatric clinic; a school medical service; a social centre which included the co-ordinating centre for supplying home help for the elderly; and a public library.

The population

In 1978, the resident population of the district was about 14,290 and consisted for the most part of immigrants from other parts of the Province of Verona and the Veneto Region as well as from other Italian Regions. The social status of the families was working and lower middle class. Many were factory workers, others were employed in the public sector or were small shopkeepers. As in other areas where there has been extensive immigration from the south, there was little social cohesion and many people lived in a difficult situation because of the conflict between their original socio-cultural background and the existential reality of their surroundings. This, in some cases, resulted in loss of cultural identity, diffidence, discouragement and generational conflicts between parents and children. This in turn led to maladjustment which manifested itself, even if not officially recognized, in the increase in the numbers of young people using habit-forming drugs.

The school medical service at the time of the experiment

The school medical service of Verona covered the school population from the age of three to 14 years. It was divided into territorial zones and in the area where the experiment took place there were about 2600 pupils distributed among four nursery schools, three elementary schools and one intermediate school. The territorial service was provided by one school doctor and one public health nurse. Centralized specialists services were available and these consisted of speech, ear, nose and throat, ophthalmic, dental, skin, cardiac, rheumatology, orthopaedic and psycho-pedagogic clinics.

The main activities of the service were concerned with:

- ☐ preparing clinical charts;
- ☐ carrying out medical examinations to establish the grade of physical and psychological development of the pupils;
- ☐ issuing certificates for exemption from physical training;
- ☐ sending children with infectious diseases or parasites away from school and re-admitting them later;
- ☐ screening for sight and hearing defects;
- ☐ inspecting environmental hygiene;
- ☐ inspecting school canteens;
- ☐ checking vaccination certificates;
- ☐ checking medical certificates of the teaching and non-teaching staff;
- ☐ controlling the tuberculin tests of children in the first and fourth year elementary and third year intermediate classes;
- ☐ vaccinating girls in the fifth elementary class against German Measles;
- ☐ carrying out periodic spot checks organized by the head of the service;
- ☐ organizing sporadic general meetings of pupils and/or parents and/or teachers to provide information on specific problems such as drug addiction and alcoholism.

Identifying the needs/problems

A critical study of the school medical service and its aims, and of the real needs of the population showed that:

a. The school population continued to be the object of the activity of the 'experts'.

b. Very often the presence of health personnel in the school was seen only from the point of view of fulfilling an obligation imposed by law. This did nothing to create dialogue and feelings of reciprocal trust, nor did it help to eliminate errors and change harmful living habits. This often resulted in an increased hostility and responses which manifested themselves in the refusal to face up to certain diseases.

c. Frequently, incorrect solutions were given to problems such as closing and disinfecting the school buildings during an epidemic of pediculosis.

d. Some of the activities constituted an inexcusable waste of time as in the case of 'hunt the child with pediculosis' or checking vaccination certificates.

e. Often health education was seen as information given from on high frequently couched in language which was incomprehensible to the recipients and without the possibility of checking its efficacy. Conferences, speeches, positive and negative commands were given which often created more problems than they solved.

f. At times the rules for prevention induced new needs, as when the statement was made that dental caries is prevented by going to the dentist twice a year.

g. The service continued to operate giving professional help in a formal, obligatory, ritualistic and paternalistic manner. Things were done to the people and not with the people. This created an enormous quantity of work and statistical data which, even though they could have been used in creating better services, remained an end in themselves. Not only did the service not provide rational answers to the real needs of the scholastic population, they sometimes actually increased the general tendency to delegate personal health care and protection to experts, medicinal products, laboratory tests and suchlike.

h. The service did not take into account the modern prevalence of chronic and degenerative pathology which is often disabling. Behaviour which is incorrect from a hygienic point of view often plays a determinant role in the aetiology of this type of pathology. It was urgent therefore to establish a process of health education that would be able to help individuals, singly or in groups, to become aware of themselves and of the various behavioural and environmental factors which facilitate or obstruct the development of disease. They needed also to be aware of the cultural and social influences that prevent them recognizing the health risks inherent in their behaviour or environment, so that they might make free and conscious changes in behaviour patterns if necessary. There was also a need to overcome the irrational attitudes of people who, while vociferously claiming that good health is a precious commodity, demonstrate a way of living aimed at its destruction. People needed to acquire the ability to decode the propaganda and cultural messages which induce needs for and a subsequent dependence on useless or harmful substances. They needed to see the human being from a holistic point of view and to remember that health is like a system that is made up of a harmonic and dynamic relationship between physical, psychological, social and spiritual wellbeing. There was need to stimulate people to fight against the modern cult of disease and the tendency to delegate health care to others and to useless medicinal products, complicated diagnostic procedures which often are unnecessary and sometimes dangerous. People needed to be enabled to influence political choices regarding the safeguarding of health and to create an anthropological health-oriented culture.

i. Health field workers and school workers initially lacked the above mentioned awareness as did the pupils. They also lacked the stimulus and desire to try to understand which technical and educational measures were needed to respond to the ever changing needs and to provide people with the wherewithal to discover the rational answer to health related problems for themselves. The health field workers did not have the sort of training that would have enabled them to 'convert' themselves in order to participate in the changes taking place in the areas of culture and health care at a national and international level. September 1978 saw the publication of the declaration of Alma Ata and in the same year the promulgation of the 833/76 Act creating the National Health Service in Italy. This Act, after laying down basic principles in its first Article, makes a list of means to these ends in Article two. The first item on this list is as follows: 'By forming a modern health consciousness based on the solid health education of the citizen and community'.

Gathering information

Information about the historical, geographical, cultural, social and economic state of the district and about the needs and existing problems was gathered. This enabled a hypothesis for a solution to be formulated.

The instruments used in collecting the data were:

a. Personal interviews with parents, teaching and non-teaching school staff, pupils, urban police, the area social worker, the parish priest, those responsible for the health services and the people engaged in the various other services in the district and whole borough.
b. Direct observation through inspections, epidemiologic research, home and area visitations.
c. The analysis of the existing demographic and epidemiologic statistics and/or of statistical data as they were collected.

A hypothesis for a solution

What follows is a hypothesis based on the analysis of the situation as it presented itself and the results of the work carried out.

The school medical service could activate a process of health education through the clinical procedures and inspections which it carries out. This would help the scholastic population:

a. to know and become aware of environmental hazards and individual and collective behaviour factors which influence their state of health;
b. to make a critical analysis of their own behaviour;
c. to correct possible errors;
d. to free themselves from cultural conditioning;
e. to stop delegating their personal health care to others and to medicinal products and suchlike;
f. to influence choices concerning health care at institutional, political, administrative and cultural levels which would provide answers to existing problems and activate health services that would correspond to the real needs of the population;
g. to create a health-oriented culture.

Planning the intervention and carrying it out

For greater clarity these phases have been subdivided into stages.

Stage 1: To increase sensitivity to the problem in those responsible for the school medical service

Some difficulties were encountered in persuading those responsible for the school medical services to accept these ideas. Fortunately organizational changes meant that some of these difficulties could be overcome.

Stage 2: Beginning a campaign for creating sensitivity to health care problems in pupils, teaching and non-teaching school staff and parents

Clinical procedures became occasions for beginning an educational process and creating dialogue with the teaching and non-teaching school staff, parents and the children themselves. This was based on the belief that no clinical procedure should be carried out on people as objects, but that people as human subjects have the right to know and choose. Apart from such circumstances as have been already mentioned above, chance circumstances such as accidents to children, the admission of handicapped pupils could also become opportunities for activating a process of health education. This process, based on the analysis of an actual situation would be automatically based on real needs and problems. Each clinical procedure became the object of a short, simple and scientific explanation before being carried out. This was for the benefit of the pupils but indirectly also for the teachers. They had previously been asked to participate and were very faithful in their attendance. These explanations stimulated a taste for further knowledge in the children about themselves and their bodies and the delicate balance present in human life and the environment which men and women frequently upset causing diseases in themselves and others.

In the third year classes of the intermediate school, the lessons on tuberculin testing were planned so that the science teacher who had been entrusted with health education and the author might be present together and work co-operatively. Each subject was approached by asking questions which stimulated the pupils to look for an answer for themselves. This in turn aroused a curiosity and a desire in them for further knowledge which affected the teachers who were sensitive to the problem and willing to do something about it. Some of these asked for help in working out a plan of study.

Stage 3: Intersystemic educational planning for parallel classes

The request for co-operation on the part of the teachers and the interest shown by the pupils made it possible to prepare a study plan which could be used in teaching individual classes and/or the combined classes of the same level. In the intermediate school it became inter-disciplinary teaching, as health education, seen as a means of forming a health-oriented culture includes historical, geographical, anthropological, medical, biological, chemical, psychological, pedagogical, political, economic and administrative aspects. The plan therefore made the discussion of subjects like sexuality and drug addiction more realistic and relevant, treating them not as a novelty which would induce curiosity only, or handling them only in formal structured lessons which have little to do with the pupils' real problems.

Keeping in mind the existing needs or problems and the willingness of the teachers, the following points were defined:

a. The groups;
b. The short, medium and long term objectives of the course;
c. The subject matter to be treated in detail;
d. The resources available;
e. The methodology to be followed;
f. The timing;
g. The evaluation of the results.

THE GROUPS
These references groups were initially made up of pupils of three second year nursery school classes, two fifth year elementary school classes and one third year class in the intermediate school.

Later, as a result of a sensitizing campaign carried out by the children themselves and their teachers, there were further requests for help and teachers and children of two nursery schools, two third year classes, four fourth year classes and one fifth year class of the elementary schools and two first and second year classes and two more third year intermediate school classes became involved. By 1981, in one of the third year intermediate school classes inter-disciplinary planning was under taken by all nine teachers involved with that particular group.

The parents became involved through the children themselves as the following example of a child in the fourth year of one of the elementary schools shows. During one of the lessons about healthy eating habits one child said, 'I ask mummy to give me a roll and some fruit for my snack, but she gives me money and I buy a sweet bun'. This involvement was of fundamental importance in avoiding conflicting educational messages that created confusion and annulled the messages themselves. At first the parents showed little interest and failed to turn up at the meetings arranged for them. The presentation of a school play at Carnival time provided a key to the solution of the problem of how to get the parents interested. On that occasion all the parents, even the busiest, were present because it was the children who were the principal actors. Why not use the same approach in health education? I put the question to the teachers who agreed that such an approach would be useful. Together we chose health education topics that could be developed by the pupils who would express what they had learnt in drawings. At the following meeting with the parents, the children would explain their drawings and if necessary the subject would be further developed by the teachers and myself. In this way the children became more than simple recipients of education, they became formidable teachers of ignorant educators.

We were careful not to arouse sentiments of judgement or condemnation of the adults in the children. We were interested rather in inculcating knowledge, awareness, critical ability, capacity for free choice and the ability to pay attention in the Platonic meaning of the expression in them. Understanding and tolerance facilitated dialogue between children, teachers and parents and reduced misunderstandings, isolation, conflict and discord.

Through their involvement the teaching and non-teaching staff came to realize that live models of behaviour meant more than the spoken word to children.

THE SHORT, MEDIUM AND LONG TERM OBJECTIVES

The syllabus for health education had one general aim which acted as a guideline for all the educational activity and other intermediate and specific objectives which were connected with the individual points in the syllabus itself.

The general aim was to activate a learning process in the scholastic population of pupils, teaching and non-teaching school staff and parents. Through this process they would grow in knowledge and awareness which would enable them to see the cultural, social and behavioural factors which hinder or help wellbeing and health. They would be able to work out strategies for the removal of factors that play a negative role in the maintenance of physical and psychological wellbeing in individuals and groups. They would come to understand that, if helped to develop personal awareness and critical and rational abilities, they would become their own masters. They would be able to decode the more or less overt external conditioning messages with which they are bombarded and to make their own choices, accepting the responsibility for the consequences. They would be able to develop hygienically correct habits, as individuals and in groups.

The intermediate and specific objectives dealt with the single subjects to be discussed. A list had been drawn up based on the problems that had been brought to light, consciously and unconsciously, by the people for whose benefit the course had been arranged.

THE SUBJECT MATTER

Subject matter refers to the single problems of health education confronted in this experiment. I will describe how these problems were dealt with according to the age of the pupils.

The content, approach and methodology used in developing the different subjects varied with the groups involved and depended on what they had already learned in previous years.

A graduated programme which included: the question of what makes for a healthy diet; prevention of dental caries; prevention of the spread of infectious diseases; and an introduction to sexual education was prepared for the children in the nursery schools.

In the elementary schools, the prevention of alcoholism, drug and medicinal abuse and accidents were included in the programme.

In the intermediate school the prevention of parasitological infestations, professional diseases and tumours were added to the above lists.

THE METHODOLOGY

The methodology adopted was as follows:

☐ a scientific method using inductive and deductive approaches which means using problems and/or real interests as a starting point and developing the subject matter by helping the pupils to deduce the relative scientific, ethical and moral principles involved;
☐ a pedagogical method which was based on group work, research, educational visits and lessons structured on maieutic principles;
☐ a method which started at the general and ended with the particular of any given subject.

THE RESOURCES

The human resources, besides myself who assumed the role of stimulus and support for the teachers, were:

☐ the teachers who with the pupils and myself developed the subjects according to pedagogical and didactic principles;
☐ the children themselves who assumed the double role of pupil-teachers.

The financial resources were made up of expenditure for films for photographs which were made into drawings and slides. On one occasion a few thousand lire were collected spontaneously by the children as an offering to some parish workers who had projected documentary films the author had acquired.

At the beginning of the venture there were no official funds available through the school medical service.

The structural resources consisted of classrooms, school assembly rooms, school corridors for preparing displays and technical laboratories in the intermediate school.

The teaching aids included:

1. documentary films obtained from public bodies such as the Ministry of Agriculture and the National Society for the Prevention of Accidents;

2. text-books which teachers and children procured for themselves;
3. questionnaires that the author had prepared and which were elaborated and discussed by the teachers;
4. short tests for the pupils in the intermediate school;
6. drawings and writings that the children produced with the help of their teachers. These became the most efficacious teaching aids in an educational process aimed at parents and children. In the case of the former this was because it called forth an emotive response which is the first rung on the ladder of learning. In the case of the children, the fact that the message had been prepared for them by other children without being structured by adults, meant that it reached them directly and encouraged them to go further into the matter and to produce something themselves.

TIMING
The timing varied according to the different teachers involved and the level of the groups, as well as the subject matter to be treated in the syllabus and the general school curriculum. Time was allotted to individual items over a period of a term, a school year or more than one year.

THE EVALUATION OF THE EXPERIMENT
This was carried out by ascertaining the knowledge acquired and by observing changes in behaviour in the various groups.

A short and medium term evaluation was undertaken using:

☐ direct observation which was registered in writing;
☐ tests, written compositions on general and specific aspects of health education, research projects and drawings that the children produced.

What follows is a summary of the results obtained in some of the subjects treated.

EDUCATION FOR A HEALTHY DIET AND THE PREVENTION OF DENTAL CARIES

☐ A large number of children came to understand the principles concerning the introduction of substances into the body and the effect they may have. This led them to change their habits and instead of eating potato crisps and various forms of sweets for their snack, they began eating bread rolls and fruit. In the school canteen, they started to eat such foods as green vegetables and fruit which they had always refused before.
☐ Parents began to understand the educational and affective errors involved in giving in to their children about what to eat and when. Some of them changed their attitude.
☐ The people employed in the school kitchen were more careful about the way they prepared the food.
☐ Pupils and teachers began cleaning their teeth after meals even at school.
☐ Some of the children who had decayed teeth asked to be taken to the dentist.

THE PREVENTION OF INFECTIOUS DISEASES AND INFESTATION BY PARASITES

- ☐ The pupils began to take more trouble over their personal hygiene and the cleanliness of their clothing. They started to bring soap and a hand towel from home for washing their hands. They stopped blocking the toilets with rolls of toilet paper.
- ☐ The children of the third year intermediate school classes began to turn up of their own accord for their buffer shots of anti-tetanus vaccine.
- ☐ The pupils in one third and three fourth year elementary school classes prepared a monographic composition with the help of their teachers on the risk of contagion from infectious diseases due to lack of personal and environmental hygiene. They then illustrated methods of prevention. The composition took the form of cartoon strips. They also prepared a series of posters about the damage caused by disease-carrying rats that live in the sewers. The cartoon strips were distributed among the families and the posters were used in an exhibition in the area.
- ☐ The school caretakers became more careful about the school cleaning.
- ☐ The school cooks took greater pains over the preparation and conservation of foodstuffs.
- ☐ Parents began to be more actively co-operative in the prevention of pediculosis.

THE PREVENTION OF TABAGISM, ALCOHOLISM AND DRUG ABUSE

The children in the nursery schools were shown how respiration is a vital act and they experienced it for themselves. They felt the difference between pure and polluted air and identified some of the polluting agents such as smoke in general and tobacco smoke in particular. They produced their own graphic representation of the number of smokers in their own families and how many cigarettes they smoked.

The children in the fifth year elementary school classes made a differential classification of substances that are useless and/or harmful to the body and those that are useful in certain circumstances and in specific quantities. They also distinguished between superfluous and vital substances. They discovered the real damage that smoking and alcohol do to their bodies. On the basis of this information, they decided that adults are very often inconsistent and should be helped. They enjoyed playing little tricks on their relatives to prevent their smoking too much. They absorbed the idea of disease caused by inconsistent personal behaviour.

The pupils of the intermediate school also became aware of economic, social, health and cultural problems connected with the acquisition and use of toxic substances. They discovered that the half-truths about the beneficial effects of such things as tobacco, medicinal products, alcohol and drugs were really half-lies. They became aware of the *clichés* and mystifying assertions made concerning them which do not help in the search for and the acquisition of knowledge, nor do they enable people to face up to problems calmly and with full awareness. The youngsters began to realize that the use of drugs does not free a person but enslaves him or her increasingly to personal habits and other people. They were able to appreciate the physical and psychological violence that people use against themselves when they do not accept their own limitations, and against others when they impose damaging behaviour on them through subtle propaganda, or by forcing others to inhale toxic substances against their will.

The parents and teachers became aware that prevention would come about through their example and not through long speeches, prohibitions and threats which might be at odds with their own behaviour. Some of them gave up smoking altogether and very few continued to smoke while the children were present.

SEXUAL EDUCATION
This subject was inserted in the wider context of cultural education thus losing its aura of novelty and mystery.

- [ ] The contents of the lessons were selected according to the effective needs of the pupils.
- [ ] The students were helped to face the existential problems connected with puberty.
- [ ] Parents were helped to free themselves from *clichés*, fears and taboos in order to be able to answer the children's questions.
- [ ] The teachers found a way of broaching the subject calmly and some of them too were freed from fears and escapist tendencies.

The verification of the hypothesis

In addition to the results already described in the section above, which dealt with the syllabus, other results were achieved.

Exhibitions of the children's work were held in the area and these spread knowledge about health education and started a process of increasing awareness of responsibility at individual and public levels. Perhaps the construction of efficient networks for water and sewerage is a tangible sign of this.

By involving the *Cassa di Risparmio* banks of Verona, Vicenza and Belluno in the experiment they began to take an active interest in the results and the branch in Belluno financed the publication of monographic texts on specific aspects of health education which were distributed free to the teachers and pupils of all the schools in the Province.

The provincial education office also became involved and they invited the author to take part in organizing and carrying out programmes of health education for parents and teachers.

Professional colleagues carried out a similar experiment in other areas of Verona and obtained similar results. These experiments were limited in scale, as those involved faced many difficulties.

Intensive courses were planned and carried out for public health nurses in other parts of the country enabling them to undertake a similar experiment in their own area. Where these experiments were carried out the results were always similar to those the author had been able to achieve.

In the light of the above the author believes that the hypothesis has been confirmed. The creation of a process of health education, which starts by educating the educators and is directed mainly at the school population, maybe the instrument with which to restore our humanity and develop a health-oriented culture.

21. Norwegians; as fit as fiddles? – A CASE STUDY

E H Endresen

Summary: The chapter presents findings from the Norwegian Health Survey (1985). The main purpose of the survey was to obtain a general and fairly comprehensive knowledge of health problems in the Norwegian population as a whole, and to reveal inequalities regarding health conditions between different groups of the population. Habits concerning different lifestyle components such as eating, drinking and smoking are reviewed. The article questions the medical understanding of health and the fruitfulness of using the topics mentioned as variables for health.

Norway and its inhabitants

The population of four million in Norway is one of the most widely scattered in Europe, with a density of only 12 persons per square kilometre. The total area of the country is 340.000 square kilometres, which is considerably larger, than for example that of the British Isles. The country stretches far up towards the North Pole. About one third of the country lies north of the Arctic Circle, and about one twelfth of the population lives there, thus constituting the northernmost sizeable permanent population in the world. The distance from the northernmost to the southernmost point is equivalent to the distance from London to Rome. The capital city of Oslo is on the same latitude as the southernmost tip of Greenland. What makes this tough country habitable is the Gulf Stream.

High mountains make transportation and communication by land both difficult to establish and costly to maintain. Important highways are closed by snow from November to April. Thus the mountains determine that nearly all the cities, and most of the people, are located near the coast, where the Gulf Stream keeps harbours ice free and relatively mild, even in winter.

Major changes in residence and economy during the last 30 years

The trend since the mid 1950s has been for people to leave the small local communities. The changing residential pattern corresponds with major changes in the national economy. Tertiary sectors are growing, while primary sectors decline. In 1960, about 20 per cent of the population worked in the primary sectors, 40 per cent in manufacturing industry and 40 per cent in services. In the mid 1980s the figures were 66 per cent in services,

28 per cent in manufacturing industry and 8 per cent in primary sectors. Norway is a member of the OECD and EFTA, but not of the EC.

The population

Of the four million Norwegians there are approximately 800,000 children (0–14 years) and 400,000 elderly (70+ years) (Statistical Yearbook 1987). Norway is a 'welfare state'. During the last 20 years national insurance has been extended to comprise a general compulsory pension scheme. The 'National insurance scheme' guarantees everyone a retirement pension and disability benefits regardless of assets or previous income. Retirement from wage labour is at 70 with optional retirement at 67–69. The increasing proportion of elderly people will have a considerable impact on health education as well as curative medicine in the years to come. Home aid and nursing services are inadequate at present, and home accidents are a serious problem among the elderly. The health services will also have to cope with chronic disease for which there is no cure. Nursing will become ever more important.

Norwegian environment and children

With a scattered population, traditionally bound to small geographical units the family has played an important part in child rearing. Role patterns of the family are changing, the number of one parent families having doubled in the period 1970 to 1980. There is a great shortage of child care facilities. Only 30 per cent of all children under compulsory school age may be admitted to the kindergartens (Royal Ministry of Church and Education 1988).

Lack of organized care is among the factors making it twice as dangerous for a child to grow up in Norway than, for example, in the neighbouring country of Sweden. The long coastline makes death by drowning a danger. Dams and ditches have often been insufficiently secured. The youngest are prone to injuries from falls, particularly from windows, balconies or steep staircases. Bicycle accidents are also far too frequent in Norway. The high number of accidents involving children made the government take action, and in 1981 the Governmental Action Committee for the Prevention of Child Accidents under The Directorate of Health was appointed. In recent years the number of deadly accidents have been reduced, but the incidence of injuries among children is still high. The National Poison Information Centre and the Norwegian State Pollution Control Authority are actively pursuing official preventive measures. Among the non-governmental organizations The Norwegian National Health Association and the Norwegian People's Aid have a long tradition of activity in this field.

Child abuse and neglect has been revealed and focused on since the 1970s. In the 1980s special attention has been given to incest and sexual abuse. Psychiatric and mental health services for adolescents are insufficient. Important work for mental health is done by voluntary organizations. Mental Aid for Children is the only non governmental organization in this field concentrating especially on children's living conditions and mental health during adolescence.

Features from Norwegian epidemiological history

Public health administration dates several hundred years back. The most important General Health Act dates from 1860, providing a basis for hygiene control in the local communities. Local health officers were extended to all municipalities, their task being to represent the national health administration and to undertake general medical service. The General Health Act of 1860 was replaced in 1982 by a new Act on Municipal Health Service.

In the nineteenth century tuberculosis swept the country, killing victims of all ages. Tuberculosis today is an historical example of a destructive condition demanding a multi-disciplinary approach to be successfully fought. What the decisive factors were is no longer under discussion. The importance of social work to increase standards of living. Improvement of nutrition and hygiene, rates the highest, followed by medical work to cure those already infected. Preventive measures at various levels, to reduce the transmission of the disease were also important. Tuberculosis was perhaps the first real task in modern times for Norwegian health education and promotion.

Seeing the conquering of tuberculosis in a health educational perspective, the work emphasized both a high-risk and a mass control – or population strategy. The mass control strategy aimed at reducing everybody's risk, those in real danger and those not in danger at all. The high risk strategy concentrated on the part of the population estimated to be in danger.

The two strategies are said to complement each other. In theory that might be so, but it is the high-risk disease oriented strategies that are given budgetary priority. What would really be of importance for future incidence might be to prevent 15 year-olds becoming high-risks at the age of 40.

This raises the question of what kind of prevention or health promotion to choose. Health promotion is to adopt a course. Which are the decisive factors influencing health today? It is said that Koch's discovery of the tubercle bacillus in 1882 obscured and turned the focus away from the 'real' causes of the disease – the underlying socio-economic factors. Without Koch's discovery, the socio-economic character of tuberculosis would have been clearer. Even in the welfare state society of Norway today this argument is still valid for a series of diseases (Waaler, 1982).

Conquering tuberculosis in Norway took almost 50 years. The disease is still not completely eradicated, but the prevalence and danger associated is low. So is the state of readiness, but all Norwegian schoolchildren are BCG-vaccinated before leaving primary school.

Glimpses from today's scenery of health or sickness

While poverty and social insecurity was the main health problem a hundred years ago, most Norwegians today enjoy the over-affluent society. In the Norwegian Health Survey (1985) the concept 'lifestyle' was operationalized to cover habits concerning:

☐ nutrition;
☐ consumption of alcoholic beverages;
☐ smoking;
☐ physical activity.

These are also topics traditionally focused on in Norwegian health education.

Nutrition

The Norwegians in general consume too much ready made and refined food, too much salt, sugar and saturated fat. The latter is especially thought to increase the levels of serum cholesterol in the blood. With regard to sugar there has been a rise in the food supply from 9 kilograms per person per year in the 1890s to 43 kilograms in 1985 (Johansson, 1987). Caries, however, has been drastically reduced during the last 20 years. In this development education has been important. The Norwegian tooth trolls 'Karius' and 'Baktus' are well known by all children in Norway. The high consumption of sugar, in ordinary and various 'light' forms such as sorbitol and xylitol, seems not to worry the health and nutritional authorities.

It is the well educated people as usual who function as the *avant garde* and consume less fat, more fruit and fibre. The 1985 health survey shows that women eat more fresh fruit and vegetables than do men. Women are also more fat-conscious, especially the youngest group. In the survey 47 per cent of the young women between 16 and 24 years of age, and 24 per cent of the men, had a low fat consumption – meaning no butter or margarine on bread, and skimmed milk only.

Coffee drinking

This has been under scrutiny during recent years. The Nordic countries have the highest consumption of coffee in the world. The average Norwegian consumes 10.5 kilograms coffee a year, compared to the English 2.5 kilograms. Eighty-five per cent of all Norwegian adults are daily coffee drinkers and the mean amount is estimated to be about five cups a day. Fifty five per cent drink filter coffee, 35 per cent boil their coffee, five per cent drink instant coffee, while five per cent use more than one method (Norwegian Report, 1987).

Coffee drinking in relation to level of serum blood lipids has been studied at the University of Tromsø and at the National Health Screening Service, Oslo. One has especially looked at levels of serum cholesterol related to ways of making the coffee in addition to the amount drunk. It seems that the boiled coffee has the strongest serum cholesterol raising effect (Stensvold *et al*, 1989).

Coffee drinking seems to be associated with socio-economic class. Men in low income households reported, for example, a considerably higher consumption of coffee at breakfast than did men in high income households, 83 per cent versus 52 per cent (Norwegian Report, 1987).

Consumption of alcoholic beverages

A general rise in personal consumption in the 1980s has also increased the consumpation of alcoholic beverages. The 1985 health survey showed consistent variations between both gender and age groups. For the frequency of drinking 'much alcohol', defined as equivalent to five half-bottles of beer or one large bottle of red or white wine or one half bottle of dessert wine or ¼ bottle of liquor weekly, the trend was that the young men, aged 16 to 24 have the higher proportion of high consumption. Forty-one per cent of the men answered that they never used alcohol, in comparison 55 per cent of the women never drank. The men in all age groups consumed more than the women.

To fight alcoholism there is a public Directorate for the Prevention of Alcohol and Drug Problems. There is also The Norwegian Temperance Alliance being an umbrella organization for several non-governmental organizations working in this field.

Smoking

The total numbers of Norwegian smokers is still high. There seem however to be some encouraging changes within certain groups. For example in the group: daily smokers aged 13 to 15 years – both boys and girls smoked less in the mid-1980s than ten years earlier. After the establishment of the National Council on Smoking and Health in 1971 and the total ban on the advertising of all tobacco products in 1975 there has been a measurable reduction in smoking among selected groups such as health professionals, especially physicians, nurses and teachers. The reduction follows the socio-economic pattern, people with no 'burn out', and people controlling their life conditions seem to smoke less. Women smoke the same amount today as ten years ago, while men have reduced their smoking in the same period.

Thirty-five per cent of the population in the 1985 health survey were daily smokers, 39 per cent of the men and 32 per cent of the women. Forty-two per cent reported that they never had been daily smokers. The figures from a comparable study 1975 gave 41 per cent daily smokers of whom 50 per cent were men and 32 per cent women.

A smoke free society in the year 2000

In the spring of 1986, five non-governmental organizations: the Norwegian Cancer Society, the Norwegian Society against Tobacco,, the Norwegian National Health Association, the Norwegian Asthma and Allergy Association, and the Co-operative Board for Health Education, presented a plan of action to achieve a smoke-free society in the year 2000 (National Council on Smoking and Health 1987).

A supplement to the Norwegian tobacco Act from 1973 was made 1988. The Act was given a new section reading:

In premises and means of transport to which the public have access, and in meeting rooms and work premises where two or more persons

are gathered, the air shall be smokefree. This does not apply to
restaurants, hotels and other establishments which serve food and/or
offer overnight accommodation.

The Act entered into force on July first 1988.

Physical activity

In the Norwegian Health Survey of 1985 people were asked if they
performed any regular physical activity during leisure time. Fifty-seven
per cent answered that they did so, while 68 per cent in the youngest group
were physically active, compared to 45 per cent among 67+ years-old. In the
older age group men were more active than women, among the youngest
this was reversed. The well educated people were more active in all groups.

To increase physical fitness, a special campaign called 'Physical exercise
for health and well-being' was carried out in the years 1983 to 1987. A wide
range of activities were initiated all over the country. The attention was
focused on groups rather than individuals, such as families, companies,
schools, groups of elderly and groups of handicapped. An important
principle was to combine campaigns in the local communities with mass
media coverage. The campaign was a co-operation between non-governmental organizations and public authorities. An additional aim for the
campaign was to work out an organizational model for health education at
the different administrative levels in the country (Sluttrapport, 1988).

Opinion on own health

The Norwegian Health Survey of 1985 was carried out during a period of two
weeks, and people were also asked to judge their own health at the
beginning of the period. Seventy-seven per cent of the total sample
evaluated their own health as very good. Even 68 per cent of the people
'with disease' judged their health to be very good, while 95 per cent of the
people without disease did so. In this question there was little difference
between socio-economic groups. Slight differences could, however, be seen
between the age groups.

Comments

These glimpses of the Norwegian lifestyle set the frame for reviewing the
conditions leading to medical consultations, drug consumption, sick leaves
and disability pensions. Musculo-skeletal diseases and coronary heart
diseases are the most frequent reasons for medical consultations. Coronary
heart disease followed by mental illnesses, require the costliest drug
consumption, but drug consumption for indigestion and digestive troubles
is also very high. The musculo-skeletal illnesses lead to most sick leaves,
while mental illnesses cause the highest total expense within the public
health insurance system.

Understanding health and illness is culturally patterned. What is regard-ed as important, the cultural values, are socially constructed. Cultural values are learned and internalized – as a kind of blueprint or guideline for ways of thinking and behaving. Cultural values are reflected at many different levels, superior ones can, for example, be seen in economic budgets, institutions built, the emphasis and priorities allocated by the government, by professionals and suchlike. It can for example be seen in the importance attached to curative medicine in comparison to preventive medicine and health education. Nearly 40 per cent of the Norwegian GNP is spent on health and social services. Thus health seems to be an important cultural value.

At the individual level cultural values are reflected, for example, in lifestyle that comprises an erroneously understood entity if regarded too narrowly. To judge health by what you eat, drink, smoke or how much you exercise, or to limit the concept of health to lack of disease, is to overlook the processes of health. These are, among other things, processes of a continuous calibration-feedback, a dialectic between form and process seen from a systemic point of view. To cultivate health is different from curing the sick. The medical curing has to date been dominated by a 'man against nature' attitude or epistemology which long ago has shown its destructive power. Processes of health have probably more to do with care than cure. Understanding, and defining, health in relation to disease blocks out the fact that processes of health may be essentially different from processes compensating for disorder (Bateson, 1979).

To understand health behaviour one must have in mind sub-cultural differences. Behaviour and health habits should also be seen as qualities associated with certain groups, their living conditions and social situations, rather than the only outcome of individual choice. Values attached to health, and the understanding and content of the concept 'health' vary. Health education/promotion will turn out rather haphazard if the basic understand-ing between sender and receiver is different.

The differences shown in various lifestyle components in the Norwegian Health Survey of 1985 had a socio-economic pattern as their major characteristic. There were marked regional differences as well. In addition there were important gender differences. The overall trend was an accumulation of unhealthy habits, especially among men in low income groups. The survey showed, for example, that teachers have the lowest mortality, while industrial workers have the highest. Teachers however, are not a particularly high income group in Norway, but the majority of teachers are women. So are most of the health promoters in this country.

From epidemic diseases, diseases of poverty, we have moved to life-style diseases – diseases of affluence. Role patterns have shifted along the way, a characteristic of today being that the feeling of closeness which creates identity and belonging (and health?) is lacking. Loneliness is put forward as a 'health problem' in many communities (Directorate of Health, 1986).

The consultation has been a major source of general health education in Norway. Advice given by doctor or nurse has been individualized and often focused on isolated risk factors, such as the serum cholesterol mentioned above. In addition it seems to be the well educated people who have taken advantage of the information given. The survey supports this theory by finding that it was the high income groups that had changed their lifestyle. It has thus been questioned whether health education increases socio-economic differences.

History shows that health promotion has to do with the allocation and distribution of knowledge. It is a challenge for future health education to provide 'healthy' knowledge – about the kind of artifacts influencing nature, processes of health. Health in this perspective seen both biologically and culturally, adjusted to cultural values such as identity, joy, suffering, meaning, in short recognized life qualities in addition to whatever was known about illness and disease. To increase equality in health the education/promotion need to stress the importance of equal access to data within a system. To reduce the socio-economic inequality in health will require political action focusing on social structure and environmental questions.

The Public Health Service

In the Norwegian system of health care and social services it is an obligation of the society as a whole to provide for every individual, regardless of social class, personal financial resources or domicile in the country:

- ☐ certainty of care and nursing in sickness, infirmity and old age;
- ☐ security against depletion of income with loss or reduction in earning capacity;
- ☐ help in circumstances of social distress.

At the central level, public health policies and operations are under the auspices of the Ministry of Social Affairs. The Ministry concentrates on policy-making, legislation and co-ordination, while the Directorate of Health aims to develop the public health system at the practical level.

The Public Health Service is composed of:

- ☐ health care services;
- ☐ social welfare services; and
- ☐ public health insurance services built up as a tri-partite system.

Public administration

This is carried out on three different administrative levels: state, county and municipality. Responsiblity for environmental questions, preventive measures, in short, standards of living including health services, rest with the municipalities.

The municipalities – independently administered units

Municipal self government dates back a hundred and fifty years. It's important to note that the municipalities are not subordinate to the counties, but separate systems with independent local administrations. The municipal council is the highest political body at the local level, consisting of representatives of the various political parties in proportion to their local strength. The municipal council appoints special committees for the various services, such as the running of local communicatons, building, fire services, primary education, primary health care, health education, social services and so forth. In 1988 there is a total of 448 municipalities in the country.

The counties: ties between administrative levels

There are 19 counties in the country. These vary considerably in size and economic basis, and range in population from about 75,000 to 500,000 inhabitants. There are two administrative systems operating at the county level. The central authority administration, consisting of senior public servants, whose offices have supervisory and control functions for the municipalities in respect of their administration, civil defence, tasks within family jurisdiction, health service and suchlike, and the county-municipal administration, which is led by the politically elected county council.

The county health administration is responsible for hospital services, including planning and the building of facilities. It also has responsiblity for child welfare institutions and for the mentally handicapped.

Municipal and county activities in general are financed through direct taxation, and through subsidies from the central Government.

Educational system

The responsibility for the Norwegian educational system rests within the same three administrative levels as mentioned. At the central level, the parliament – the *Storting* has, as the legislative and levying power, the overall responsibility and authority for the schools. Through legislation the *Storting* stipulates the overall aim for the schools, the structure and organization, responsibility for the running costs, administration, finance and so forth. The county covers upper secondary schools, while the state is responsible for the universities and institutions of higher education. The primary and lower secondary schools which require adapted education for all children up to the age of 16 are the responsiblity of the municipalities (Royal Ministry of Church and Education 1988).

No separate health educators

There are no separate health educators in Norway. Traditionally, health education has been part of everyday work for doctors, nurses, physiotherapists and suchlike.

To overcome the medical domination in the field, the concept 'health promotion' is now more commonly used than 'health education'. Neither concepts are delimited nor clearly defined. Some principles for action have been put forward in the Ottawa and Adelaide charters, but the concept 'health promotion' and the subject area remain unclear apart from the overall purpose of a 'Healthy Public Policy' (Ottawa Charter, 1986) (Adelaide Charter, 1988). The principles of the Alma Ata Declaration and the 'Health for all' movement are still mainly words of honour given very little budgetary priority (WHO, 1985).

Non-governmental organizations and health education

The NGOs (non governmental organizations) have always played an important role in Norwegian public health work. The oldest of them dates its origin a hundred years or more back, fighting tuberculosis by nation-wide social networks. Tasks were manifold: to be mentioned is the building of more than a hundred sanitaria and nursing homes for the diseased. Special homes for children living in a contaminated environment were built as well, emphasizing hygiene, nutrition and education to give them a more healthy future.

Health education and health examinations were among the main tasks for the NGOs from the very beginning of their work. Another example is the nation-wide network of local clinics providing health screenings, vaccines and suchlike, for small children, and later an organizing ante- and post-natal care for women. The NGOs have in many ways been pioneers in public health work. Ideas and practical ventures, initiated and paid for by the NGOs have very often in Norway become part of the municipal health services.

The role of the NGOs are looked upon rather ambiguously. Their experience and willingness in voluntary work is highly needed at times of budget reduction. However, the changed role patterns, especially for women, where they total more than 60 per cent engaged in employment, makes it more difficult to recruit new members. Of women between 30 and 50 years a total of 85 to 90 per cent are employed (Statistical Yearbook, 1987). Women behind the core group of the NGOs previous engagement and activities seldom have any leisure time at all. This has given the NGOs severe recruiting problems.

There are however encouraging signs towards new ways of thinking in health promotion. In the recently held second International Conference on Health Promotion in Australia the following was said about the role of non-governmental organizations: 'Voluntary work is important because it is unbureaucratic and impatient; it mobilizes the public and can influence politicians and decision-makers'. In this work there is an important lesson to remember from the epidemiological history – the necessity for unpredicated thinking, co-operation between organizations – governmental as well as non-governmental ones, between the sectors and with long range policies and long term evaluation.

The Co-ordinating Board of Health Education – SOHO

The first introductory meetings of the Co-ordinating Board took place in 1979. By 1988, 28 different organizations, approximately half of them NGOs, are members of the Board. The secretarial function is placed within the Directorate of Health, Ministry of Social Affairs.

Similar Co-ordinating Boards of Health Education are now being established in the counties. The Boards of Health and Social Welfare are administratively responsible in the municipalities.

A separate Division of Health Education since 1986

In 1986 the Division of Health Education was established as a central unit under the National Health Screening Service. The staff in 1988 numbered five. According to plan the unit will be extended and the staff doubled in the coming years. The commission of the Division is mainly to be an advisory and clarifying unit for the Directorate of Health and to serve as a consultative organ for the municipalities, counties and non-governmental organizations.

References

Adelaide Charter (1988) Healthy public policy strategy for action *Second International Conference on Health Promotion*

Bateson, G (1979) *Mind and Nature* Bantam Books

Directorate of Health (1986) Helseopplysning i en kommune

Health Survey (1985) Central Bureau of Statistics of Norway

Johansson, I (1987) Kosthold oq helse, Noras-rapport

National Council on Smoking and Health Draft Act of 18 December (1987) Supplement to the Norwegian Tobacco Act of 9 March 1973

Norwegian Report 1987 Coffee information

Ottawa Charter (1986) *First International Conference on Health Promotion*

Royal Ministry of Church and Education and Royal Ministry of Cultural and Scientific Affairs (1988) Report to OECD, Reviews of national policies for education

Statistical Yearbook (1987) Central Bureau of Statistics

Stenmarck, S (1988) The role of non-governmental organizations in mobilization for a healthy public policy *paper presented at second International Conference on Health Promotion, Adelaide*

Stensvold, I et al (1989) The effect of boiled and filter coffee on serum cholesterol and triglycerides (to be published) National Health Screening Service, Oslo

Sluttrapport for fysisk aktivitet for helse og trivsel (1988)

Waaler, H T (1982) Tuberculosis and socio-economic development, *Bulletin of the Int. Union Against Tuberculosis* 57

WHO (1985) Targets for health for all. Regional Office for Europe

22. Health education in Finland – AN OVERVIEW

H Vertio

Summary: In the last decade, the scope and purpose of health education in Finland has widened from being just about health care. Many sectors and groups are involved. Particular *foci* for funding are smoking and alcohol education. Many voluntary bodies are active in health education and have numerous links with the authorities. The activities of the voluntary bodies are co-ordinated by the Finnish Council for Health Education. Health education is part of the school curriculum. Trends in health education are tracked by a variety of methods. Evaluated research is increasing. Particular projects of a very diverse nature are described in this chapter.

The Organization of health education

Health education in Finland has progressed from being mere health care to being the concern of many sectors, groups and people. The national co-ordination of health education has been entrusted to the National Board of Health, which founded an office for that purpose in 1976. This has laid relatively more emphasis on the word 'health', though 'education' has continued to be very much to the fore. The new wording opens up new potential and definitely widens the scope and purpose of health education work. Although the office for Health Education has mainly worked with smoking control policy, it now covers all aspects of health education. It has a regular staff of 10, half of whom hold university degrees. In health care, the office is in direct contact with a network of people in all the Finnish health centres and hospitals (some 450 in all, most of them nurses). Only 10 per cent of these are full-time health educators. They have a demanding task: to act as health education co-ordinators between the various sectors and experts in their local areas. They are trained by the central office, supplied with material and resources, and give each other mutual support. Nevertheless, they work for their local health centres and are not governed by any central body.

The Council of Health Education operating at national level consists of leaders and experts from different sectors, voluntary organizations and the media. This council also has a counterpart at health centre level. The local co-ordination groups are mainly concerned with planning.

The National Council issued a recommendation for health education for the period 1984 to 1988. This is a five-year plan giving detailed proposals and models for all sectors of health education. There is a specific plan for health education, to be updated every five years. Most of the local co-ordination committees have made their plans more or less accordingly.

The funding of health education

The resources for health education are hidden in the budgets and almost impossible to find. However, the contact persons at the health centres share the opinion that money is not the main problem: it is the lack of faith among health care people and the traditional tendency to preach that still haunts health education. The national budget has allocated approximately 11 million Finnish Marks for health education in 1989 for the express purpose of reducing smoking. This is something like 0.1 per cent of the total state health care budget, which is in turn around eight per cent of the total national budget. This does not mean that health education has to exist solely on this; it is indeed included in all planning and therefore gets its main resources elsewhere. The prevention of drinking, that is, temperance work, does, however, have a budget of its own amounting to more than 60 million Finnish Marks, because of its long tradition in Finland.

Health education by voluntary bodies

The first voluntary organizations in the field of health education were founded in Finland over a century ago, though no organization has ever been established exclusively for this purpose. Health education is an integral part of their work, as with schools and health centres. The work of the non-governmental organizations is more informal and practical than that of the public organizations. They are primarily concerned with promoting the health of their members but sometimes extend their objectives to the entire population.

The voluntary organizations have traditionally engaged in experimental activities that have, after a period of assessment, been transferred to the public administration. The majority of the modern health education methods used in Finland – including maternity and child care –were first introduced informally on limited scale by a voluntary organization. Private groups have also initiated special training programmes for health educators and still maintain institutes for this purpose.

There are numerous links between the private bodies and the authorities which mostly share the same objectives. They have a tradition of organizing campaigns, attempting to influence public opinion and decision-makers, and informing the public of health risks, diseases and the importance of adopting a healthy lifestyle. In the past two decades, however, the voluntary organizations have introduced more carefully-planned long-term programmes, including more sophisticated methods and evaluation. More careful study is being given to the target groups, their features, needs and expectations. The complex nature of many health problems has, furthermore, prompted private groups to join forces: more and more joint programmes involving either several voluntary organizations and/or the authorities are being carried out.

The voluntary organizations do not aim to make a profit. They produce and sell services and themselves finance about half their activities. This is why they are sometimes called the 'third sector', standing as they do in between the authorities and the commercial groups. Their other most important source of income, covering the rest of their budget, is the Finnish Slot Machine Association, which they own jointly with the State. This company has a monopoloy over all slot machines, entertainment and music machines. Its net annual income is distributed between public health, child welfare, leisure pursuits, and services for the aged and the handicapped.

In 1962, the leading private organizations decided to establish the Finnish Council for Health Education to improve co-ordination between them. The Council then applied for membership of the International Union of Health Education and was recognized as a national committee. By the end of 1987, 70 national organizations had joined the Council. Since 1974, the Council has annually published a catalogue of health education materials assessed and recommended by a committee. The 1987 catalogue reviews some 800 items: posters, leaflets, slide and tape programmes, films and booklets.

Health education in schools and colleges

Health education is part of the Finnish school curriculum. Over the past few decades the volume of health education has, however, been diminishing under pressure from many new subjects. Under the new legislation, health, unlike physical education, does not enjoy the status of an educational target. It is incorporated into many subjects on the curriculum, mainly environmental studies, biology and physical education. Colleges teach a subject called health education, or rather health information. Some new experiments are being carried out to test comprehensive means of including health promotion in schools. Health education is growing and acquiring a more closely-defined status in vocational training.

Research and evaluation

It is often said that health education is important, that it should receive more resources, and that it should be more effective.

To achieve its goals, health education needs a wide variety of information. It must be constantly aware of the climate in society and the community and the rating of health in the opinion of the public. This means that health education needs information broader in scope than mere health data. Even so, it must have comprehensive health data too – on diseases, the use of services, trends in the health sector and so on. Of particular importance to health education is information on behaviour – smoking, drinking and drugs, nutritional habits, levels of exercise, risks and safety. Obviously, this information alone is not enough; it is also essential to anticipate developments.

Here in Finland the National Institute for Public Health collects behaviour in an annual study. This takes the form of a postal questionnaire to which there is always a good response (80 to 85 per cent). A larger study consisting of personal interviews is also made every five years by the Institute of Social

Security. The National Board of Health requires more speedy methods of measuring the climate, so the Central Statistical Office conducts telephone enquiries twice a year. Some issues of interest such as the level of smoking and the manufacture of tobacco products are subjected to even greater scrutiny. The State Alcohol Monopoly keeps an equally close check on the consumption of alcohol.

It is often demanded that health education should be effective, yet it is extremely difficult to produce reliable and accurate data to prove it. All studies supported by health education resources should carry a built-in evaluation of an appropriate style. The results of public health measures may not be evident for many years and even then they may be open to criticism. Every major health education project in Finland today is in fact evaluated. There is still however, a lack of research into policies: what effects do policies have? Some attempts to answer this question have been made with reference to smoking control. Finland has a relatively new and explicit health strategy that might be a very interesting target for policy analysis and evaluation. Research into health education and promotion has not found a home at any of the Finnish universities, though there is a chair in health education at the University of Jyvaskyla. Research is carried out at all the universities and at the Urho Kekkonen Institute in Tampere. The research tradition is growing slowly, perhaps more slowly than the change from health education to health promotion.

Health education publications

The National Board of Health and its Office for Health Education publish two health education series, one for research reports and the other for statistics and other reports. About 20 dissertations on health education have been published since 1975. Reports are sometimes also published in the University series particularly in Jyvaskula University. Most of the publications are in Finnish, but the *Yearbook of Health Education* contains English summaries of all reports and the same applies to reports in the research series.

Future trends in health education

There are several indications of a shift towards health promotion. It has become evident that health education must be backed by decisions and conditions promoting health. On the other hand people have often expressed their faith in health education, rather than in such measures as price policy or penalties. Health education may thus be viewed as a means of health promotion.

Health education is sometimes accused of being patronizing, but there is a strong move towards new approaches that are more comprehensive and that make allowance for a person's life situation and his or her ability to cope with life. This suggests that health education is becoming more subjectively oriented than it used to be. Instead of concentrating on toxic substances, health education promises to be more interested in helping people to cope with life, or make their own decisions. Some of the future trends only exist on paper. Many things can affect the development of health education. In many countries of Europe the administrative resources for health education have been cut, but in Finland there is strong support for health promotion and education.

Health education initiatives and projects

Mother and Child Health Care Centres

The network of Mother and Child Health Care (MCH) centres constitutes the backbone of Finland's health education. This network was created in the 1940s, and by the 1950s there were already 6,000 MCH centres. The work of these centres was mostly counselling, by nurses and midwives, but many regular check-ups were included, to teach mothers how to take good care of their children. The amount of health education passed on in this way is inestimable, but it has often been said that the results can be seen in the diminishing infant mortality figures. This is obviously true, although allowance has to be made for changes in living conditions over the same period. The centres have meant security and help for the majority of Finnish women and nowadays men, too, as the system is working towards greater family orientation and counselling.

The North Karelia Project

The North Karelia Project is possibly the best-known health education project in Finland. It was initiated at the beginning of the 1970s to discover why so many Finnish men die at an exceptionally young age of cardio-vascular diseases. This was even more marked in North Karelia than in other parts of the country. The risk factors were defined as being high blood pressure, high serum cholesterol and smoking. Health education was planned accordingly and centred around the health care system, with regular check-ups and intensified care efforts. The project took the form of a study, which permitted evaluation of the results although less attention was paid to the process. The publicity of the project was considered important for two reasons: coherence increased in the region and the resources for the project became easier to tap. The results of the project are well documented and have been discussed on numerous occasions. The evaluation of trends in the health of North Karelian people continues.

Smoking control policy

Many European countries tightened up their smoking control policies in the mid-1970s. In Finland, the work of an endless succession of smoking committees finally resulted in a proposal for smoking control legislation. This proposal was comprehensive and health-oriented. After a year of wide and deep-going public debate Parliament passed a Tobacco Act in 1976, 15 years after the first demands for strong measures. The timing was opportune. The control policy was based on hard epidemiological facts and its four cornerstones were health education, restrictions, research, and product control. Health education took the form of the channelling of resources to (mainly voluntary) organizations via the media, and the intensification of activities in schools and the health services. The health authorities were made responsible for co-ordinating health education, research and evaluation.

Analysis of the development of health care with reference to smoking reveals a clear trend from lung cancer and other diseases to seeing smoking as a social problem. The importance of keeping a close check on trends in society, not only the prevalence of smoking, has become evident. So, has health education been successful? There is some evidence that it has counteracted the price policy and had some effect, but the results are so often obscured by numerous other factors.

The 'Man 2000' project

'Man 2000' was the name given to one of the largest co-operation experiments organized by the authorities and voluntary organizations in 1986. It was financed by the National Board of Health, the Ministry of Social Affairs and Health and the State Alcohol Monopoly. The project had the following aims: to help men to cope, to test a mass media project for adults, and to improve practical co-operation between different interests. The media campaign had three peaks: the start, May Day and Father's Day. Evaluation of the project revealed that this approach sparked off wide public debate touching on every possible theme connected with men or health. Most of the comments came from women. The critics accused the project of intruding on men's privacy, of making men child-like softies. Judging by the feelings expressed in the debate, the project touched on some sensitive areas in society and may also have had an effect on people's health.

The 'Health on canvas' competition

In 1987, the Office for Health Education, *Folkhalsan* (a voluntary health organization) and one county government ran a very special competition. This was an art competition restricted to one county and only five invited artists, who were asked to express in painting their thoughts on health. As a result five paintings were produced, all different, but they did have certain elements in common. The most striking feature was perhaps the balance present in them all. These works of art were then duplicated and displayed at all the health centres in the county. Next it will be the turn of poets.

The healthy cities

'Healthy cities' is a WHO project that has quickly become a movement. Three Finnish cities were immediately interested in the idea in 1985, and five more have seriously considered the idea of developing the health of the city. The health of the city here means more than the health of its citizens, for the project is concerned with health promotion. One of the main principles has been the participation of the people. Another has been social support and a third equality. How can these principles be applied to produce healthier cities? Each of the cities involved has devised its own plan of action, but they all make use of meetings, training and information. The project is still in progress but is becoming more one of understanding and networking. The results of such work could and should be measured, but they cannot be evaluated in the same way as conventional projects. What is needed are new indicators, greater subjectivity, more policy analysis and more elasticity.

23. Health Education in Wales – AN OVERVIEW

J Griffiths

Summary: As a result of discussions which took place during the early 1980s, it was decided to establish a demonstration programme in Wales with the aim of reducing the incidence of cardio-vascular disease in that country. At that time Wales had among the highest figures of mortality and morbidity due to cardio-vascular disease in the world. With a population of some three million, its own language and identity, the challenge to reduce the incidence of cardio-vascular disease amongst the general population was not an insignificant one. The Welsh Heart Programme or as it came to be known Heartbeat Wales, was established on 1 March 1985 for a five year period. This chapter describes the background to the programme and its activities especially those directed at young people. The activities of the programme were broadly based and centred upon seven headings, these included school based curriculum developments, policy development, educational programmes involving parents in the home, the use of other networks such as youth clubs and youth organizations, and attention to the macro environment.

The chapter then describes the creation of the Health Promotion Authority for Wales, which has, as one of its main programmes the Welsh Heart Programme. The article also looks at the significance of the new national curriculum which is intended to be implemented in the near future. An outline is provided of some of the proposed future activities and the point is made repeatedly of the close co-operation and communication that exists between the central organization, namely the Health Promotion Authority for Wales and the regional statutory organizations, namely the county councils and the district health authorities. Close co-operation is also occurring between the Health Education Authority in London and the Health Promotion Authority for Wales. Future proposed activities are described briefly and it is hoped that the reader will gain an impression of the current levels of activity in health education and health promotion that are occurring in a variety of different settings throughout the Principality of Wales.

Introduction

The Principality of Wales has a population of some three million people, its own language and its own national identity. As part of the United Kingdom it is governed from Parliament in London. However it has its own Secretary of State who is a member of the Cabinet and its own Government Department, The Welsh Office which has responsibility for overseeing many of the activities of Government within Wales.

There are eight counties in Wales each of which has its own elected body, the county council. At a more local level are the thirty seven district councils. The county councils have responsibility for the provision of education within their county. To do this each has established an education authority comprised of elected representatives, who through the director of education are charged with providing an education service for the community they represent.

For children between the ages of five and sixteen education is compulsory. Those between the ages of five and eleven will attend a primary school and those between the ages of eleven and sixteen a secondary school. There are approximately eighteen hundred primary schools and two hundred and seventy secondary schools in Wales. In some schools the process of education occurs through the medium of the English language, in others through the medium of the Welsh language while some are bilingual.

Health service provision in Wales is achieved through the family practitioner committees and nine district health authorities. Each health authority has a health education department, which is responsible for providing expertise and resources for health education and health promotion in the area served by the authority.

Background to the Welsh Heart Programme

The following extract is taken from the document entitled Take Heart. This document was produced as a consultative document on the development of community based heart health initiatives within Wales and sets the scene for the activities of the Welsh Heart Programme.

The early history

At its Colloquium at Llandudno in May 1981, the Health Education Council (HEC) declared its intention to devote increased efforts and resources towards health education and health promotion in Wales. Coronary heart disease prevention was acknowledged as an important priority area in the Principality.

Shortly afterwards in December 1981 the report of the Welsh Medical Committee's Working Party on Cardio-thoracic Services in Wales was published. It recommended the development of a co-ordinated programme for the prevention of cardio-vascular disease in Wales, comprising:

1. Mass prevention by education and alteration of living habits in the community;
2. Specific measures in high risk subjects, with screening programmes to identify and estimate the degree of risk in symptomless subjects and patients with known cardio-vascular disease.

The report was received by the Welsh Office, who recommended that discussions should be held with the Health Education Council with a view to developing a major preventive programme.

Subsequently in 1983 the HEC outlined its plans concerning coronary heart disease prevention. The HEC proposed that it should develop a pilot project and concentrate resources and effort in a single region over a five year period. Lessons learned in the development of a regional strategy could then be applied to other parts of the country. After discussions with the Welsh Office and others, Wales was selected as the designated region and the programme was given the provisional title of the Welsh Heart Programme (WHP).

Having informally consulted within Wales, the HEC drew up provisional outline proposals for a five year community-based heart-health programme. These were widely distributed for comment to district health authorities, professional bodies and other interested groups, and drew a substantial, encouraging and helpful response. A document outlining the final proposals that emerged from the consultation process was published in 1984.

This document outlined the broad strategy that should be adopted and specified aims and objectives for the WHP concerning smoking, diet, raised blood pressure, exercise, stress, and first aid. The HEC emphasized the importance of assessing the effectiveness and efficiency of the interventions undertaken. The intention was to use Wales as a 'test-bed' for developing an overall strategy and a variety of component projects. These could then subsequently be applied elsewhere in Britain. Evaluation would mostly take the form of action research, studying the implementation process itself.

The Health Education Council recognized that the effectiveness of the WHP would depend very largely on the wholehearted support and co-operation of the various organizations, professional groups and individuals concerned. These included such bodies as health authorities, family practitioner committees, education authorities, occupational health services, voluntary bodies leisure services, commerce and industry.

Ultimately, the WHP's success would hand on its capturing interest and enthusiasm of the general public. The HEP proposed that the WHP should be promoted to give it a strong identity throughout Wales. This would provide 'agenda-setting' for the component projects. The mass media messages should emphasize the benefits of health living; both in terms of immediate gratification and long-term health. The campaign should take account of the cultural and social differences in the various parts of Wales. Broadcasting and printed matter should use the Welsh language as appropriate. Maximum use should be made of local radio and newspaper to augment local efforts. The campaign should be devised and funded by a central directorate acting on advice from those in the field (WHP, 1985).

The Central Directorate's primary role is to develop a community based programme involving close and regular contacts with a wide range of statutory authorities, professional organizations and voluntary bodies. The HEC envisaged that component projects should be devised, selected and developed over the first year of the WHP. In the main these projects should be locally based, operating in a variety of settings (such as schools, adult education centres, places of work, primary care) and involving a variety of health education techniques such as one to one counselling, group work, printed material, audio visual aids and health promotion events (WHP, 1985b).

The development of the Young People's Programme

The WHP was formally launched as Heartbeat Wales on March 1985. Jointly funded by the Welsh Office and the Health Education Council, it was administered through the University of Wales College of Medicine. Since then it has initiated a wide range of national and local projects and programmes. One of the major problems that confronted the WHP upon its establishment in 1985, was the lack of information concerning the health knowledge and attitudes and health behaviour of young people in Wales, and the nature and extent of organized health education in Welsh schools. An initial priority therefore was the development and implementation of two surveys. The first focused on the lifestyle patterns of the young people in Wales, the second on the organization of health education in schools. The purpose of these surveys is twofold, firstly, to obtain baseline information so that changes can be monitored over time and, secondly, to assist in the development and targeting of health promotion programmes. For further information regarding these surveys the following documents should be consulted: The Welsh Youth Health Survey (1986); The Health Promoting School (1987).

These surveys were followed by a series of educational initiatives and the development of class-room materials for use when health education topics were being taught. As many of the lifestyle elements associated with an increased risk of cardio-vascular disease have their origins in childhood and adolescence, the development of a youth health project has been an important theme within the WHP. Key areas are smoking, nutrition, physical activity, and alcohol abuse. In developing a strategy for the young people's programme it was decided to make this broad based rather than specific to schools or any one setting. The following activities and areas of approach were identified as a result:

☐ School based curriculum development;
☐ School based organizational and policy development;
☐ Mass communication through television, print and so forth;
☐ Professional training;
☐ Educational programmes involving parents;
☐ The use of other networks such as youth clubs and voluntary youth organizations; and
☐ Macro environment, for example the supply and promotion of tobacco or alcohol products.

It must be stated here that many of these activities were in existence before the establishment of the WHP. However, it must also be said that the establishment of the WHP provided a much needed impetus and focus for them. As can be seen from the above list, many different groups of people have been and are involved, including teachers, health education officers and other health professionals, local education authority advisers, school governors, parents and youth workers.

Current activities

School based curriculum developments

IN THE PRIMARY SCHOOL SETTING
The major dissemination activity in primary schools is currently centred on the HEC/My Body Project (MBP). This project, developed in the UK from the

American Berkeley Project, is designed for use with nine to eleven year-old pupils, although it has been successfully used in the early years of secondary education as well.

The MBP is 'cross curricular' in nature and its health education message deals mainly with the issue of smoking and its effect on health.

As a result of the carefully thought out dissemination strategy based upon the one developed at the MBP centre in Sheffield, many schools in Wales are now using the project. A key component of the dissemination of the material has been the development of an in-service training package for teachers. Staff from the WHP, health education officers from the District Health Authorities health education units and local education authority advisers have all been involved in organizing and running training sessions for teachers. Such training provides the teacher with the knowledge and skills required to teach the materials effectively; it gives them the opportunity to explore the full potential of the material and to overcome any anxieties that they may have regarding it; it provides the opportunity to give encouragement and it provides an insight into the methodology, the approaches and possible further developments of the material or in a supportive environment.

In addition to promoting the dissemination of the project, the WHP has sponsored the development of additional material for the MBP. In Dyfed Local Education Authority, a group of teachers with the support of the Pembrokeshire Area Education Officer have produced materials which will be utilized in a nutrition and healthy eating pack. This pack is further supported by the development of computer software in the micro-electronics Unit of the Welsh Joint Education Commiteee. In Gwynedd, additional material on fitness and exercise is being developed. This is occurring in the health education unit of Gwynedd Health Authority and shows the collaboration that can take place between the various statutory organizations and the WHP. Both of these packs have been designed as extension material to the original project, both however can be used independently of the project as projects in themselves.

Such has been the success of the dissemination of the MBP that in one authority in Wales, namely Powys Local Education Authority (LEA), every school now possesses a project pack and at least one person from each school has attended an in-sevice course. In South Glamorgan LEA a similar picture is being achieved and the other counties are following close behind.

The tremendous impetus given to the dissemination of the MBP by Heartbeat Wales shows that the WHP is keen to utilize existing material rather than spend lengthy periods of time developing new but nevertheless similar material itself. However, it was felt that all primary schools in Wales would not be prepared to use the MBP, as its cost makes it a relatively expensive item for small schools. In conjunction therefore with the British Heart Foundation and the HEC as it then was, Heartbeat Wales commissioned the production of the new primary school project called Health At Heart (HAH). This project which will be published early in 1989 deals with each of the main cardio-vascular disease risk factors and it will be available at a considerably lower price than that of the MBP.

IN THE SECONDARY SETTING

In the secondary sector of education several projects are being actively disseminated. These include two which deal with the issue of young people and smoking. The first, the family smoking education project, is designed for use with eleven and twelve year-old pupils. Whilst the second, the smoking education for teenagers project is used with twelve to fourteen year-olds. The latter project uses the concept of discussion groups and aims to provide young people with the skills they need to prevent themselves from starting to smoke. Many teachers of physical education have attended courses in which they examine the role of exercise for health and a package of materials is being produced to support these courses.

In the South Glamorgan area, Heartbeat Wales has sponsored the production of a secondary school heart health pack. This material, designed for children in the middle years of their secondary school education, is being produced by a health education officer for schools who is an ex-teacher and who is funded by Heartbeat Wales. The LEA and the district health authority's health education department have worked closely together in the production of this pack.

Research is being carried out among teachers to identify their knowledge and attitudes towards lifestyle issues and data from the Heartbeat Wales youth survey and is also being used to identify the issues which the material to be produced ought to address. The project not only involves the development of material for the classroom but also the development and adoption of school policies on smoking and healthy eating and the important element of parental involvement.

Once the material has been tried and evaluated it will be available for use throughout Wales. The completeness of this package, in that it deals with policy, practice and classroom material, will make it an extremely valuable component in the youth programme.

Also occurring in the South Glamorgan area is the trial of a concept which it is hoped will be eventually extended throughout Wales. It involves the local ambulance service in training older pupils in the county secondary schools in the techniques of cardio-pulmonary resuscitation. These pupils in turn train younger pupils. The training process is monitored and regularly checked to ensure that standards are being maintained and upheld. To date several thousand pupils have been trained.

Game for Life is a consumer education pack that has been produced as a result of the efforts of the trading standards department of Mid-Glamorgan County Council. The district health authority through its health education department in co-operation with Heartbeat Wales developed the section on healthy lifestyle which puts health education for older teenagers firmly in the context of 'everyday life'.

The levels of health education

With so much activity occurring one of the questions that needs to be answered is whether the teachers of Wales are involving themselves in health education and whether the process is occurring successfully. To answer it a survey was carried out in 81 of the secondary schools in Wales. Seventy-two of the 76 schools that responded reported that health education was currently taught and a further two 'had future plans'. Fifty-nine of the schools reported that they had a planned programme of health education – a planned programme being defined as either a specific health education course or a specific component of a more broadly based personal and social education course or a plan and co-ordinated programme integrated into existing subject areas (*Health Education Journals*, 1987).

COLLEGES OF FURTHER AND HIGHER EDUCATION
For older young people who are either in their last years of compulsory education or who have gone on to higher education, Heartbeat Wales is encouraging the establishment of smoking cessation groups. These groups, using material developed by Dr Ann Charlton of the Cancer Research Campaign (WHP, 1987) can offer support to those young people who have started to smoke and who now want to give up.

The health education model

The model of health education based upon the education system, is that of the spiral curriculum, which builds on what has been done before. For example, the smoking education programme has elements which appear in the primary school setting, the secondary school setting and in colleges of further and higher education. The package involves providing younger children with information about the dangers of smoking, older children with the information, skills and self esteem to resist pressure and finally, adolescents who have started to smoke with support that will help them to stop smoking. Such an approach takes into consideration the childrens age, and state of development. It seeks to provide information and stimulate response in a planned, co-ordinated manner that is developmental in approach and appropriate to the children's needs at different stages in their schooling.

Policy development

AT THE LEVEL OF THE LOCAL EDUCATION AUTHORITY
The development of health education policies both at the country-wide level as well as at the individual school level has been an important part in the development of the health education strategy for Wales. Heartbeat Wales has recommended that each local education authority devises and develops guidelines and/or a policy statement for the role and teaching of education for health in its education establishments. Such policies are now being drawn up and are being developed as a result of discussions between the representatives of the teaching profession, the officials of the local education authority, with advice from the district health authorities health education unit, Heartbeat Wales and other key professional groups such as the drug advisory teachers.

Such policies give added impetus to the adoption of health education programmes in the schools, give added credibility to the concept of health education and give added justification for the necessary time and resources to be allocated to education for health. The policy, as part of the official education authority curriculum policy, would place education for health on the agenda for each of the schools within the authority. Such a policy needs to consider the overall principles of education for health – what subject matter to include, how to achieve organizational changes that might result from adopting a policy, the level of provision of in-service education for teachers and the proportioning of resources, to name but a few.

AT THE LEVEL OF THE INDIVIDUAL SCHOOL

At the individual school level it is imperative that the activities and ethos of a school do not undermine what is being taught as good practice in the classroom. For this reason it is essential that each school has a clearly defined health education/promotion policy and that each school takes its responsibilities as a health promoting community seriously. Examples of particular issues that are currently being addressed are:

a. The school smoking policy and this includes staff as well as pupils;
b. The schools healthy eating policy.

A school smoking policy needs to look at the following issues. Firstly, so far as pupils are concerned, are they offered counselling or support when they admit to smoking or are caught smoking on the school premises, or are they simply punished for breaking school rules? The majority of schools forbid pupils smoking, yet very few offer counselling or cessation groups for those who want to give up. For pupils, smoking is often perceived as being an 'adult' activity, yet in these days when many adults are giving up smoking, smoking cessation groups could be promoted to young people as also being an adult 'activity'. Heartbeat Wales therefore is encouraging all schools to have a written policy on pupils' smoking and that this should be distributed to pupils and parents as the pupils enter the school in their first year. Such a policy may well forbid pupils smoking on the premises and have clearly stated consequences for those who break this rule. But it would also show that the opportunity and support for those who wish to give up smoking is provided by means of smoking cessation groups and counselling methods.

So far as the staff are concerned, Heartbeat Wales, by collaborating with a wide range of organizations, is looking to support and facilitate the development of smoking policies in workplaces in the principality. To be successful, smoking policies must recognize both the rights of the non-smoker and the needs of the smoker. Organizations such as the Trades Union Congress in Wales, Action against Smoking and Health in Wales and the British Institute of Management are actively supporting this process. For the school this means the development of a clearly identified policy with 'no smoking areas' but with perhaps one smoking area where there would be no contact with pupils. The successful development of such a policy depends upon discussion between all concerned.

In addition, teachers must be aware of their responsibilities as exemplary role models. It is important that those who wish to smoke do not do so where they can be seen by the pupils. We are also recommending that all the places visited by parents when they visit a school, for example, the entrance area, and reception area should be designated as no smoking areas and that they should be clearly sign-posted to that effect. In other words, anyone visiting the school should be under no misapprehensions that they are in a 'no smoking' area. In one LEA in Wales this principle has been applied very rigorously and schools are 'no smoking' areas twenty-four hours a day. This means that groups using school facilities outside normal school hours also have to conform to this rule which means that the children in the school should never be able to smell or see the remains of smoking practices.

A school smoking policy will probably only directly affect a minority of those who either work in or attend the school. While this minority may not be an insignificant one, the numbers influenced by a healthy eating policy may well be greater. For such a policy to be effective it needs to address the situation within the school's canteen and dining room as well as the school's tuck shop.

As a result of close co-operation between Heartbeat Wales and the school meals organizers in Wales, a healthy eating policy for schools has been developed and implemented. The overall aim of this policy is 'to help pupils choose and eat a healthy diet'. Three specific areas are contained within the above aim, firstly, pupils' awareness of the concepts behind eating for health and how receptive they are to the foods on offer. Secondly, the nutrition needs of the pupils and how these can best be met and thirdly, the budget controls under which the school meals service operates. One of the specific objectives of the policy is stated thus: 'to increase awareness of the healthier foods amongst staff, pupils and parents and as a consequence of this, increasing the uptake of the healthier foods amongst the groups mentioned' (WHP 1987). Evidence exists that where the policy has been fully implemented, the uptake of healthy foods has increased and the implementation of the policy is being well received by staff and pupils alike.

It is also of the utmost importance that the healthy eating policy adopted by a school or college is reinforced by what is taught in the classroom. The close co-operation of teaching staff and the school meals organizers/school cooks will clearly enhance this process.

THE ROLE OF THE SCHOOL MEDICAL SERVICE

During its school career a child will come into contact with the school medical service, that is, school doctor and school nurse on several occasions. When the child's class or year group are being routinely screened or immunized, for example. This provides an ideal opportunity for the medical service to offer advice and counselling on lifestyle issues, especially those of smoking, healthy eating and the importance of exercise. Such advice is already being offered in some circumstances, but the advantage of having it as an integral part of the screening process is that every child will have the opportunity to listen to the advice and guidance of an expert, that is not a school teacher. This is an important point as some children have negative views towards school and do not readily accept the information provided by their teachers.

It is through the adoption of school based policies, for example, the school smoking and healthy eating policy that many of the young people of Wales are brought into contact with organizational strategies designed to promote good health. It is the responsibility of all concerned in health promotion to ensure that the full potential of these policies is achieved.

Professional training

TEACHERS

With so much activity in health education and health promotion occurring, it is vitally important that the expertise of professional groups involved in delivering the messages is as up to date as possible. For this reason Heartbeat Wales has been extensively involved in the training of the professional groups concerned. Such training is necessary for two main reasons, firstly to provide teachers with the knowledge that they need concerning the issues they are involved with and secondly as a result of the teaching methods recommended to be used in some of the topic areas which may well be unfamiliar to the teachers concerned. Such methods include role play, the correct use of trigger films and discussion groups and also the organization of discussion groups.

STUDENT TEACHERS

Heartbeat Wales is also promoting the use of the health education authorities' initial teacher education course in those colleges and institutions with teacher training courses that are currently not dealing with the issues of health education and health promotion. We are also encouraging such colleges to provide a compulsory health education course for all students on initial teacher training courses.

GOVERNORS

A further key group for whom training has become a priority is that of school governors. The Education Acts of 1986 and 1988 have made several important changes in the way schools are governed. If health education and health promotion is to remain a high priority for schools, then it is imperative that governors are provided with a background knowledge of the issues involved and also some practical experience on how these issues can be tackled. Governors come from a wide range of backgrounds, they might include parents, nominated representatives of the local education authority, teachers, the head teacher of the school as well as representatives from local business and commerce. To help these individuals come to terms with their responsibilities relating to health education, Heartbeat Wales has commissioned the production of a resource pack. This pack will be disseminated through a variety of different means but it is hoped that all governors in Wales, will within the next year to eighteen months, come into contact with the material and thus have a better understanding of what health education actually involves.

PARENTS

The involvement of parents in the education of their children in health education (and thus their own education as well) is a vital component of the Heartbeat Wales youth strategy. As well as the school governors' pack which suggests to governors that they might involve parents in the lifestyle education of their children by, for example, inviting them onto working parties or by hosting a materials and content evening, when new and sensitive areas of the curriculum are being developed. It is also intended that all materials currently being developed will, wherever possible, include an element of parental involvement. This is being achieved by including work that the children can do at home with their parents, providing information leaflets for parents and by seeking to involve parents in special activities in schools, such as health weeks. Such a 'health week' enables health to receive a very high profile. The school canteen for example produces only healthy food, assemblies and other lessons are devoted to health issues, exercise activities are made available both in normal physical education time and during periods set aside for extra-curricular activities. The organization of sponsored fun runs and suchlike with the proceeds going to charities involved in health promotion and health care and parents being involved in as many of these activities as possible, provides an opportunity for parents to become aware of the issues that their children are confronting in school.

Mass communicaton through TV and print

A children's health club called Pulse is currently being piloted in four of the local education authorities in Wales. It currently has a membership of two thousand children. To become a member of the club, each child has to sign a pledge not to smoke. Once they are members they receive three magazines a year. The content of the magazine covers issues relating to health, for example, eating healthily, exercising and not smoking. Within the magazine there are sections that invite the children to write in response to the articles they had read, to send in competition entries and produce reports about health issues in their locality. The children also receive a membership card that in some areas enables them to gain reduced admission prices to leisure facilities as well as obtaining reductions in price on articles bought in sports shops.

The pulse project maintains the Heartbeat Wales policy at producing all material bilingually. This policy is particularly well identified in the work that Heartbeat Wales has undertaken with the press and media. Several television series have been co-produced with local TV companies. These are also being used by schools in their health education teaching programmes, a development that Heartbeat Wales is encouraging. In addition it is proposed to produce articles for inclusion in magazines read by young people. These articles will be along the theme of healthy lifestyles and will seek to encourage their adoption by the young people of Wales. Many radio, TV and newspaper interviews have been held and members of the organization have been able through such interviews to convey the messages relating to healthy lifestyles to the population of Wales as a whole. Clearly such articles are also being read by the young people of Wales and this method of making the information available to them reinforces strongly the work being undertaken in schools and colleges.

Youth clubs and voluntary youth organizations

The production of material suitable for use in youth clubs and other settings where young people meet both formally and informally has long been a high priority. These materials include items on the risks associated with smoking, smoking cessation groups, the importance of exercise, healthy eating and sensible use of alcohol. In line with the development of this material, Heartbeat Wales has recommended that youth clubs and youth organizations adopt both a smoking policy and a healthy eating policy that is similar in nature to those described in schools. These will ensure that there are clearly identified areas where smoking is permitted and areas where it is not, it will provide support for those who wish to stop smoking, and it will provide an environment in which healthy eating becomes the norm. The adoption of these policies by youth clubs and youth organizations will again enhance the work that is being undertaken in schools and will provide the young people of Wales with many opportunities to experience a health promoting environment.

In conjunction with these materials and policy development, training sessions have occurred for youth leaders and organizers which have provided them with background information and have enabled them to become familiar with the material and policies that they are seeking to use and implement.

Supporting the macro-initiatives

All the activities previously described for young people complement and support the other initiatives of Heartbeat Wales, targeted at the adult population. These initiatives include the promotion of 'no smoking' areas in public places; the development of smoking policies in the workplace; the monitoring of the voluntary code on tobacco advertising; the establishment of links with the food retail organizations leading to food labelling schemes and the promotion of healthy options in shops, cafés, restaurants and canteens; the promotion of leisure activities in order to encourage and motivate people to exercise regularly and the use of the media to carry health promotion messages into people's homes. Each of these has at least an indirect affect on the young people of Wales and will enable them to see many of the health promotion issues which they have been learning about in school, being dealt with in a much wider context.

The creation of the Health Promotion Authority for Wales

Initially Heartbeat Wales was established as a five year demonstration programme, funded jointly with the Welsh Office and the HEC. However, on 1 April 1987 a new authority was created to replace the HEC. The new Health Education Authority maintained many of the Health Education Council's activities with the major difference that it no longer had responsibility for health education in Wales.

In Wales a separate body was established by the Secretary of State. The

Health Promotion Authority for Wales (HPAW) as it is now known, has incorporated the two major health education/promotion initiatives which were in existence prior to 1 April 1987, namely the Welsh Aids Campaign and Heartbeat Wales. Funded directly by the Welsh Office the HPAW has responsibility for health promotion throughout the principality, covering all relevant issues. Heartbeat Wales is one of the new authority's major programmes and all the activities previously described are continuing apace with the added benefit that the time scale for some now stretches beyond the end of 1990.

The HPAW is currently identifying its future activities and is devising a strategic plan. Issues that are likely to be included within the strategic plan include, cancer education, the sensible use of alcohol an HIV education programme and lifestyle issues particularly those relating to coronary heart disease.

The establishment of the HPAW is an indication of the importance attached to health promotion in Wales by the various bodies concerned. Building on the links established between Heartbeat Wales and the various statutory and voluntary organizations, the new authority is continuing to ensure that health education and health promotion gain increasing importance and priority in the workings of those organizations. That this is being achieved is shown in the increasing levels of health education and health promotion throughout the principality.

The national curriculum

A major challenge facing health education in the future is the implementation of the Government's national curriculum. While health education is identified as an important element within the curriculum, its place is seen in the context of a cross curricular theme. The recent publication of the science working groups report however, gives some cause for optimism as it identifies many opportunities for health education within the science curriculum. Health educators and the HPAW are mindful of their responsibilities in ensuring that where these opportunities exist, they are utilized to the full. This has implications for the resourcing of health education, and it is to be hoped that sufficient resources will be found by the organizations involved to provide additional classroom material to meet the demand, and especially a sufficient level of in-service education for teachers and other professional groups who come into contact with children, so that their expertise and knowledge is adequate for the task.

The Master of Science Degree in Health Promotion

The HPAW, through the Institute of Health Promotion (IHP), (the IHP is part of the University of Wales College of Medicine but is funded and staffed by the HPAW) is offering a Master of Science Degree in Health Promotion. Such a degree provides an opportunity for those involved in health education/health promotion, to study in greater detail the philosophy, principle and processes of health promotion. They are then expected to use the knowledge and experience that they have gained in their own sphere of activity. The IHP is also hoping to organize differing courses meeting the needs of other professionals in health education/health promotion in the future.

Conclusions

Health education in Wales received a considerable boost from the creation of Heartbeat Wales. For the first time Wales possessed a national health education programme (albeit only considering cardio-vascular diseases) with its own identity and character. Under the leadership of Professor John Catford, progress was rapid and the evaluation process which occurred as part of the programme has shown a high level of awareness amongst the general population and increase in levels of activity in all settings especially in education establishments. By working in close co-operation and collaboration with statutory and voluntary organizations, a high degree of unanimity has been achieved which has considerably enhanced the overall process.

The establishment of the Health Promotion Authority for Wales has further benefited health promotion in the country and has given it a more permanent basis. As a wider range of issues are dealt with in the future, the foundation already laid through the activity of Heartbeat Wales will provide an excellent platform on which to build.

References

Health Education Journal (1987) The health promoting school organization and policy development in Welsh secondary schools *Health Education Journal* **46**, 3

The Welsh Heart Programme (1985a) Heartbeat report number one *Take Heart* pages 6 and 7

The Welsh Heart Programme (1985b) Heartbeat report number two *Take Heart* pages 7 and 8

The Welsh Heart Programme (1987) Healthy eating policy for schools in Wales

24. From theory into practice – Lose Weight Wales – A CASE STUDY

H Howson

Summary: We were faced with a challenge: The Pulse of Wales showed that approximately 43 per cent of people in Wales were overweight or obese. Yet in the clinical survey results, where clinical researchers weighed and measured individuals, it was found to be almost 50 per cent. This was shown to be well above the national average.

At any one time it is estimated that approximately 65 per cent of the population are on some form of diet to help them lose weight, yet they seem to get nowhere on a permanent basis.

For two years the Heartbeat Wales Nutrition Programme (HWNP) dealt specifically with promoting healthy eating in the community. However, when the clinical results emerged there was a need to address this target group specifically. It was also a 'new face' on which we could promote the healthy eating messages which were in danger of losing impact.

As a result the Lose Weight Wales (LWW) campaign emerged. This had to create public awareness of the problem and then encourage and support individuals and groups to do something about it. It also had to clarify that we were promoting a healthier way of eating on a permanent basis. We sought to address our challenge and achieve our objectives in a variety of approaches involving industry and commerce, as well as the health sector. This was as part of an overall health promotion package for the people in Wales.

Introduction

Heartbeat Wales was set up as a five year intervention programme to reduce the incidence of cardio-vascular disease. The HWNP has played a major role in helping to reduce the risks by encouraging a healthy varied diet. The 1985 Pulse of Wales survey results, which covered over 22,000 households, was able to identify current dietary trends as well as other indicators on nutritional knowledge and general attitudes towards health. This highlighted some of the problems with which we were faced and provided some guidance as to where we ought to be directing our resources.

The Heart-beat Wales Nutrition Programme

The HWNP has for over two years pioneered a variety of approaches to improve the dietary patterns of the Welsh population as a whole. These initiatives varied from developments at macro level with major food retailers to intervention at more local levels with community and voluntary groups, offering practical advice and guidelines, towards healthier eating habits. The programme has sought to promote healthy eating messages while addressing the issues of supply and demand. In the past mistakes have been made amidst the general enthusiasm to give advice and promote health messages, without ensuring that individuals are able to follow this action through. For example, we may encourage individuals to partake in the healthy eating messages, but unless they can interpret and purchase the food in the store or the canteen the time and effort invested is wasted.

The HWNP recognized this concept early in the programme and sought to work with the food and other industries in order to help facilitate changes at household level. The programme has liaised with the major food retailer Tesco to undertake a food labelling system, nutrition information for customers, health fayres, as well as nutrition training for staff along with improved in-house catering facilities. It established close liaison with the Meat and Livestock Commission to introduce new methods of grading and cutting, to produce leaner meat, and consider ways of communicating this to the public. Collaboration with the major milk supplier, Unigate, to promote the sale of skimmed and semi-skimmed milk at doorstep delivery was also shown to be effective as a means of changing food purchasing patterns.

The significant role of caterers in effecting changes in food consumption was also recognized. This led to programmes providing both 'hands on' experience within catering establishments and the development of a menu labelling system for use in catering outlets of all kinds. The Heartwise menu scheme was a comprehensive package providing guidelines and resources for caterers at all levels and was disseminated widely.

School meals policy guidelines were also developed in order to encourage the promotion and uptake of 'healthy' meals by children. This encompassed recipe and menu analysis, staff training, the development of support materials as well as corresponding curricula materials and liaison programmes with the teaching staff.

We had also recognized the importance of working closely with the media to reinforce our efforts and to help communicate and enhance our messages. A ten week series of television programmes entitled *When the Chips are Down* perused our 'mission' to convert the Welsh people to adopt a healthier approach to eating. This was systematically enhanced with media support from local radio stations and the regional newspapers.

A time for change – the evolution of Lose Weight Wales

The term 'healthy eating' became almost an everyday word that was in danger of becoming ineffective in making any further progress towards change. While faced with this dilemma the clinical survey results, 1988, were published, showing us that we were dealing with a population who not only ate an unhealthy balance of foods, but ate excessive amounts and took very little exercise to counter this effect. As a result we were faced with a population where nearly 50 per cent was overweight or obese. Of this, within the age group of 18 to 65, there were more overweight men than women, yet more obese women than men. It was at this stage that we recognized the need to consider targeting this group specifically and so LWW evolved. The LWW campaign provided an answer to some of our concerns. It provided a slightly different vehicle by which we could promote our healthy eating messages, while tackling the problems of overweight. We were able to link a number of initiatives already developed into this campaign, as well as developing new approaches and a new identity to help deal with the problem. It also allowed the opportunity to clarify misconceptions about diets and dieting and promote a sustained, healthier way of eating on a permanent basis, avoiding faddy, short term or very low calorie diets. It also enabled us to include messages to increase physical activity in a balanced context with food consumption.

The aim of the LWW campaign was to encourage people to achieve their ideal weight for height and maintain this by adopting healthier eating habits. It was important to recognize that while it can be relatively easy to achieve a weight loss, it is much more difficult to maintain this 'ideal' weight. Therefore the time scale was crucial and had to take account of this at the planning stage. The campaign was to last 18 months to encompass two summer periods and one Christmas. These are key receptive periods for the messages being promoted.

Firstly in the lead up to the summer, from Whitsun onwards, people are planning holidays and are therefore more concerned about 'baring all' in their swimwear. Secondly in the post-Christmas period when individuals recognize their excessive eating and drinking and the need to make New Year's resolutions to redress the effects of these acts of gluttony.

The objectives identified at the outset were as follows:

1. Through a variety of staggered media events to help raise public awareness of the need to maintain the correct height for weight.
2. To provide individuals and groups in the community with the motivation and skills necessary to achieve weight loss and maintain their correct height for weight.
3. To provide appropriate guidelines and information on weight loss to achieve both short term and long term weight-loss goals.
4. To develop a variety of resources that will help both individuals and groups to attain their correct height for weight.
5. To provide the healthy eating and general lifestyle messages as part of the LWW campaign.

The launch of Lose Weight Wales

Before we could launch a campaign we needed to establish an identity. The LWW title and logo were adopted after much consideration. In doing so we tried to include the concept of the heart, but change the image of previous Heartbeat Wales materials by using a yellow colour and a tape measure pattern to form the heart shape. This also linked in with the corresponding artwork for the planned TV series.

LWW was launched in the first week of June. This launch was preceded by the release of the clinical survey results highlighting the current weight problems in the principality.

The launch of the campaign needed a high public profile and it was recognized in the early stages of planning that a television series would provide this. Although approximately 65 per cent of people are thought to be continually dieting there had, to date, been no television series concerned with this topic. With this in mind we were able to negotiate with BBC Wales the joint production of a six week television series to coincide with our launch, in early June, entitled *The BBC Diet Programme*.

The television series was intended as 'light entertainment' and involved a variety of celebrities as well as ten key volunteers who were followed throughout the series. The series presented the key messages in a light-hearted, amusing way that encouraged viewers to watch. The programme timing was also important to viewing as it followed a popular 'soap' programme and from our early unofficial results, it is claimed to have even topped the viewing figures for some of the programmes.

The joint launch and publicity leading up to the programmes and start of the LWW campaign generated considerable public and media interest. As a result of the high profile we were also able to achieve considerable newspaper coverage and a long-standing Radio Series on the same theme. Having raised public interest and the profile of LWW we now had to provide on-going support for those who needed it, as well as maintain interest and enthusiasm.

The support resources

In the planning stages we identified the key support resources for this programme. In the past, lessons had been learnt from high public profile campaigns falling short because of the lack of support for the messages they promoted.

With this in mind a number of resources were developed for both individuals and groups within the community. Firstly a self-supporting information pack, The Healthy Eating Guide to Losing Weight, providing the key message for individuals wishing to address the problems for themselves.

This package contains sections covering planning and preparation for weight loss, healthy eating guidelines, diet plans, recipes as well as advice on exercise, shopping and eating out. It also provides ideas for gaining and winning support and includes a 'contract' that can be signed by a partner on the way to achieving his or her target weight. It was planned to provide the packs to support the television series, but as momentum was increasing the BBC, in conjunction with Heartbeat Wales, decided to produce a book entitled *The BBC Diet Book*. This included more detailed information and was distributed through our networks for sale as well as through the television series itself.

Secondly it was recognized that people lost weight through informal group contact. These were individuals who often needed some support from friends or colleagues at work, but who would not consider joining a more formal weight-loss class. Therefore there was a need to produce guidelines for those people wishing to adopt this method and so 'Guidelines for Setting up your own Weight Loss Group' was produced. This was disseminated to a variety of both lay and professional groups. With this package we were able to provide the correct, consistent information, present ideas as to how they may put this into practice as well as presenting ideas for running a group, group support and weight maintenance.

Thirdly the need to provide group support for people wishing to lose weight was also addressed. The importance of linking such behaviour change into an overall 'lifestyle' context was crucial and often omitted from commercially developed classes. The Look After Yourself class, which offers a 10 week course for adults, on exercise, stress and relaxation and various health topics, provided an excellent basis from which to work. Look After Yourself also recognized the need to revise methods of marketing the course, as the philosophy behind it was often difficult to grasp by the general public, who were confused as to what to expect.

The LWW Look After Yourself courses were developed by taking the health topic section over to weight loss issues. This involved programme planning, tutor training, piloting and evaluation of the course as well as marketing them as part of the LWW campaign. We had to ensure that enough classes were established to meet the demands though in some more rural areas this was not always possible.

The possibility of negotiating with commercially run slimming groups was also considered. If this was to be taken forward we needed to ensure that the messages and mechanisms which they followed were sound and fitted in with the LWW philosophy. There was the advantage that they had already established a considerable network system throughout Wales for dealing with weight loss groups throughout the principality. However, our first priority was to try to meet the needs with the Look After Yourself groups. Other miscellaneous support materials were also developed. This included a leaflet for general distribution, The Simple Guide to Losing Weight, which highlighted the other support materials that individuals could send for.

Also badges, fridge stickers and t-shirts were made available throughout the campaign.

LWW and the commercial sector

The 18 month programme established strategically planned activities throughout this period to enhance the campaign, and help maintain momentum. This involved collaboration with a number of organizations and target groups to help achieve our objectives. This was achieved by planning programmes with commercial organizations, many of whom we had already established collaboration on healthy eating initiatives. LWW provided another means by which we could re-establish the original liaison, providing a new and fresh approach towards healthy eating.

We were able to link the Lean Choice Scheme which we had established with the MLC, to promote leaner cuts of meat in butcher shops, with the campaign. The term 'lean' enabled this to tie in well. This was to be extended in the autumn along with a series of cookery demonstrations linked with British Gas (Wales). The theme Let's Talk Lose Weight Wales, was adapted and highlighted healthy and exciting dishes that were low in calories. They were run in six venues throughout Wales, with audiences of approximately 200 people. The joint liaison with our voluntary groups and networks helped make the communication with interested bodies easier.

The extension of this into British Gas as a workplace initiative, and as part of their display materials in local gas showrooms, illustrates the benefits of working with such bodies in helping to promote health throughout the community. Unigate, the major milk retailer in Wales, were also involved in the campaign in a number of ways. They jointly produced a leaflet promoting both the campaign generally and the purchase of skimmed and semi-skimmed milk, at doorstep delivery. This took the campaign into thousands of households, inviting them to participate in the campaign by changing their purchase of milk to the lower fat version and offering prizes as an incentive. We were also able to involve milkmen themselves in LWW and utilize them as door to door outlets for the purchase of the *BBC Diet Book*. Milk floats carrying the LWW logo also enhanced their involvement and extended the profile of the campaign within the community.

The liaison with Tesco's was well established and it was a natural extension of the nutrition programme to involve them in LWW. This was primarily in the distribution of materials, promotion of low calorie products, and the in-house activities of staff joining the campaign.

Other options to work with retail chemists were also explored and provided an ideal opportunity to extend their role in the field of health promotion. It also enabled LWW to be taken into smaller communities bringing it into closer contact with individuals.

Involving the voluntary sector

The networks of voluntary organizations in the principality were also another prime target group for the campaign. Liaison with those networks were well established and this helped in the dissemination of the campaign materials and the 'group' pack in particular. This provided guidelines for existing groups who could take on board LWW and set up their own informal support sessions. This also provided such groups with the opportunity to participate with a health promotion activity that they could measure to some extent, and one that many of them had already some previous experience of.

For those who were particularly interested to find out more, workshops were offered to allow an opportunity to discuss the issues and the implications of losing weight and clarify any misconceptions. Such organizations as the Women's Institute (WI), Ladies Circle, Young Farmer's Club (YFC) and many others provided ample opportunity to extend the campaign.

LWW in the workplace

The existing programme for health promotion in the workplace encouraged industries to adopt policies addressing issues such as smoking, health screening and catering. The programme already worked closely with 18 major industries and liaised generally with other industries throughout Wales.

This included considerable involvement with both the TUC and the CBI and provided a platform for the extension of LWW. On-going discussion with the TUC, to consider options for this, are underway and the Make Health Your Business award, organized jointly with the Confederation of British Industry (CBI), highlights 'ideas for action' and includes references to joining the LWW campaign. The next major initiative planned for the New Year is to launch LWW into industry and encourage their participation. This may be achieved by targeting both the individual and group pack at occupational health, personnel or health and safety representatives. It is anticipated that we will follow these up in six months to reveal the participation and total weight lost for each industry. Suggestions and incentives to lose and maintain ideal weight may include: raising money for a local charity, or £1 for 1 lb lost from the employer, the provision of an exercise bike and other leisure facilities even a shower at work. The package will outline the programme, providing guidelines and ideas for action in the workplace. This may range from the provision of weighing scales to the establishment of support groups or even exercise sessions at lunchtime. This will also allow interested individuals the opportunity to attend a workshop for further details.

By launching this in the New Year we will be able to play on the fact that many people will have overeaten and drunk to excess during this period and will generally be more receptive to this information.

The Healthy Hospital initiative provides a similar mechanism to extending this into the National Health Service (NHS) workforce. We are already aware of some health authorities adopting a policy not to employ overweight nurses and this campaign and the resources will provide them with the opportunity to support such decisions and be seen to be actively involved in a health promotion activity. A variety of contact points are open to us in its dissemination and these could include occupational health staff, chief administrative medical/nursing officers and general managers.

The primary health care team

The primary health care network is one of particular importance as it provides key points of contact with individuals within the overweight category. It is well known that information or advice given to patients by their general practitioner (GP) has a greater chance of being followed through than by other individuals or professionals. We needed not only to build on this, but to offer clear concise guidelines on weight loss for the GP to use with his patient. The individual weight loss pack provides this and further group support is also suggested for those who need it, in the form of Lose Weight and Look After Yourself Courses. Each GP practice has been circulated with details of the campaign forewarning them of the timescale and materials being developed. They have also been sent materials for use within their practice and directly with their patients. They will be encouraged to consider, in conjunction with their practice nurse, or primary health care facilitator, the possibility of establishing a weight loss group within the practice.

Other health professionals such as district health education officers, dieticians and health visitors have also been kept updated with the information and invited to participate wherever possible or applicable. Many dieticians are using the materials as part of their on-going weight reducing clinic resources.

Timetabled as part of the campaign is a conference aiming to up-date health professionals and other interested individuals. This will cover the basic fundamentals of assessing over weight and the reasons behind it, and the psychological and practical aspects of applying theory into practice. Traditionally Heartbeat Wales has been concerned not only with changes at policy level, but the methods by which we can see changes in both lifestyle and health status to help achieve our goals and ultimately improve the health of the Welsh population.

Measuring its effect

In establishing such a campaign we need to measure its effectiveness in achieving the goals identified at the outset. This will be achieved by process evaluation and hard data looking at changes in the body mass index. It is too early in the programme to be able to draw any conclusions yet as we are only six months into an 18 month campaign. However, we have received some feedback indicating the success of the television series and of the support packages that were sent out. For the period of the programme and just after we had sold 8000 BBC Diet Packs at three pounds each. The response from the general public and the media have been overwhelming and we have informal feedback that the TV series has topped the viewing for one of UK's most popular soaps. Such is the success that the BBC are networking a repeat of the series in the New Year. We also established a five month radio programme on Losing Weight for Wales.

We can also monitor the number of Lose Weight/Look After Yourself classes established and enquiries from individuals and groups for these, along with requests for further leaflets and resources.

At a different level we will be able to measure changes in the body mass index as well as acquire interim measures from the Omnibus and Welsh Health Promotion Authority survey. Here we will be able to assess awareness and other parameters of change. Questions will also be built into health and other professional surveys including the GP Survey, to provide us with more detailed information. We also have over 200 individuals who participated with the TV series that we will be able to monitor retrospectively along with those individuals who have written in for packs and other resources.

We are only a few months into the campaign, but we are already seeing that considerable interest is being shown. Our challenge still has to be achieved. In this case the 'proof of the pudding will NOT be in the eating', or in how much weight is lost, but in how people who join LWW can achieve and perhaps more importantly maintain their ideal weight for height, whilst establishing healthy eating habits on a permanent basis.

25. Health education in England – AN OVERVIEW

K Tones

Summary: An effective health promotion service within a nation requires a synergistic relationship between public policy-making and education. In recent years England has moved towards this position and is currently beginning to seriously address the implementation of WHO's HFA 2000 goals through health promotion and the healthy cities initiatives. This chapter has attempted to provide an overview of the contemporary health education scene and its historical antecedents.

England has a central Health Education Authority which launches mass media campaigns and supports the critically important infra-structure of interpersonal health education delivered by professional and lay health educators. Its system of health education is special in that each district health authority has a health education or health promotion unit employing specialist health education staff whose role is to support, stimulate and co-ordinate the activities of the interpersonal infra-structure mentioned above. Major features of the work of these 'agencies' have been described and in particular the work of schools, primary health care and community development. Despite a limited presence in the workplace, the non-existence of patient education in hospitals and the threat to health education in schools posed by the new national curriculum, the future looks reasonably bright. Health promotion appears to be popular with central government – often for the wrong reasons – and the slow growth of health education units continues. Important developments in primary care will hopefully transfuse into the acute sector; community health projects with their outstanding potential for addressing the major health problems of disadvantaged people will receive a major boost from newly established local authority units in the pursuit of healthy cities.

Health promotion and education for health

Before attempting to review the current status of health education in England, it is advisable to clarify a few terms. Apart from the fact that health education means different things to different people, it is virtually impossible to provide a meaningful analysis without first considering the symbiotic relationship between health education and health policy which is at the centre of health promotion. A detailed discussion of this is beyond the scope of this chapter. However, before considering the main ways in which health education is delivered in England, an attempt will be made to succinctly describe how different approaches to health education contribute to health promotion.

Figure 25.1 below views the promotion of health (and the avoidance of disease) as the result of three major influences: the lifestyle choices made by individuals, the social and physical environment in which individuals live and work and, last and arguably least, the medical services.

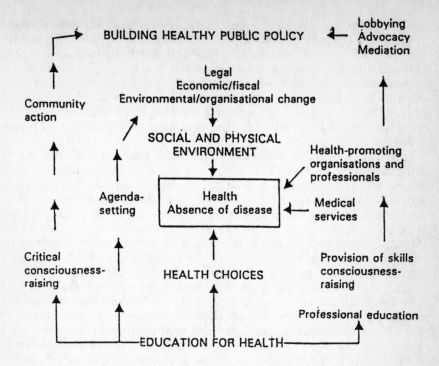

Figure 25.1 *The contribution of education to health promotion* (Tones, 1987)

Health education has traditionally been concerned to prevent disease (at primary, secondary and tertiary levels) and promote the 'proper' use of health services by influencing health choices. More recently this kind of approach has been condemned as 'victim blaming' while, at the same time, the creation of a healthy environment has been urged as a more effective and ethical alternative. The social-structural change involved in creating such an environment requires what the Ottawa Charter (WHO 1986) describes as Building Healthy Public Policy which influences the environment by means of legislative measures which include among other things selective taxation and an injection of money designed to mitigate the unhealthy effects of poverty and deprivation. The creation of health promoting public policy will depend on the normal processes of political influence – the Ottawa Charter singles out lobbying, advocacy and mediation. However, the substantial funding and political will required to achieve most major public health initiatives will not be forthcoming without equally substantial pressure from the public. This pressure will be exerted to a greater or lesser extent as a result of education. The creation of healthy public policy has been associated with a 'new public health' movement; health education which contributes to the new public health differs from traditional, individually-focused education in its concern to energize the public and bring about environmental change.

The new health education is shown in Figure 25.1 as having two strands.

the first paves the way for change by its agenda-setting function. A classic example of this is provided by various road safety campaigns which sought to persuade individuals to wear safety belts in cars. While this traditional variety of health education had only limited success in achieving this goal, it was undoubtedly successful in 'agenda setting', that is raising the issue with the public to the extent that government was willing to take the electoral risk of enacting legislation which infringed individual freedom and might well have alienated potential voters without the awareness raising function of health education.

The second strand is politically much more problematical: it seeks to stimulate public awareness through the process of critical consciousness raising which is designed to lead to community action. Such action is supposed to pressure government to carry out actions which are not merely inconvenient but often ideologically unacceptable: for instance the alienation of powerful lobbies such as the tobacco and alcohol interests. One of the standard means of delivering such education – community development – will be mentioned below in relation to other strategies for delivering health education. For the present we will note the final role played by health education as delineated in Figure 25.1, namely 'professional education'.

Professional education includes the traditional provision of training for medical services personnel to help them fulfil their health education role vis-à-vis their patients and clients. Within the context of contemporary views of the role of health promotion (see for instance WHO 1987) a new function is identified. As part of the general thrust to demedicalize health, WHO is concerned to generate awareness of the importance of 'inter-sectoral collaboration', that is the ways in which a wide range of professionals contribute to health promotion. A new 'professional education' function is therefore concerned to raise awareness of how, say, town planners, housing managers, trades unions and the like might carry out their potential health promoting responsibilities.

It should be noted that within this all-embracing model of health promotion there will frequently be tension between approaches which are here depicted as complementary. Some intimation of this is apparent in the earlier reference to 'victim blaming' and one of the more obvious conflicts between the proponents of different approaches to health education centres on the distinction between a 'preventive model' which seeks to prevent disease by changing individuals' behaviours and a 'radical model' which is concerned primarily to create social change through the process of critical consciousness raising mentioned above. An analysis of different approaches may be consulted elsewhere (French and Adams, 1986; Tones 1981). For present purposes the general distinction between a preventive 'medical model' and an 'educational model' should be borne in mind as this has some relevance in considering the historical development of health education in England.

Historical aspects

A detailed historical analysis is, of course, beyond the scope of the present article and only a few salient points will be discussed here in order that the contemporary scene may be set in an appropriate perspective. In fact the origins of English health education are many and varied. It is self evident that some form of health education has existed from the earliest times – ever since some humans had sufficient consciousness of their condition to show concern for their well being and others were pretentious enough to advise them how to achieve and maintain it.

At one level, health education might be said to operate whenever the provision of information (in formal or informal fashion and with or without a deliberate intent to influence) has led to changes in social structure or individual practice which have, in turn, resulted in the enhancement of wellbeing or the prevention of disease and disability. Such a definition is too all-embracing and vague for present purposes and the more 'ideological' descriptions of health education and health promotion presented earlier must be supplemented by a more technical definition which will be used as a basis for future observations in this chapter. Accordingly, health education is viewed as a deliberate attempt to promote health-related learning. This involves a relatively permanent change in capability or disposition and might thus comprise the acquisition of knowledge and understanding; the clarification of values, a development of or change in beliefs and/or attitudes; the achievement of competence in psychomotor or social interaction skills. Such learning may or may not result in changes in behaviour or lifestyle; if it has been effective it should always result in enhanced decision-making capabilities.

It should be apparent from the above definition that the stance adopted by the author is an 'educational' one, that is that health education should at any rate strive to foster voluntaristic choice – even if it often falls short of such a counsel of perfection. It might be argued that this approach is individualistic – and indeed it is. This is not to deny the importance of the socio-economic and physical environment in health promotion. However, *individual* attitudes, values, knowledge, beliefs and skills are at the root of community movements and political activism. Health education is therefore fundamentally concerned with individual learning – whether it is concerned with lifestyle modification, the facilitation of decision-making or has more radical socio-political aims.

Although a detailed discussion of the ethical basis of health education cannot be entertained here, it is worth underlining the distinction between health *education* and other related more coercive tactics such as propaganda or indoctrination. While the former is essentially a voluntaristic process in which the learner retains control and has insight into what is happening to her or him, the latter situation is deliberately manipulative and the means of influence may well be subservient to the health promoting ends. Historically, propaganda and pamphleteering rather than education for choice seem to have characterized early health promotion efforts. Sutherland (1987) states that the first *formal* reference to health education *per se* in England was apparently made when the precursor to the Health Education Council and Health Education Authority was established in 1927. This Central Council for Health Education (CCHE) was concerned to promote the '. . . science and art of healthy living . . . in accordance with . . . principles of hygiene . . .' Its goal was that of '. . . safeguarding public health and

preventing disease . . . by *health education* (author's emphasis) and propaganda.' It will be noted in passing that prior to the efforts of Dr Goebbels,
'propaganda' did not generate the kind of opprobrium it does today in
educational circles.

Perhaps the most significant early health propaganda is associated with
the great public health movement of the 19th Century and its 'sanitary' goals
– clean water supply, clean air, sewage disposal, light, improved housing
and the attack on poverty – are too well known to merit further elaboration
here. In relation to the current scene in England, we should however,
remind readers of the emergence of the medical officer of health (MOH)
from the great sanitary movement. Until 1974 the MOH was appointed by
the local authority (that is democratically elected local government) and
vested with security of tenure. The latter point is of especial importance
considering the political sensitivity of many of the environmental health
measures which had to be taken in the interests of public health. In short the
MOH could agitate for unpopular health promotion measures and irritate
the rich and powerful without fear of losing his job. Again, until 1974, the
health education officer, a peculiar feature of the English health education
establishment, was to a large extent created at the whim of the MOH and
responsible to him.

Since the earliest years, the public health nurse or health visitor has been
at the forefront of health promotion and the prevention of disease. Her
major weapon has been health education. As Sutherland (1987) points out,
their origin may be traced to the Manchester and Salford Sanitary Association's employment of '. . . women of the working class to visit poorer
people and teach them the laws of health as early as 1862. In 1890
Manchester Corporation agreed to pay the salaries of six of the city's
fourteen health visitors.' The importance of the health visitor in relation to
primary medical care and community nursing will receive further comment
later.

It is patently obvious that the school is of paramount importance in health
education and it is to be expected that they will have played a major role
during this century. Sutherland (1987), however, asserts that very slow
progress was made and '. . . health propaganda remained on the periphery
of professional interest'. Certainly little change was apparent between 1901
and 1951 despite a series of publications on health, hygiene and health
education. The content of these make interesting reading – especially in
relation to the debate about education versus propaganda.

The first production appears to have been a Syllabus of Hygiene for the
Training of Teachers in 1907 followed in 1928 with a 'Handbook of
Suggestions on Health *Education*' (author's emphasis) in 1928 hard on the
heels of the establishment of the CCHE. Sutherland provides a revealing
summary of aims from the Board of Education's new handbook:

> If children learn at school to keep themselves clean and tidy, to eat
> wholesome food, to keep their classrooms, corridors and playground
> free from litter, to keep the windows open, to see that the lavatories and
> closets are properly used, they are likely to carry these habits into
> practice when they leave school, and in this way will not only assist the

health departments in their task but also do much to build up the health and secure the wellbeing of the community.

By the time that the 1956 version (Ministry of Education, 1956) of the handbook had been published, the mix of morality and public health had, to some extent, been influenced by new epidemiological realities such as smoking, drug misuse, accidents and the like. The didactic flavour was still in evidence in 1968 (Department of Education and Science, 1968). This more recent handbook pointed out how 'In a modern community everybody needs to know and follow the rules of healthy living in order to keep well.' Teachers had '. . . a unique opportunity of giving young people the training in matters of health which they need.' Its 18 chapters comprised five on 'major health topics' – such as 'cleanliness' and 'movement and rest'; four were on 'community health' and the remainder related to general organizational matters. It was not until the 1977 version that the 'hygienic' flavour was to give way to the epidemiological-realities created by the chronic degenerative diseases and the implication of individual lifestyle in disease and premature death. Perhaps the continued marginalization of health education in schools has in part been due to the phenomenon of the 'sabre toothed curriculum' – the tendency of curricula to reflect past concerns rather than present needs.

There is almost unanimous agreement that one of the key influences on modern English health education was the publication in 1964 of the Cohen Report (Cohen Committee, 1964). A detailed review is not possible here but suffice it to say that it added the impetus needed to create the beginnings of an integrated health education service. Although this has hardly yet been fully achieved, considerable progress has been made and this can be traced to the influence of the Cohen Report. Two especially significant developments were the emergence of the Health Education Council and an expansion in the numbers of health education officers.

The Health Education Council was established in 1968 and replaced the former CCHE which had carried the banner of health education since the 1920s. Whereas CCHE had been funded by local authorities and voluntary bodies, the Health Education Council (HEC) was formed as a limited company with a chairman and 'governing' members appointed by the Secretary of State for Social Services. It was in fact a QUANGO (Quasi Autonomous Government Organization) in that it received its financial support from government while retaining a degree of independence. A full and interesting history of HEC has recently been published by Sutherland (1988), and the following comments on HEC's contribution to English Health Education will of necessity be sketchy. First it must be said that unlike its recent replacement, HEC was responsible for health education in Wales and Northern Ireland as well as England. During the 19 years of its existence, its contribution to health education has been considerable. Apart from its national (and arguably less important) function of providing mass-media based campaigns, HEC has made a lasting impact through its policy of meeting the needs of a wide range of health professionals for education, training and general support. It acted as a catalyst for many developments, sensitizing workers to their unrecognized potential health education functions and providing resources for those who fully acknowledged their role. It provided pump-priming and funding for major education and training initiatives and the current academic base of health education in England is almost completely due to the initiatives of HEC's council and officers. In addition to providing training and support for all of the delivery strategies described in Figure 25.3 below, it developed the research base of health education and, together with its support of academic establishments, has made a major contribution to the theoretical underpinnings of the subject. These important influences are nowhere more apparent than in HEC's support of school health education.

The Cohen Report, which was not charged with the task of considering the education sector, nonetheless emphasized the paramount importance of developing a strong school base – and, incidentally, continued the trend whereby health professionals ascribed more importance than teachers to the schools' potential for health promotion. Indeed the tendency to view the schools as another wing of preventive medicine exemplifies well one of the important philosophical polarities mentioned earlier – the tension between preventive medical and educational models of health education. However, to return to HEC's contribution to the schools, Cohen's recommendation was vigorously heeded and it is undoubtedly true to say that HEC, during the final years of its reign, made a bigger contribution to curriculum development than any other organization. Indeed, since the demise of the Schools Council, it probably generated a larger number of curriculum projects in health and social education than in all other subject areas combined.

It is perhaps too early to comment authoritatively on the reasons for HEC's replacement by the Health Education Authority (HEA) in 1987. What is clear is that the HEA is organizationally much more closely wedded to the National Health Service as a special health authority and is thus more directly under the control of the Minister. It has been speculated that HEC's demise had something to do with its irritating habit of disagreeing with government views about the measures needed to improve the nation's health and the kinds of educational methods which were most appropriate to attaining those goals which both HEC and government both believed to be important. In the context of later discussions, it is worth observing that a significant point of disagreement had been over the use of mass media. HEC had increasingly adopted a view that mass media were not a panacea which could be used, for example, to eradicate drug misuse: interpersonal education through schools, health professionals and community development were considered to be more important. For these reasons – and in common with most expert opinion – a media based heroin campaign was considered inappropriate. Government was therefore obliged to develop and operate its own programme. The validity of this step is beyond the scope of this discussion and is considered elsewhere (Tones, 1986): the point is made here to emphasize the significance of independence in the context of an increasing recognition of the political dimension to the 'new public health'. Indeed HEC's departure from the public scene was not undramatic and coincided with what has been described as an almost underground publication of a document which provided evidence of the increasing gap in health status between the privileged and underprivileged social classes in the UK (Whitehead, 1987).

Then and now

Before shifting the perspective from the past to the present, it is illuminating to ponder on the changes which have taken place in philosophy and approach of health education. Perhaps the most intriguing phenomenon is the way in which the wheel has almost turned full circle (although perhaps a curricular spiral might be a more appropriate geometrical analogy). The progress of health education in many ways mirrors the progress of medicine as viewed by influential epidemiologists such as McKeown (McKeown, 1976). In the 19th Century the major problems were poverty-related and environmentally initiated infectious diseases. Medicine was incapable of handling community health problems and remained ineffectual until the mid 1930s. The major improvement in public health which had occurred by the time medicine had begun to acquire the means of combating disease was due to the public health measures mentioned earlier – better nutrition, population control, sanitary measures and suchlike.

The kind of health education accompanying the early improvements tended to be propagandist – and it is interesting to note Sutherland's (1987) reference to the *Times'* comment about the General Board of Health's zealotry, 'We prefer to take the chance of cholera and the rest than to be bullied into health.'

With the increasing recognition that the 'magic bullets', which were then available to deal with the rapidly disappearing problem of infectious diseases, were less appropriate for the newly recognized problems of chronic degenerative disease, health education shifted its focus. In the face of opposition and indifference from acute medicine, preventive medicine sought to absorb health education as a device which might be used to prevent the incurable and cope with the intractable. It would of course achieve this by influencing unhealthy lifestyles. Health education was now less concerned with raising awareness and campaigning for social action but almost entirely preoccupied with acquiring techniques to persuade individuals to modify their behaviour. Health education as employed by medicine (as opposed to the continuing 'educational' tradition occasionally found in schools and educational establishments) was less propagandist but still manipulative and concerned with 'persuasion'. In England this approach probably reached its highpoint with the publication of *Prevention and Health, Everybody's Business* by DHSS (Department of Health and Social Security, 1976).

The present picture portrays a resurgence of interest in the use of education as part of the armamentarium of the 'new public health'; we now need to raise public consciousness about a new range of environmental and social pathogens and generate a political movement to foster a healthier society – akin to the efforts of the 19th century reformers. Health education is the energizer of the new public health. It is, however, much less likely to be propagandist and more inclined to respect the principle of voluntarism –

to facilitate informed decision-making and empower action. Consideration of recent WHO documents on health promotion reveals a new focus for health education whose main features may be summarized as follows:

1. it is less concerned with preventing *specific* diseases; more concerned with promoting generally healthy life styles and promoting feelings of wellbeing;
2. it is more concerned to provide *support* for healthier lifestyles than with exhortation and attitude change;
3. it is concerned to avoid victim-blaming and with raising critical consciousness about environmental conditions and stimulating community and government action;
4. it is not concerned to create *compliance* with medical prescriptions but with promoting collaboration and co-operation between medical practitioner and consumer; it is less concerned with promoting 'proper' use of health services than with 're-orienting' the services to meet consumer needs;
5. it is, above all, concerned to *empower* communities and individuals; to promote greater self reliance and control. Health education seeks to facilitate choice not to coerce into healthy choices defined by others; a major goal is, therefore, to remove barriers to healthy choices.

These changes in orientation and the debate and argument which conflicting philosophies generate are apparent in most contexts in England where health education is delivered. One of the more interesting conflicts is that which often characterizes the differing viewpoints and philosophies of the present government's emphasis on the enterprise culture when compared with the emerging philosophy of health education which is summarized in the five principles listed above. On the one hand government has a firm commitment economically to efficiency and cost effectiveness which leads it to support individually focused preventive health education efforts which it assumes will reduce the 'unnecessary' demands made on the hardpressed national health services. On the other hand the health promotion movement emphasizes the importance of collective rather than individual efforts to remedy the plight of the under privileged whose unhealthy condition is deemed to result from social and environmental factors. At the same time right wing government is ideologically committed to the notion of individual responsibility: if the poor and unemployed are unhealthy, it is their own fault – they should change their unhealthy habits and even unhealthier value systems. The radical current of health promotion would assert that it is the society which is unhealthy: some would insist that it is the enterprise culture which harms your health not the unenterprising individual. There is insufficient opportunity here to explore these matters further nor is there time to comment on the myth that effective prevention ultimately saves money. For present purposes it should merely be noted that these debates operate as a continuing undercurrent to the delivery of health education. Two further illustrations will be provided before offering an overview of current provision in England. The first of these picks up the new public health theme.

One of the more interesting aspects of health promotion in Britain has been a kind of resurrection of the MOH who, as we have seen, has been considered historically a key figure in improving public health by addressing environmental hazards. The last four or five years have witnessed an increasing interest on the part of local authorities – that is politically elected authorities – in health matters. This movement has been inspired in large part by general opposition to central right wing government and an associated concern to address the health problems of the deprived and disadvantaged and in part by the 'undemocratic' nature of local health authorities which, at the same time as being unresponsive to local needs have been obliged to represent the philosophy of central government. Whatever the merits of these assertions, an increasing number of local authority health units have emerged – often having a close relationship with local authority environmental health departments. Apart from the political drive to address the recalcitrant problems of poverty and disadvantage, they have proved to be a major stimulus in attempting to achieve the inter-sectoral collaboration central to health promotion and are typically at the centre of WHO's Healthy Cities initiative. They differ from the situation in which the MOH found himself in that they lack the same security of tenure and cannot therefore make unpopular political decisions with impunity. There is also a suggestion that the wholehearted adoption of health promotion's drive to demedicalization might have led to a distrust of all professionalism – including the necessity to acquire the knowledge and skills which are essential to the effective and ethical practice of health education. More recently we are also witnessing increased collaboration with the health service at district level in pursuit of WHO/HFA 2000 and healthy cities. A related movement can be seen after the demise of the Health Education Council. Rightly or wrongly, as indicated earlier, the new Authority (HEA) was expected to be less able to address politically sensitive issues. As a result we have seen or rather, are seeing, the birth of a new organization, the Public Health Alliance. This is an independent and voluntary body which aims to attract wide range of lay and professional members whose major concern is to fearlessly confront the political issues inherent in the new public health.

A rather similar kind of confrontation has been observed in recent time between government and the education sector. Apart from the reaction of teachers, unions and educationists generally against increasing centralization of control, a direct clash of philosophy between government ideology and those interested in the so-called 'softer' areas of the curriculum – especially personal and social education – is apparent to even the casual observer. In order to clarify the nature of this tension, we will pick up the story of the development of health education in schools that was introduced at the beginning of this chapter.

As mentioned earlier, the 1977 version of the *Health Education Handbook* (Department of Education and Science, 1977) was more closely geared to epidemiological realities than earlier books (its 14 chapters included one on Health, Preventive Medicine and Health Education, a second reviewed the relationship between health education and the health services and a third focused on biology and health education. The remaining chapters reviewed what are often called the diseases of affluence; alcohol and drug misuse, dental health and suchlike). However, only one year later a working paper produced by the Health Education Committee of HM Inspectorate (Department of Education and Science, 1977) demonstrated the significant shift away from the medical model which had been occurring steadily in recent time. Not only did it place greater emphasis on values and attitudes but it also underlined the importance of personal and social factors – interpersonal relationships, self esteem and decision-making capabilities. In other words the almost inextricable relationship between health education and Personal and Social Health Education (PSHE) was in process of recognition. More recently, a survey by Jones (1987) has demonstrated unequivocally that in a majority of secondary schools the most common way of teaching about health matters was in the context of Personal and Social Education (PSE). Again, a detailed exploration of the issues is not possible here; they have been more thoroughly examined elsewhere (Tones, 1988). However, Figure 25.2 opposite provides the author's analysis not only of one way of conceptualizing the symbiotic relationship of health education and PSE but also how another recent concern in school health education – the notion of the health promoting school – may be operationalized. Not surprisingly, the general thrust towards health promotion, HFA 2000 and the acknowledgement of the supremacy of environmental influences on health have all caused some re-thinking and to some reinvention of ideas about the impact of the school culture and environment on staff and pupils' health. Although the hidden curriculum has long been seen to be an important influence on learning, health promotion has given it a higher profile and urged teachers and planners to deliberate the structure of the social and physical environment of the school so that it complements rather than militates against the achievement of health and the prevention of disease!

Since variety has characterized the English education system it would be totally misleading to suggest that Figure 25.2 opposite actually represents the situation obtaining in most English schools. It does, however, represent the author's attempt to offer a model of the kind of curriculum arrangement towards which PSHE has been moving in recent years. As such it acknowledges the following developments: the importance of collaborating with parents and taking account of the environment of the home and local community (the 'parallel curriculum'); the importance of the hidden curriculum, for example of the quality of school meals and the inter-personal relationships existing between staff and students; the importance of facilitating decision-making and increasing empowerment; the synergism of lifeskills teaching and social education which make up PSE and the role of the latter in supporting 'mainstream' health education; the relevance of 'healthskills' teaching, for example the re-direction of lifeskills teaching to provide students with the capabilities for resisting pressures to smoke, take illicit drugs and indulge in other unhealthy activities. Organizationally, PSHE is seen as an overlay of specialist teaching which is supported by a contextual curriculum which comprises the standard curricular subjects. It should also be noted that social education (a key part of PSHE) has the radical function of having students critically examine their environment – whether this be in school or in the broader community and society. This

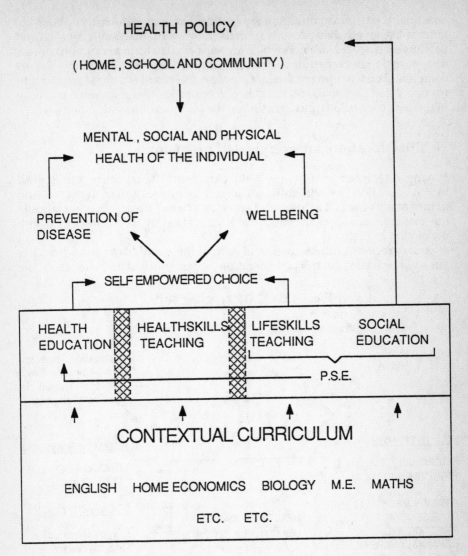

Figure 25.2: *The Contribution of Personal, Social and Health Education to Health Promotion*

consciousness-raising exercise should be supplemented by providing young people with the lifeskills which will enable them to take action to develop healthy public policy and the motivation to do so.

It should be clear from Figure 25.2 then that PSHE represents a keystone in the health promoting school. At the time of writing health educationists in England have therefore been alarmed by the threats to this critically important curricular subject which have been posed by the Government Educational Reform Bill. This Bill, which is currently in process of enactment, pays scant attention to health education – which is supposed to emerge like an ethereal phoenix from the new traditional, subject-based and cognitively oriented subjects which are supposed to form a common core for a new national curriculum. Personal social education is notable for its complete absence from curriculum plans. A rearguard action is being fought to ensure that personal, social and health education maintain some presence in the new curriculum and to maintain the impetus of recent initiatives.

Health education: an overview of provision

Having attempted to provide a developmental perspective on English health education, we will now seek to give an impression of the extent and nature of provision. To this end, Figure 25.3 below describes schematically the major means of delivering health education in the context of health promotion in England.

Space precludes full discussion of each of these and, since the school has already received quite full consideration, comments will be made about the

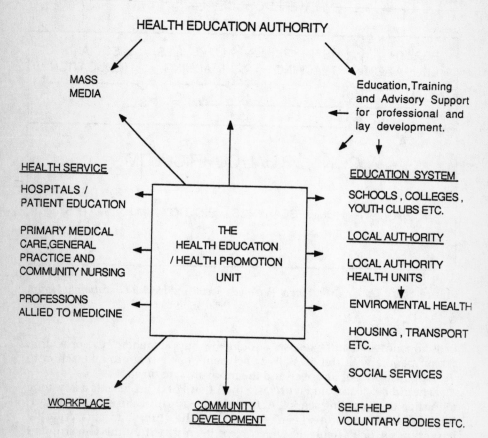

Figure 25.3 *Strategies for delivering health education in England*

delivery of health education within the National Health Service and in the less formal context of community.

First, though, it should be noted that mass media are shown as one significant strategy for delivering health education. Some reference has already been made to the role of the HEC in national campaigns and the differences in opinion between government and the HEC over the role of mass media in achieving certain health goals. The new Health Education Authority is now firmly charged by government with the task of media campaigning – especially in connection with the AIDS programme. No further observations about the use of mass media will be made here except to assert the principle that although useful for agenda-setting and supporting integrated programmes, they are not a panacea. Indeed, without a coherent programme of inter-personal education backed up by broader health promotion measures, they are often an irrelevancy (Tones, 1981, Tones *et al*, 1988).

Health education and the NHS

Although much space could be profitably devoted to health education in the hospital and the associated activities of patient education and counselling, discussion here will be severely curtailed for two reasons: the first is lack of space in which to do justice to such an important subject and the second is that patient education is virtually non-existent in England. Apart from specialist settings – such as ante-natal classes and situations where some education is essential, for example in the control of diabetes – hospitals in general and curative medicine in particular have registered zero interest. Although explicable in terms of professional myopia, this lack of concern is surprising in view of the alacrity with which many American health maintenance organizations have adopted health education. The hospitals' attitude is even more inexplicable considering the comprehensively documented evidence of failures in communication and compliance and the success of anticipatory guidance in improving the prognosis for a wide range of medical interventions.

By contrast, it is pleasing to note the not inconsiderable progress made in the context of *primary* medical care. Increasing interest has been shown by general practitioners and members of the primary health care team (health visitors, district and practice nurses and others working in alliance with the GP). General practice has increasingly recognized the realities of the burden of disease in developed countries, acknowledging the importance of chronic conditions, the need for early diagnosis of curable disease and the psycho-social determinants of what have been in the past labelled as 'trivial' complaints and the human misery which often leads patients to take their self limiting and often incurable conditions to their doctor as an excuse for more general counselling and consolation. Above all in subscribing to the notion of 'anticipatory care', GPs have legitimized a broader health promoting/health education role. It would be foolish to assert that all doctors have adopted health education with unbridled enthusiasm but innovators and probably the 'early majority' (to borrow terms from Communication of

Innovations Theory) have modified practice to a greater or lesser extent. As Fowler (1983) has noted:

> A philosophical change is required to take on board the roles of teacher and active interventionist. But a generation of doctors . . . whose education and training had been oriented towards pharmacological magic, cannot easily forsake the magician's wand of medical services and the patient's concern with instant remedy rather than future health . . .

Various productions of the Royal College of General Practitioners have provided legitimation for anticipatory care and prevention. The first of these published in 1981 encapsulates the new philosophy:

> . . . anticipatory care emphasizes the union between prevention, care and cure; it includes the concepts of disease prevention and health promotion; it can be applied to problems which cannot be resolved by diagnosis and treatment or even understood in terms of disease at all . . . Final responsibility lies with patients, but they need to learn how to promote their own health, to prevent diseases and to use health services. General practitioners are in a position to help them to learn and to stimulate their sense of personal responsibility (Royal College of General Practitioners, 1981).

This clarion call received further elaboration in a series of publications related specifically to the control of arterial disease, to family planning, to the prevention of psychiatric disorders and to the promotion of child health.

Community development

While there is evidence of limited GP involvement in broader community health promotion strategies, it is perhaps more reasonable to expect these initiatives to be taken by other people. Figure 25.3 above shows community development as one of the major ways in which health may be promoted through education. Again the problems of space constraints limit discussion here and a more thorough analysis of community-wide initiatives and community development in particular may be found elsewhere (Tones *et al* 1988).

Community development or community organization as it is sometimes known has, in Bivins' (1979) words, been for a long time '. . . an old and reliable grassroots approach to health education, identified in the 1940s'. It has, however, assumed greater significance with the rise of health promotion, the notion of primary health care and WHO's recognition that the achievement of HFA 2000 will not be possible without facing up to the mental, physical and social health conditions of the poor and disadvantaged. Community development offers perhaps the one key strategy for attaining this difficult goal. The essence of the strategy is well outlined in Ross' definition:

> Community organization . . . is . . . a process by which a community identifies its needs or objectives, orders (or ranks) these needs or

objectives, develops the confidence and will to work at these needs or objectives, finds the resources (internal and/or external) to deal with these needs and objectives, takes action in respect to them and in so doing extends and develops co-operation and collaborative attitudes and practices in the community (Ross and Lappin, 1967).

The fundamental goal of the approach is self empowerment, it involves, (Kindervatter, 1979) '. . . People gaining an understanding of and control over social, economic, and/or political forces in order to improve their standing in society.' It is highly political and corresponds to one of the essential functions of the model of health promotion adumbrated in Figure 25.1. For these reasons the major thrusts of community development are likely to be informal: not only is it undesirable for community workers to be seen to be too closely associated with the 'establishment' – the power base in society – (otherwise they risk losing their credibility) but also such an association is politically problematical. Community development therefore tends to be associated with various projects funded by charities or local authorities on a short-term basis. Frequently they will be helped by health education units and, increasingly, by local authority health units whose political nature make it not merely possible but perhaps inevitable that they become involved. In England a wide range of community initiatives exist and have flourished during recent years. In 1984, the London Community Health Resource listed some 200 community health projects.

It will be seen from Figure 25.3 that the workplace has been shown as a strategy for delivering health education and has been located in the community sector generally. This has been done in order to distinguish workplace from the formal education system and from the recognized system for the delivery of health care. Its *modus operandi* is, however, typically very different from that of community development: indeed in many ways it might be said to be antithetical. It could also be argued that self help groups differ from community development and this would be true insofar as they are merely ancillary to and cheaper alternatives for health care within the national service. On the other hand many such groups have a major self empowerment goal and may be firmly located within community development. By contrast the major task for workplace health promotion generally – at least in North America – appears to be that of creating a healthy workforce in order to save money on health insurance and increase productivity and profit. In England, very few initiatives exist – possibly because the availability of a national health service reduces the need for cost containment induced by health insurance premiums. Probably the most widespread scheme of workplace education is one which owed its origin to the Health Education Council's Look After Yourself (LAY) Project. Originally designed for use in the context of adult education, this project focuses on those activities which enhance fitness and reduce the risk of cardio-vascular disease. In short, workplace education is still in its infancy in England and receives scant attention in this chapter for the same reason that patient education has had to be dealt with in a cursory fashion. The author's view is that health education *about* work is as important as health education delivered through the workplace. This is discussed elsewhere along with a review of the extent of worksite health promotion in the UK (Tones *et al*, 1988).

Perhaps the most interesting feature of health education in England has been left until last. Prior to the incorporation of health education into the national health service in 1974, medical officers of health were at liberty to appoint health education officers. Several such appointments had been made during the 1960s and the Cohen Report, together with the stimulus provided by the newly formed HEC, resulted in a steady growth in their numbers. Today, district health authorities are expected to have a health education or health promotion unit and their role and function will now be briefly described.

The first point worthy of note is the way in which these units have begun to change their titles from health education to health promotion. In part such a move might be construed as a cosmetic exercise designed to add glamour to the service but in many, if not most, instances, the change in nomenclature represents an increasing interest in the development and implementation of health policy. Since the publication of the Kirby Report (Department of Health and Social Security, 1981), which analysed the role of health education officers (HEOs) and their training needs, the general function of a health education unit has been one of catalyst, co-ordination and consultancy. HEOs' duties do not normally involve face-to-face education nor direct contact with the public. Rather they seek to generate action in other health professionals – to make them aware of their potential health education function and motivate them to realize their potential for promoting health and preventing disease through communication and education. Their consultancy role consists of providing support and advice for these professionals – and for lay and informal health educators – in making their health education activities more effective. The consultancy role includes the provision of training and education.

The co-ordination role is self evident. The health education unit has been shown in Figure 25.3 in a central position: ideally HEOs will support *and* seek to co-ordinate health education within a locality. Typically this could involve supporting a national mass media initiative with local media work in addition to efforts directed at galvanizing inter personal education. The units are unique in the NHS in that they provide links not only with the public and between health service staff, but also provide for contacts with the education sector – for instance by stimulating curriculum development in school and making resources available. They also may have close contact with local government organizations – in some cases via the local authority health units.

Where a unit has elected to become a health promotion unit, its catalyst/consultancy/co-ordination role will be extended to include the wider range of advocacy, lobbying and mediation functions listed at the beginning of this chapter. In practice this might be revealed in attempts to initiate healthy eating policies in schools or non-smoking policies within the health authority, its clinics, hospitals and other premises.

In 1987 a survey of the impact of management changes in the NHS on health education units indicated that there were some 809 HEOs/HPOs in posts (Robinson, 1987). Some of these were short term posts created to deal with ad hoc problems such as drug misuse or AIDS. A generally accepted recommendation which was formalized in the Kirby Report was that there should be one HEO per 50,000 population. A report produced by the Health Education Training Advisory Group (HETAG) of the Health Education Authority has recommended that there should be one HEO/HPO for every priority area of work – however defined – in addition to a chief officer and deputy. In a typical authority priority areas might include: schools liaison; NHS liaison; workplace liaison; community liaison; AIDS; nutrition; CHD prevention; drug misuse. Administrative and technical support staff should be provided *pro rata* and an operational budget of 10 pence per head of population (1987 prices) should be allocated. Needless to say this level of provision is rare – but the 1987 survey mentioned above showed that the mean size of HEO staffing was of the order of 5.1 per health education unit.

The centrality of the HEO/HPO role is predicated on a truism: the all embracing, ambitious goals of health promotion will only be achieved when each country, or geographical entity within it, operates a well co-ordinated and coherent programme of health promotion which incorporates the synergistic relationship between policy and education identified at the beginning of the chapter and which involves the full range of complementary strategies presented in Figure 25.3.

References

Bivins, G cited in Lazes, PM (ed) (1979), *Handbook of Health Education* Aspen Systems Corp, Maryland

Cohen Committee (1964), Health Education, Report of a Joint Committee of the Central and Scottish Health Services Councils, HMSO, London

Department of Education and Science (1977) *Health Education in Schools* HMSO, London

Department of Education and Science (1977) *Curriculum 11–16: Health Education in the Secondary School Curriculum* HMSO, London

Department of Education and Science (1968), *A Handbook of Health Education*, HMSO, London

(1976) *Prevention and Health: Everybody's Business* HMSO, London

(1981), *Health education: the recruitment, training and development of health education officers*, Report of a Working Party of the National Staff Commiteee for Admin and Clerical Staff, DHSS, London

Fowler, G (1983) 'The opportunity for preventive medicine in general practice', in Pritchard, P (ed), *The Practice Nurse and Prevention*, Report of Two Study Days for Practice Nurses, Oxford Regional Health Authority

French, J and Adams, L (1986) From analysis to synthesis: theories of health education, *Health Education Journal* 45, 2, pp 71–71

Jones, A (1987) *Health Education and the Secondary School Curriculum: A Report for Health Education council*, Health Education Unit, University of Southampton, Southampton

Kindervatter, S (1979) *Nonformal Education as an Empowering Process*, Center for International Education: Amherst, Mass

McKeown, T (1976) *The Role of Medicine: Dream, Mirage or Nemesis?* Nuffield Provincial Hospitals Trust, London

Ministry of Education (1956) Health Education, Pamphlet No. 31, HMSO, London

Robinson, Y K (1987) *Health Education Promotion in the NHS Post Griffiths*, Health Education Authority, London

Ross, M G and Lappin, B W (1967) *Community Organization: Theory Principles and Practice* Harper and Row, New York

Royal College of General Practitioners (1981), Health and prevention in primary care *General Practice* 18, RCGP, London

Sutherland, I (1987) *Health Education: Perspectives and Choices* (Chapter 1), National Extension College, Cambridge

Sutherland, I (1988) *Health Education – Half a Policy: the Rise and Fall of the Health Education Council* National Extension College, Cambridge

Tones, B K (1987) Promoting health: the contribution of education, Paper presented at WHO Consultation on Co-ordinated Infrastructure for Health Education, WHO, Copenhagen

Tones, B K (1981) Health education: prevention of subversion ? *Royal Society of Health Journal* March 1981, pp. 114–117

Tones, B K (1986) Preventing drug misuse: the case for breadth, balance and coherence *Health Education Journal* **45**, 4, pp. 223–230

Tones, B K (1988) The Role of the School in Health Promotion: The Primacy of Personal and Social Education, *Westminster Studies in Education* (forthcoming)

Tones, B K (1981) The use and abuse of mass media in health promotion in Leathar, D S, Hastings, G B and Davies, J K (eds), *Health Education and the Media* Pergamon, London

Tones, B K, Tilford, S and Robinson, Y K (1988), *Evaluating Health Education: The Meaning of Success* Chapman and Hall, London (in press)

Whitehead, M (1987), *The Health Divide: Inequalities in Health in the 1980's* Health Education Council, London

WHO (1986) The Ottawa Charter for health promotion, *An International Conference on Health Promotion, November 17–21, Ottawa* Copenhagen, WHO Regional Office for Europe

WHO (1987) *Health Promotion: Concept and Principles in Action, A Policy Framework* Copenhagen, WHO Regional Office for Europe

26. Involving parents in health education – A CASE STUDY

G Combes

Summary: The chapter begins by looking at the historical origins of parental involvement and identifying present policy recommendations. Six models of parental involvement are described: consultation; information meetings and open days; parents groups and workshops; school and classroom involvement; home support; and parent-school-community links. The strengths and weaknesses of the different models are discussed. A discussion of the wider context covers: understanding the blocks to involvement (which the author feels can be considerable); finding out parents' views; identifying different approaches; re-thinking the professional role; and training issues. The author stresses that parents' experiences of health education cannot be isolated from their involvement in, and experience of, the rest of the school.

Introduction

Health issues have always been centre-stage for schools as issues that are potentially sensitive with parents. They can be possible sources of controversy or difficulty which require careful handling. Parents may, for instance, have strong views about what schools should or should not be teaching their children about drugs or sex. They may also be concerned about school meals, or safety in and around school, and feel that they have some right to challenge the school about these concerns. Schools then have the sometimes difficult task of balancing parents' opinions, which may themselves be quite divergent, with their own professional judgements about what is in the best interests of the children. It is also recognized that children's health is strongly influenced by the home, and that schools therefore need to take due consideration of this in their teaching. Given these observations, involving parents in a variety of ways – for instance, in classroom work, in decisions about the curriculum, in learning about health themselves, in supporting the school's work – is unavoidable if schools want their work in health education to be effective.

This chapter begins by setting the scene for current interest in involving parents in health education, by looking briefly at the historical origins of these ideas, and identifying present policy recommendations. A detailed overview of different initiatives of involvement in health education then follows.[1] The second half of the chapter attempts to set these initiatives into the wider context of general home-school relations, arguing that parents' experiences of health education cannot be isolated from their involvement in and experience of the rest of the school. Through a discussion of these wider issues, a number of key questions are raised:

How far can and should parents become involved?
What kind of involvement would be most beneficial to parents, staff and pupils?
Is partnership desirable or possible?
What are parents' views about their role in school?
What are some of the pitfalls in working with parents and how can they be avoided?
How can schools begin to work more closely with parents?
What implications are there for teachers' professional role?
What are the implications for the school's role in the community?

There are no straightforward answers to these questions, but they are significant areas for debate, which it is hoped, will provide a useful framework within which to consider the practical experience of schools.

Involvement in health education

Background

Over the past ten to twenty years in England and Wales, there has been increasing interest in, and acknowledgement of, the need to involve parents in their children's education. This has found expression in the policies of both national government and local education authorities, and at the local level with individual schools seeking greater participation with the parents of their pupils. Beginning with the Plowden Report in 1967, partnership between parents and schools has been highlighted as a major contributing factor to children's educational development. The Court Report (1975) noted:

There is no better way to help children than to help their parents to share in their growth and development.

The idea of partnership was more clearly identified in the Government White Paper *Better Schools* (Department of Education and Science (DES), 1985):

At that stage (when the child starts school) parents and school become partners in a shared task for the benefit of the child. The school discharges its part of the task more effectively if it can rely on the co-operation and support of the parents in pursuit of shared objectives.

Exactly what such a partnership with parents might mean in practice has been much less clear than the acknowledgement of its importance. The Hargreaves Report (1984) however, did attempt to outline a model of good practice, which included the need for: clear and regular communication to parents; open days; explanations about educational practice; increased parent governors; home-school councils to promote involvement and solve difficulties; small group parent-teacher associations; making the school welcoming to parents. Elsewhere, partnership is often talked of as an important goal, but one which in practical terms seems open to very wide interpretation. How many schools for instance, claim to have good relations with parents on the one hand, while decrying poor turnout to parents' meetings or parents' lack of interest in the school on the other hand? A major study in progress at the National Foundation for Educational Research (NFER) is exploring in detail different forms of involvement in schools across the country (Jowett and Baginsky, 1988).

More recent legislation has moved the debate away from partnership with parents towards parent power. The 1988 Education Act (DES, 1988) provides for the opting out of a school from local authority control, based primarily around parents' votes. The potential for direct parental influence on both the curriculum and the organization and running of the school is greatly increased by the provision of this option and other changes in policy. There is legislation for increased parent representation on governing bodies to 50 per cent; the requirement for an annual parents meeting (DES, 1986a) from which resolutions passed must be considered by the governors; and plans for devolving financial management to individual schools.

Within this wider context of the development of ideas about parental involvement in schools over the past twenty years, involvement specifically in health education has been increasingly encouraged. The HMI curriculum document, *Health Education from 5 to 16* (DES 1986b), acknowledges the central importance of parental influence on health in its opening paragraph:

Education for health begins in the home where patterns of behaviour and attitudes influence health for good or ill throughout life and will be well established before the child is five. The tasks for the schools are to support and promote attitudes, practices and understanding conducive to good health. Insofar as they are able to counteract influences which are not conducive to good health, they should do so with sensitive regard to the relationship which exists between children and their families.

In its concluding paragraphs, the report highlights parental co-operation as one of five major pre-requisites for successful health education in schools:

. . . the encouragement of parental co-operation so that between them, parents and schools are able to provide a sound basis for children to make informed choices and take increasing responsibility for their own health.

Particular emphasis is currently placed on involving parents in decisions about sex education, which is often the most controversial and sensitive part of health education for both parents and teachers. It is also one arena where some schools in the past, have felt that parental views are more important than professional views about the need for sex education, and have consequently operated informal opting-out procedures. Controversies about what is, may be or should not be taught in sex education have also raged in the local and national press for some years, and successive governments have had to contend with pressures from all sides and in all directions.

For all these reasons, considerable effort has been put into developing procedures that are designed to enable schools to take account of both professional judgements and the often wide-ranging views of parents. The HMI Report (DES, 1986b), recommends that for sex education, schools:

☐ will need to seek and give weight to parents' views (even though responsibility for the curriculum does not lie with parents);
☐ should inform parents of their policy on sex education with great care, to include:
  – an outline of the programme;
  – teaching approaches used;
  – materials used;
  while stressing the balance and objectivity of teaching;
☐ should be ready to discuss fully and sensitively with parents, any particular concerns;
☐ should keep their teaching of sex education under continuous scrutiny in the light of parents' views.

These recommendations might apply equally well to the development of any health education programme, whether or not it includes sex education. They do not, however, go as far as suggesting that parents' views should inform and direct schools about exactly what they should be teaching.

Clearly, many schools fall short of these practices, as confirmed by a recent survey of parents' views about sex education (Allen, 1987). This survey found that only 11 per cent of parents had been invited to their child's primary school, and 14 per cent to their secondary school to hear about their work on sex education. Overall, only 5 per cent had actually attended such a meeting. The report also confirmed that many parents want information and involvement. More than half of the parents interviewed welcomed the idea of meetings about sex education, although a significant one-third minority did express little interest.

Overview of involvement in health education

In 1985, the HEC: Health Education for Slow Learners Project at Bath University, sent out national publicity about its work on parental involvement in health education, and requested information from schools about their own work with parents. From over 200 replies, 50 schools were invited to contribute reports for publication in a handbook (Health Education Council, 1987) covering a wide range of work in special, primary and secondary schools. The following overview of initiatives involving parents draws on this research, along with other published sources and the author's experience of working with schools in Birmingham.

CONSULTATION ABOUT THE CURRICULUM AND TEACHING MATERIALS
Quite a number of schools replying to the original request for information,

were consulting parents about the health education curriculum, often particularly about sex education. One middle school used a consultation questionnaire devised by the Health Education Unit, University of Exeter, UK, which consisted of a straightforward list of 45 health themes. Parents were asked to rate how important they felt each theme was, with a view to its inclusion in the curriculum. Similar questionnaires are available for use with staff and students, so that all opinions can be considered in reviewing or drawing up a health education curriculum. Another school adopted a somewhat different approach, by inviting parents to an open forum to discuss proposals for a health education course which were outlined in a discussion document circulated prior to the meeting.

This approach recognized the need to raise parents' awareness about the issues, through group discussion, before asking for their opinions about priorities. Without this, some parents may, quite understandably, have unrealistic expectations of what schools can achieve, for instance expecting a drug education course to prevent their child taking up illegal drug use. Conversely, parents can be anxious that schools are too influential in other areas such as sex education. These anxieties may derive more from biased or selective media reporting in recent years, than from most schools' actual practice. Therefore, if consultation with parents is to be a meaningful procedure which truly values their opinions, parents will need to be able to make *informed* choices. This in turn requires opportunities for parents to hear about and discuss the aims for health education and the views of other parents and staff.

The special school which held the open forum took consultation one step further: following the forum, a modular health and sex education course was set up, and parents were invited to view the teaching materials and to discuss with staff which module would be most appropriate for their child to take. Thus parents were involved in both the wider process of curriculum development and the detailed decision-making about meeting their own child's needs. Although such close consultation and individualized learning might be very difficult in mainstream schools where staff-pupil ratios are much higher, there is the potential for greater consideration of individual needs by working in small pupil groups which are based on their needs in health education rather than their ability or age.

Many schools consult or inform parents solely about the teaching materials they use. Previewing materials with parents before their use with students can aid the school's selection of appropriate resources. It also helps to reduce the potential for parental anxieties and concern when students talk at home about the videos they may have watched at school or activities followed in a health education lesson. Children's unintentional selective reporting to their parents, such as 'we watched a film about how to make a baby', will result less often in a hasty trip to the headteacher, if parents are already familiar with the teaching materials used. An added advantage is that parents will also be better able to talk to their child or answer any questions at home. One middle school extended this idea by having the videos used in sex education available for home viewing. Parents were informed of which videos would be used on what dates, and were encouraged to borrow them beforehand.

Figure 26.1 is a written statement by a group of parents about their views on sex education. The group, all mothers, attended an adult education course for unwaged mothers with young children, based initially in a primary school. Their statement was compiled after much discussion, partway through the course. It conveys a depth of understanding of both their own children and the dilemmas facing schools in teaching sex education. Schools might view such contributions from parents in two distinct ways: either as important views, among many, which feed into their debate about the curriculum; or, as the foundation on which decisions about the curriculum are based.

INFORMATION MEETINGS AND OPEN DAYS

Many schools reported holding meetings for parents, where pupils' work in health education was displayed, or where parents were informed about a particular health issue. Head lice infections and how to deal with them is a common cause for concern among parents of primary age children. Schools felt that myths and misinformation about head lice still abounded, and that infections in school could be dealt with better if parents and staff had a common understanding of treatment procedures and prevention. At the second stage, drugs were the focus of meetings for some schools, with parents expressing the need for accurate information about legal and illegal drugs, and an opportunity to talk about what they could do at home to reinforce the school's work.

The main purpose of these kinds of meetings is for schools to inform and communicate with parents. Individual parents may well benefit by increasing their understanding of what their child does at school, or by expanding their own knowledge of health issues. The underlying message that the school is responding to parents' concerns is also important. However, there are limits to the scope of such meetings. Parents may feel themselves to be on the receiving end of 'good advice', which in the arena of health, is always open to debate. Many parents find it much harder to question such advice or express their own opinions in a formal meeting, than in a smaller discussion group or workshop. The recognition of these difficulties, and of a high level of general interest in learning about and discussing health issues, has led some schools to set up workshops and groups for parents.

PARENTS' GROUPS AND WORKSHOPS

Quite a number of primary and special schools had developed workshops for parents, where they participated in activities similar to those followed by their own children, in various curriculum areas including health education. Schools planned these workshops in the belief that parents are interested in the content of the curriculum and the teaching methods used, but that both have changed considerably since most parents were themselves at school. Parents' understanding of both the school's approach and their own children's work can often be greatly enhanced by this approach.

Other schools, particularly special schools, set up workshops for parents because they felt that parents needed an opportunity to consider and discuss their own children's needs in relation to health education. Many

How we think sex education should be taught

Sex education should happen at home for junior age children, because not all children are ready to take in the information.

Without the context of a loving relationship children may find the clinical details of intercourse a shock. A film or pictures of naked people in intimate positions might shock or repel them.

The subject needs more careful and subtle preparation than school has time for. It needs a one-to-one relationship to help a child understand sexual intercourse in its context. The deeper meaning of sex should be stressed.

but

Maybe it is a mistake to leave all this till secondary school. When they are little children, they accept information about sex as part of the normal fascination with bodies. By the time they are older it will seem frightening or disgusting or dirty. Also what about those parents who have not got the knowledge, the vocabulary or the inclination to tell their children about sex? Should those children just be left in ignorance?

It is a mistake to assume kids will 'pick it up'. What they pick up from magazines or television might give a wrong emphasis or not give really accurate physiological information. If it is left too late, say till Secondary School, it may be dangerous or frightening. For instance, ignorance about periods can make first signs of bleeding seem like the onset of serious illness or girls fear having done something wrong.

The complexity of sexual relationships is not the only complex thing in life – they learn about complex things in politics and on the news and they ask about them. When they are still quite young they should be told about sex if they ask about it – not have it saved up till they are in secondary school. Boys should be taught more about periods, about women's bodies and contraception.

What we see as the problem for schools

There is a difficulty about using TV programmes or films: the school can't research every family to know what they have told their children; some children could come from homes where the subject is avoided and say, nudity is not allowed, so such programmes would be very shocking to children like that.

There is a problem of misinterpretation: your child may come home with a garbled version of what she or he has seen and been told in a sex education lesson and you go up to school saying 'You've been telling our kids to sleep around'.

Can you be sure to get a 'good' teacher to introduce the subject? Some might be embarrassed, some might do it badly. Their hang-ups or their over-free views of sex might come across. On the other hand you can rely too much on a video or film when such programmes need sensitive follow-up.

Ignorance is a vicious circle: If you don't know, you think the wrong things or you don't know the right vocabulary *so* you can't find out for yourself *so* you can't solve your own ignorance. The school has to ensure children are equipped with knowledge *and* the means to find out what they may need to know in future.

What we would like to see

Small group work with children

Close consultation with small groups of parents

A more rounded view of sex as part of life, not an isolated or over-exaggerated part.

To get the film or video and let parents see it first and explain how it will be prepared for and followed up together in home *and* classroom.

by the 'Out of the House Group'
A women's self-help and communication group
Birmingham, May 1986

Figure 26.1 *One group of parents' views about sex education*

parents of children with moderate or severe learning difficulties experience difficulties with their child during adolescence. They may face very practical problems in helping their child to understand and manage body changes during puberty, such as coping with periods or wet dreams. Talking with other parents in a small group can help to allay fears and anxieties as well as providing a forum for the exchange of ideas, experience and practical tips. Some parents may also find it hard to come to terms with their child's development into a young adult, which brings with it the desire for independence and participation in adult activities. It is particularly important for students with learning difficulties that home and school have shared aims, and are consistent in the kinds of health-related information and skills developed with students.

Difficulties with adolescence are by no means confined to particular groups of students or parents. One secondary school set up a six week course for parents, based on the workshop materials *Parents and Teenagers* (Open University, 1982). A range of activities were used to increase parents' awareness and knowledge of teenagers' development and aspirations; to explore ways of communicating more effectively with them and to look at ways of dealing with particular problems. Parents were encouraged to learn from one another's experience and provide mutual support. The school also took this as an opportunity to inform parents about their work with students on personal development, and explore with them how this might support better relations at home.

Although many parents' groups and workshops are clearly linked to the school's curriculum and pupils' work in health education, some groups are set up primarily for the parents themselves, as a supportive forum in which they can discuss and learn about health issues. The reasons for initiating this kind of work vary. Some schools feel that parents need educating because they are in some way ill-informed or 'inadequate', and that the task of the school in educating children about health will be made easier if parents themselves are better educated. These schools tend to set the agenda and direct the groups according to their own ideas about what parents need. In contrast, other schools begin with the view that parents' own concerns and agendas are legitimate and correct starting points for a parents group that exists primarily for the parents themselves. Here the school sees itself as a resource for the community, with parents' groups having the dual role of providing support for parents and a channel through which the local community can influence and participate in the school.

The Spon Gate Mums' group (Braun, 1987) set out to provide an environment where women could find friendship and support and gain confidence in their own ideas and experience. It was hoped that if the mothers' confidence increased, they would be better equipped to work with the school as equal partners in their children's education. The group met for discussion and activities based on the parents' own interests around the theme of parenthood, put together and led by a facilitator.

SCHOOL AND CLASSROOM INVOLVEMENT

Many schools have traditionally looked upon parents as a valuable source of expertise which helps them in providing as broad and varied a curriculum as possible. Within health education, teachers may draw on parents' professional experiences through talks or visits where parents may be shopkeepers, cooks, hairdressers, doctors, nurses and so on. Parents' personal experiences also make a valuable contribution, particularly in the areas of pregnancy, birth and childcare, disability, and historical perspectives on health.

Several schools reported inviting parents into school to take part in a lesson or activity. One infant school regularly involved parents in cookery lessons, with parents preparing and eating the meal alongside their own children. Through parents' contributing recipes and ideas for meals, both they and their children learnt about and experienced a wide range of diets and foods. Another school invited parents to a home economics lesson, as a means of establishing informal contact, while at the same time giving pupils an opportunity to practise hospitality skills.

Classroom involvement of parents in a health education course appears to be less common. The three schools reporting in the handbook (Health Education Council, 1987) on this kind of involvement all felt that it offered one of the best opportunities for parents to understand and support their children's work in health education, and for teachers to ensure that their teaching was both relevant and sensitive to students' home backgrounds, values and lifestyles. In addition it can help to raise the status and importance of health education with the pupils, who also know that their parents will be well-informed and better able to talk over the lesson later on at home should they wish to do so.

In several schools, parents have worked on projects aimed at helping and informing other parents about health issues. A group of parents and staff at one junior school made a video about home safety, following several serious home accidents. Parents and children performed in the video which was set in the local community. At an infant school, a parent-staff group compiled a *Children's Health Handbook* giving information and advice about common childhood ailments and a directory of local health-related services. The booklet has been used widely by both parents and staff.

HOME SUPPORT FOR HEALTH EDUCATION

While not all parents have the time or opportunity for such close and direct involvement in their child's school, many can and do support various aspects of health education at home. Several schools had devised activities and projects with a significant amount of home-based work. One secondary school collected information about students' diets and exercise levels through a daily diary, with a view to reviewing the curriculum. Parents were invited to add their written comments to the completed diaries. This served in some instances, to raise their awareness about their children's lifestyles:

> This project has shown me that my daughter takes little exercise out of school hours and that her diet leaves a lot to be desired with regards to sweets and crisps.

One primary school produced packs for children to work on alongside an adult at home, on the themes of food, television and play. Although originally devised to increase conversational skills and widen children's vocabulary, children were also gaining from learning about the health-related themes alongside their parents. 'Family-work' in some primary schools in Flanders, Belgium (Geirnaert, 1984) involved parents and children in project work at home, which was designed to inform parents about school work on health education, and to gather health-related information for the teachers on which to base class work.

One special school gained very practical and committed home-based support from some of its mothers, where students went on home placements in order to learn first-hand about childcare and home management. This scheme required careful negotiation and debriefing with the mothers and students concerned, to ensure that it was a valuable learning experience for students and a manageable activity for the mothers.

A second special school followed up the visit of a pregnant mother to the class, by home visits once the baby was born, to monitor and observe the baby's progress and talk with the mother about caring for the baby at home. Finally, many schools experienced home support for health education in the form of parents sending in materials such as family photos, birth cards and injection records to contribute to classroom work.

PARENT–SCHOOL–COMMUNITY LINKS
Quite a number of schools reported activities and events around health themes, designed to draw parents and the local community into the school for joint work with pupils. One large secondary school ran a three-day conference for parents, pupils and governors at which a large number of local helping and health agencies ran workshops. Health days and health weeks are also becoming increasingly popular in Birmingham schools, with schools seeking to raise awareness about health among parents and pupils through fun and stimulating activities and events. Some schools have also offered blood pressure testing, fitness tests, and information and advice about nutrition, safety, dental health and drugs to parents and the local community.

The pros and cons of involvement

From an educational perspective, parental involvement is considered to be important because it can enhance children's educational development and contribute to the realization of their full potential. Numerous studies have demonstrated the positive effects on children of involvement in a wide range of initiatives. While the direct links to children's development are clear for some initiatives, for example parental help with reading schemes, or curriculum design taking account of parents' views and experiences of children's needs other initiatives appear to have a more indirect impact. Seeing parents involved in school may serve to validate the importance of school for many children, and the effects of this on motivation and attitudes to school may be equally or more important than the details of a particular initiative. Within this context of parental involvement supporting children's education, there are various specific benefits for parents, staff and children, summarized in Table 26.1. These include some benefits specific to health education, but also many more general benefits.

PARENTS

* their role in children's education acknowledged and validated
* feel more confident in broaching potentially embarrassing or sensitive topics with their child
* views help to shape the curriculum
* school becomes more accessible to them
* increased understanding of what is done at school and why
* increased confidence in approaching teachers
* benefit from learning about health
* increased confidence in parental role
* fears and aspirations understood
* opinions and views valued and listened to
* increased contact and friendship with other parents
* learn from other parents, share problems
* reduced isolation for parents at special schools

PARENTS AND TEACHERS

* shared aims and goals and understanding of these
* shared approach to sensitive issues and problems
* reduced misunderstanding, fear and conflict
* know each other as people
* widens horizons of staff and parents and breaks down social barriers
* school practices may be modified and improved

PARENTS, TEACHERS AND PUPILS

* greater consistency between home and school becomes possible, eg. health messages and practices
* early detection and solution of problems

PUPILS

* questions at home may be better answered
* confirms parents' support for and interest in education
* see parents and teachers working together
* input from and contact with other adults
* parents can support work at home
* increased motivation

TEACHERS

* increases teachers' knowledge of and sensitivity to home life and cultural background
* helps to provide a more complete picture of the child
* able to act on areas of concern to parents
* specific skills and expertise contribute to the curriculum
* helps to prevent schools being isolated institutions
* increased understanding and response to the needs of the community

NB. This table has been compiled from interviews with parents, and comments from teachers on in-service training courses. It simply lists those benefits most frequently mentioned, without attempting to distinguish their relative importance.

Table 26.1 *Who gains and how?*

The prospect of increased parental involvement can raise fears and doubts for many teachers. Recurring themes include: some parents being too demanding at the expense of other parents or pupils; others expressing minority views vociferously; parents bringing undue pressure to bear for change; a fear of conflicting or irreconcilable views among parents or between staff and parents; over-reactions to sensitive issues; reactions based on ignorance or prejudice; some pupils not liking to see their parents at school.

Although many of these fears are understandable, few, if any, problems that do arise are insurmountable where the school as a whole is committed to working with parents. Greater involvement can itself reduce the likelihood of such problems occurring, because of the increase in under-standing between parents and teachers, that involvement can bring. An alternative perspective on the rationale for parental involvement is that if schools fail to take due account of parents' views, parents will send their children to school elsewhere. The overriding advantage of parental involve-ment then becomes one of ensuring a viable future for the school.

Difficulties that may arise

Problems can arise when parents become more involved in a school, particularly if they are involved in classroom work or in parents' groups that meet during school time. One area of difficulty can be how both parents and children react to one another at school. One of the mothers at Shawfold School had expressed anxiety about her child misbehaving or showing her up at school, and several of the mothers in the 'Out of the House' group (Combes, 1986) felt that for this reason it was better to be involved in classes other than your own child's class. Staff at Shawfold also felt that there were sometimes difficulties over whether staff or parents dealt with children's discipline while on school premises.

In running parents' workshops and groups, common problems may be dominant or vociferous individuals, or parents who may be shy or embarrassed to talk in a group. Structured activities which allow contribu-tions from everyone, and which get parents working in pairs or small groups can help to overcome both these problems and establish group ground rules whereby everyone has the chance to participate.

Teachers may also experience difficulty where parents' behaviour or attitudes appear to contradict the teacher's approach to health issues with the children. Parents' smoking was an issue at both Corley and Shawfold Schools:

were parents to be allowed to smoke in class, while children were not allowed to smoke anywhere in school?
would the pupils interpret this as condoning smoking?
would the parents be put off from getting involved in classroom work if they weren't allowed to smoke?

Similarly at Shawfold, one teacher who was increasingly encouraging parental involvement found herself in a difficult position when inviting parents to a home economics lesson. Work on nutrition was to be displayed and pupils were to provide tea and healthy snacks for the parents. One mother, unable to come on the day, sent in a box of chocolates for the occasion. The teacher wanted to value this mother's support and contribution, but felt that the chocolates would undermine the nutritional aims of the afternoon. The issue was resolved by sending a note home to thank the mother and explain that the chocolates were to be kept as an end-of-term treat.

How staff themselves relate to parents is crucial. A patronizing manner, or criticisms of parents' lifestyles or attitudes to health can create difficulties, as illustrated by these comments from parents and staff at Corley:

Home school support worker:	After the first time (attending a health education lesson) some of them weren't going to come again – they hadn't liked the way the teacher treated them or spoke to them.
	They can be afraid of being put on the spot. That did happen a few times, when the teacher asked them what they did at home – like what foods they gave their children, and that was after she'd talked about right and wrong foods. Another time she asked round the parents 'Do you know where the liver is?' and no-one knew and they were all embarrassed.
Parent:	The teacher was a bit domineering – she made me feel uncomfortable.
Parent:	Yes, she treated us like she does the kids, like we don't know anything.
Home school support worker:	She said 'What do *you* do? Do *you* give your child sweets?' in a demanding sort of way. But everyone knows that sweets aren't really good for your teeth.
Parent:	She wanted to know what we give them to eat – well, to me that was being nosy. We didn't have much discussion either – she did most of the talking.
Home school support worker:	When it comes down to it, the personalities of the staff are so important, they determine whether it'll succeed or not.

Inevitably parental involvement in health education raises the possibility of a clash of values and cultures between home and school. Effective working with parents and children therefore means finding ways of educating for good health which do not undermine home experience but which build positively on existing knowledge, attitudes and lifestyles.

Wider issues

Work on involving parents in health education takes place within the wider context of a school's general relations with its parents. It is important to examine this wider context, since it will exert a significant influence on any specific scheme. Health education teachers who are enthusiastic about the value of involving parents, but who fail to consider its context within the school, may face unnecessary difficulties. They may also fail to appreciate significant reasons for these difficulties and retreat into the time-honoured defence of blaming parents for their lack of interest. This section raises some of these wider issues which need careful consideration by schools wishing to develop their links with parents.

Understanding blocks to involvement

Blocks to involvement can arise at any point in the process of parental involvement. First there is a need for clear and appropriate two-way channels of communication between school and parents, which are often sadly lacking. Then there is a range of practical difficulties which parents may face in actually getting to the school. Once at the school, its ethos and environment are crucial in making parents feel welcomed and valued. The attitudes of staff and parents to one another, and their perceptions of one anothers' roles will also strongly influence the success of any initiative. Some of the specific blocks that may be important are summarized in Table 26.2. The significance of these wider factors is well-illustrated by the experience of Whittington Oval School in Birmingham. Staff were encouraged during staff development sessions to identify possible blocks to parental involvement. Their views early on, that the school communicated well with parents and was welcoming and open to them, were challenged as a result of discussions with parents who felt there was much to be improved. As a result, a staff working group developed four strategies for improving communication:

- ☐ a termly Newsletter, written and produced both by and for staff and parents;
- ☐ noticeboards to display information and news, and signs to help visitors find their way round school;
- ☐ regular surgeries run by governors, through which parents could make suggestions and complaints;
- ☐ a small staff-parent liaison group to develop further parental involvement in the school.

It is important to emphasize the significance of this last point – the need for parents themselves to contribute to making decisions about their own involvement in a school. Failure to do this can represent a major block to long-term successful involvement.

Finding out parents' views

Many schools begin by thinking that they know what parents' needs are, and set up an initiative accordingly. Very often though, there is a mismatch between teachers' and parents' perceptions of these needs. Parents may not, for instance, need to learn about health issues, still less want to. Instead they may need to build their confidence in dealing with health matters with their children, and want support from other parents and the school in this. There is a very real danger of schools adopting a patronizing attitude to parents, by making decisions as professionals that exclude the views of those they wish to involve. Consultation is not, however, always an easy process. Past experience of the school will colour parents' aspirations – there

Communication
* one-way channels, school to parents;
* written communication full of jargon, wordy and impersonal;
* no home visiting;
* lack of multi-lingual communication (verbal and written);
* lack of information about curriculum and teaching methods;
* personal contact from school only if child is naughty, problematic or injured – lack of positive feedback;
* parents unsure how to make their views known to the school;
* parents' views and opinions not routinely sought.

Practical difficulties experienced by parents
* lack of time because of work or family commitments;
* young children to look after and no crêche at school;
* lack of transport, or money for transport;
* large catchment area of some schools makes them inaccessible to many parents.

School environment and ethos
* lack of welcome or feeling welcome;
* no reception area or staff to welcome parents;
* unsure where to go, lack of signposts around school;
* rigid appointment system to see staff;
* formal atmosphere.

Staff attitudes
* lack of time to work with parents;
* parental involvement seen as threat to professional role;
* patronizing manner;
* knowing what's best, without consultation;
* fear of 'difficult' parent;
* attitudes of support staff, eg. dinner helpers, caretaker.

Parents' attitudes and perceptions
* schools felt to be unfamiliar environments with different approach since own school days;
* memories of own schooling influencing attitudes to own child's school;
* feelings about child's progress may influence willingness to be involved, eg. feeling judged by teachers according to the success of their child;
* perception of class or cultural differences between staff and parents (see also Combes and Craft, 1986);
* cultural traditions working against involvement;
* feelings generated by coming into school.

Table 26.2: *Possible blocks to parental involvement*

may be a need to raise awareness of what the possibilities for involvement might be in order to stimulate thinking beyond past and present experience. Consultation about involvement in health education needs to acknowledge wider issues relating to involvement in the school. Parents are unlikely to restrict their thinking to a specific curriculum area. They are likely to be as concerned about how the school communicates with them if their child is experiencing difficulty, as they are about what is taught in a health education course.

A good starting point for consultation in many schools is to find out what parents currently think about the school. Beginning with what parents already know and experience is likely to generate a wider and more confident response, than asking about the potential for future involvement. It also helps to set a very real agenda of parental likes, dislikes and issues, which a school can use to develop their work. Figure 26.2 gives a taste of the kinds of issues that parents may raise. More detailed discussion and reports of parents' perspectives on schools can be found in Combes and Craft (1989), Mori (1987), Braun and Combes (1987), Combes (1986), National Consumer Council (NCC) (1986) and Woods (1984). Finally, when schools consider when and how to consult, it is important that they remember that the process of consultation tends to raise expectations among parents, who will want to see action by the school. Failure to meet these expectations can create disillusion. Parents therefore need to be informed of the purpose and potential of consultation.

'I think most parents are really concerned about how their children learn.'

'But we're not threatening, we just want to know what they're doing and why. We know the whats, but we want to know the whys, I think that's what they have to explain'. (Braun and Combes, 1987).

'They want to help with painting the pool or painting the walls or making curtains but I don't think as far as the actual working or running of the school is involved, I don't think as a parent you are encouraged to have anything to do with it.' (NCC, 1986)

'The attitude of the teachers is 'You know nothing about it. You're only the parents' and it's a bit of oneupmanship as if they're the clever ones; they know best.' (NCC, 1986).

'I think we should have some way of expressing our view to the teachers as to what we, the parents, feel that the children should be learning.' (NCC, 1986)

'When I go into my child's school, I feel helpless, I can't change anything I disapprove of.' (Combes, 1986)

'I think they could tell parents everything and they'd soak it up. I think we're very eager to learn and very shy of asking–we don't even know what the right questions are. We go in and say 'How are they getting on?', we're stumped, we don't know what to say after that.' (Combes, 1986).

Figure 26.2 *Some parents' views on their involvement with schools*

Identifying different approaches

In setting clear aims and objectives, it is important for schools to think about what they can realistically hope to achieve, given their particular circumstances and history. It is useful to identify where they currently are in their relations with parents and where they hope to go. An aid to this, is the continuum of involvement outlined by Braun and Combes (1987). They identify a continuum based on the balance of power between parents and schools, with four key points on the continuum. These are classified according to how far parents are involved, on whose terms, and how the school views parents:

Parents are:

receivers   – parents seen as needing information or education themselves (for example talks on health topics);

helpers   – schools ask for help when needed, but usually on non-
professional matters (for example help with swimming or
organization of class activities);

contributors – parents seen as an essential part of their child's education, but schools initiate and direct the parents' contributions, for example mother and baby visit to talk about
childcare; parents involved in project work at home;

partners   – parents and teachers make equal contributions and
decide together about the children's education, for example joint negotiation of health education curriculum.

A fifth point on this continuum could be added, where parents are seen as
customers or clients (as enshrined in recent legislation). The school's role
then becomes meeting parents' needs. For health education this would
mean basing the curriculum on parents' views about it.

The classification of parental involvement in primary schools by Torkington (1986) similarly identifies the balance between and weight given to
parents' and teachers' contributions as crucial: she distinguishes a parent-
centred approach in which parents are valued as equal partners, from a
school-centred approach in which the parents' role is to support the school,
and a curriculum-centred approach in which parents' role is to help
teachers, who are the experts, to develop their child's skills.

It is important to think carefully about the differences between parents as
partners and parents as clients or customers. The latter raises the very real
prospect of schools being directed and controlled by parents. Are schools
primarily a public service accountable to the public they serve, and teachers
public servants? Whilst any move to increase accountability is to be
welcomed, it is important to remember that the clients are the children, and
only through them are the parents clients. Education, including health
education, should serve the best interests of the child, which can surely be
best achieved by both parents and teachers working together in a close and
equal partnership.

Movement towards a parent-centred approach or a partnership with
parents, may require schools to rethink not only their view of parents' role
within education, but their view of their own role in the community. Schools
may then come to view themselves less as a focus of the community, serving
and shaping community needs, but more as a community resource in which
schools work both with and within the community to define and meet that
community's educational needs.

Rethinking the professional role

The idea of a partnership between schools and parents can seem to threaten
teachers' views about their own professionalism. Many teachers may feel
that they have far greater experience and knowledge on which to base

decisions about education than the subjective experience of parents, whose views are often based on their relatively restricted experience of their own children. The notion of partnership, however, does not seek to undermine the importance and value of teachers' experience and training. Instead it seeks to enhance it, by combining parents' specific in-depth experience of their own children, with teachers' broader experience of children in general – a powerful combination. If professionalism means seeking to work in the best interests of the child, then teachers cannot avoid working towards this kind of partnership with parents.

In relation to working with parents in health education, teachers may also need to rethink their role as the expert holders of knowledge. In discussing the Spon Gate Mums' group Braun (1987) argues that:

> . . . if health educators were more honest about the level of doubt and uncertainty surrounding their 'expert knowledge', they might have more credibility (with parents) not less, as many currently feel.

In this group, the mums were not on the receiving end of 'good advice' about parenting. Instead they contributed their experiences and feelings about it, and were in some senses allowed to create their own knowledge. This, Braun notes, involves a view of professionalism based not on knowledge but on skills – in this case the skills to facilitate personal development (including acquiring knowledge) through a group.

This perspective on the professional role leads away from viewing some parents as 'inadequate', 'deprived' or 'needing to learn about health', towards a focus on valuing and using creatively the widely-ranging experiences and values which parents can bring to health education. Thus involvement in health education would not undermine their lifestyles and values, but use these positively in creating possibilities for personal change and development in relation to health. Parents are then a resource and an aid to health education with pupils, rather than a source of potential difficulty. This does however require a sensitivity of teachers to lifestyles and values which may often be very different from their own. It also requires an acknowledgement of the constraints on choices about health which very many people face, in order to avoid presenting choices or opportunities for change that may not in reality be equally available to everyone. This in turn necessitates skills of both listening to what parents say about their lives, and imagination to enter into dialogue about areas where health is open to change.

Training issues

Opportunities to discuss these and other issues in staff development sessions are essential if schools are to move forward in their thinking about the potential and practice of parental involvement. Ideally all staff should be involved, given the importance of the influence of wider school organization on particular initiatives involving parents. The value and organization of staff development has been discussed in detail elsewhere (Braun and Combes (1987), Combes and Lloyd (1988)). A range of useful ideas for working with staff are included in Combes and Craft (1989), Braun and Combes (1988), De'Ath and Pugh (1986) and Long (1986).

Concluding remarks

Having discussed a range of views about the benefits of involving parents in health education, and having set a wide range of initiatives into the wider context of a school's relations with parents and the local community, it is important to conclude with a few observations about the process of change in schools. Work in Birmingham suggests a tendency among teachers to both over-estimate what is achievable within a given time and set of circumstances, and under-estimate the power of the *status quo* and possible blocks to involvement. It is important to recognize that time will be needed to create a climate that nurtures change within the school and convinces parents of the school's genuine desire for involvement. Schools will also be at different points on the continuum of involvement, which will influence the perceptions and feelings of both staff and parents. If, for instance, a school has viewed parents largely as 'helpers' or 'receivers', it may well experience difficulty if parents are suddenly requested to participate in curriculum decisions. As with many teachers, parents may have neither the experience, skills nor confidence to do so, and it may be inappropriate to ask them to do this without first providing opportunities for them to gradually build their skills and confidence. If parents seemingly fail to respond to invitations to participate in curriculum decisions, it may be more to do with these factors than a lack of interest. Identifying realistic expectations is therefore important if both staff and parents are to find greater involvement a positive and rewarding experience. It may be that both a school and its parents need to work through the different levels of involvement in order to build up success, as steps towards the longer-term aim of partnership.

Change is inevitably often a fairly slow process, and one which may involve failures as well as successes. Failures can be useful learning experiences which can also contribute to future success. It is important to remember that no single strategy will be appropriate or attractive to all parents and that there will always be some parents who have no wish to be involved in the school. The number of parents involved is far less important than the quality of those parents' experiences. The common cry of disaster 'but only five turned up and we invited fifty' can prevent a critical examination of the involvement of those five. Again, the oft-heard cry of 'but the parents we really want to see don't turn up' as a preface to abandoning an initiative, diverts attention away from assessing the value of the work for those who did turn up.

It also begs the question of whether all parents' involvement is equally valid and valued, or whether there is an underlying judgement about some parents needing it more than others. Regrettably, schools have always been more successful at involving their middle-class parents, as highlighted in the NCC study (1986) where only 16 per cent of parents in professional and clerical occupations had had no contact with their child's school, compared with 48 per cent of parents in semi and unskilled manual occupations. This demands a long hard look at possible blocks to involvement, and feedback from all parents about how they experience the school.

Keeping the momentum of parental involvement going, is also an issue. Many schools experience less long-term involvement than initial interest among parents might suggest they could expect. The pace of change is often slow, but better gradual change arising from parents and staff working together to make realistic decisions, than massive change which cannot be sustained over time and which depends on the power of individual personalities.

There may be unexpected outcomes (both positive and negative) but these may be as valid and important as those originally expected. It may be that the specific health value of involving parents in health education is much less important in the long run, than its contribution to good home-school relations. Thus at one school which worked with parents out of a concern for their pupils' health, the staff pointed to improvements in pupils' hygiene and dress, and increased attendance at medicals, as indicators of the success of their work. The parents however, found the health issues relatively insignificant. Of greater value to them was that they felt more self-confident, that their relations with the school had improved, and that they felt a greater sense of being valued by and belonging to the school. While judgements about the success of any work on parental involvement must ultimately rest with the parents themselves, the benefits highlighted by these parents are particularly interesting. It is almost paradoxical that what the parents felt were very significant changes and benefits (a sense of being valued and belonging to the school, of confidence in approaching staff), are in reality the very minimum that all parents have a right to expect from a school – schools, which after all, belong to and exist, not for teachers, but for children and their parents.

Notes

1. This chapter draws on the author's work as research officer on the HEC: Health Education for Slow Learners Project, which researched parental involvement in health education. Subsequent experience as Schools Health Education Adviser in Birmingham has involved running in-service training courses on working with parents, and working closely with individual schools to develop their links with parents.
2. The 1986 Education Act further extended parental influence on sex education by conferring legal responsibility for developing a policy on the schools governing body (in consultation with the school and wider community).

References

Allen, I (1987) Education in sex and personal relationships, Research report 665 Policy studies Institute, London

Braun, D (1987) Spon Gate Mums' group: supporting mothers of young children, CEDC, Coventry

Braun, D and Combes, G (1987) Parental involvement: what are we preparing teachers to do? *Community Education Journal* 6, 2 24–28

Braun, D and Combes, G (1988) *Working with Parents: A report of a teachers' development group working in Birmingham*. Distributed by Martineau Education Centre, Birmingham

Combes, G (1986) Transcript of discussions with the Out of the House Group, Birmingham (Unpublished)

Combes, G and Craft, A (1989) *Special Health* A professional development programme in health education for teachers of pupils with mild or moderate learning difficulties, HEC: Health Education for Slow Learners Project, Health Education Authority, London

Combes, G and Lloyd, J (1988) Working with teachers *Community Education Network* **8**, 7, 4

Court Report (1976) *Fit for the Future* HMSO, London

De'Ath, E and Pugh, G (1986) Working with parents: a training resources pack, National Children's Bureau, London

Department of Education and Science, (1985) *Better Schools* White Paper, HMSO, London

Department of Education and Science, (1986a) *Education (No. 2) Act* HMSO, London

Department of Education and Science, (1986b) *Health Education from 5 to 16* Curriculum Matters 8: an HMI series, HMSO, London

Department of Education and Science, (1987) *Sex Education at school* Circular No. 11/87, DES, London

Department of Education and Science, (1988) *Education Reform Act* HMSO, London

Geirnaert, M (1984) Parents' involvement in health education in primary schools. *Paper presented at a National Conference on Health Education and Youth, Southampton University 24–29th September 1984*

Hargreaves Report (1984) *Improving Secondary Schools* Inner London LEA

Health Education Council, (1987) Health education for slow learners project, Parents, schools and community: working together in health education. Distributed by Community Education Development Centre, Coventry

Jowett, S and Baginsky, M (1988) Parents and education: a survey of their involvement and a discussion of some issues *Education Research* **30**, 1, 36–45

Long, R (1986) *Developing Parental Involvement in Primary Schools* Macmillans, Basingstoke

National Consumer Council (1986) *The Missing Links between Home and School: a consumer view* NCC, London

Open University (1982) *Parents and Teenagers* Harper and Row, London

Plowden Report (1967) *Children and their Primary Schools* HMSO, London

Torkington, K (1986) Involving parents in the primary curriculum *Perspectives* **24**, 12–20

Woods, P (1984) *Parents and School* SCDC/Welsh Consumer Council, Cardiff

27. Survey methods as a stimulus to health education in schools – A CASE STUDY

J Balding

Summary: Two survey methods are described, namely: **Just a Tick**, a method for discovering priorities for a school programme according to the attitudes of, for example, parents teachers, children, health care professionals and governors, and **The General Health Related Behaviour Survey**, a method for discovering priorities for the school curriculum according to the reported levels of behaviours by the pupils/students, over a wide range of activities.

The use of either method raises awareness of health education in the school community and enhances its status. The **attitudinal** surveys (HEA Schools Health Education Unit, 1985) raise the level of excitement and are ideally suited to provide a vigorous agenda for debate amongst staff, parents, children, governors and any combination between these groups. The **behaviour** surveys (HEA Schools Health Education Unit, 1987) give far more precise data than the attitudinal ones and serve to provide reliable data on which to base decisions on timing of courses in health and social education and to provide relevant content; they also provide guidance in the selection of appropriate methods to be adopted for the courses and lessons taught.

The **attitudinal** surveys are available for use in schools of all types and all ages of children. Surveys have been carried out in secondary schools and their feeder primary schools which enable the planning of a continuous programme from age five to age 16 or beyond. The **behavioural** surveys have been developed for use with children/students between the ages of 11 to 19 years of age. A version for use with younger age groups is being developed.

A service to support the use of the survey methods by schools is currently available from Exeter University. Hundreds of schools have used either one or both of the methods and significant data banks have accumulated to support wider research. The Health Education Authority (HEA) have provided major funding to support the Health Related Behaviour Survey Service to Schools from 1983 until the present.

Introduction

Within the United Kingdom most primary and secondary schools have given a lot of attention to the social education and the health education components of their curricula. The influence that the school life experience has on the social development of young people is substantial. For school staff to examine their programme of courses and also the way they organize their schools (at the beginning and end of the school day, at lunch time and between lessons, on school trips, for school meals provision, and indeed for any aspect of the declared or 'hidden' curriculum), reliable information on the way people feel about the programme and the school and reliable information on what the young people are doing makes a sensible base from which to plan or review their programme and policy.

The attitudinal surveys, Just a Tick

These surveys are based on a check list of topics of potential importance in the school curriculum in connection with health and social education. At present, in 1988, there are 43 topics for consideration for the primary school and for secondary schools this list is extended to 49 topics. The list for the primary school use can be seen in **Tables 27.1** and **27.2**, the

					Boys		Girls	
		Par	Tch	HCP	Yr 3	Yr 4	Yr 3	Yr 4
1.	How my body works	8	6	2	17	24	23	26
2.	Staying Well	30	14	17	29	27	20	22
3.	Immunisation(injection and drops)	31	30	27	41	41	42	40
4.	Illness and recovery	40	38	39	27	27	27	28
5.	Talking with doctors, nurses, dentists	26	40	23	43	43	42	43
6.	Care of hair, teeth, skin	8	4	2	14	16	6	6
7.	Care of eyes	18	11	14	9	9	17	19
8.	Care of feet	21	15	17	37	35	28	32
9.	How a baby is made(human reproduction)	14	22	13	13	12	10	9
10.	Menstruation (periods)	15	22	6	42	39	20	12
11.	Food and health	19	7	9	10	10	15	18
12.	Drinking alcohol	26	37	27	18	20	38	36
13.	Glue-sniffing	11	34	23	33	25	31	27
14.	Smoking	12	22	11	24	20	23	24
15.	Physical fitness	7	17	16	2	3	7	7
16.	Understanding the needs of handicapped people	24	21	36	33	36	19	16
17.	Understanding the needs of old people	26	22	37	24	23	12	11
18.	Health and social services	43	43	43	38	39	37	40
19.	Safety at home	12	7	8	8	7	5	5
20.	Safety in traffic	1	1	1	7	8	15	20
21.	Water safety	2	2	5	4	4	4	4
22.	First aid	17	31	22	6·	5	2	2

Table 27.1 *Rank order positions (out of 43) of topics numbered 1 to 22 from data processed from 10,208 parents, 639 teachers, 230 health care professionals, and 6,940 boys and girls aged 9, 10 and 11 years (junior/middle school age range 8–12)*

					Boys		Girls	
		Par	Tch	HCP	Yr 3	Yr 4	Yr 3	Yr 4
23.	Family life	34	28	25	18	16	12	12
24.	How to cope with being separated from your parents	38	39	39	14	11	8	7
25.	Death and bereavement	40	41	41	11	16	11	16
26.	Why people worry	42	41	42	39	42	41	40
27.	How boys and girls behave	31	36	29	35	32	34	33
28.	Differences in growth and development	23	31	21	26	27	26	20
29.	Getting on with boys and girls the same age as yourself	22	20	26	18	20	22	24
30.	Understanding people with different coloured skins or different religions	15	9	14	38	36	32	30
31.	Feelings (love, hate, anger, jealousy)	24	19	19	14	13	18	15
32.	Bullying	8	12	19	18	15	38	37
33.	Feeling good about yourself	36	27	32	23	25	32	29
34.	Making up our minds	31	29	38	31	34	28	33
35.	Being honest	2	3	2	11	13	12	12
36.	Being responsible	4	5	7	30	31	23	23
37.	Spare time activities	35	33	30	3	2	8	10
38.	Being bored	38	35	33	36	36	35	33
39.	Caring for pets	37	26	34	1	1	1	1
40.	Vandalism	6	16	12	27	30	38	39
41.	Stealing	5	10	9	31	32	36	37
42.	Pollution	26	17	34	18	16	28	30
43.	Conservation	20	12	31	4	5	3	3

Table 27.2 *Rank order positions (out of 43) of topics numbered 23 to 43 from data processed from 10,208 parents, 639 teachers, 230 health care professionals, and 6,940 boys and girls aged 9, 10 and 11 years (junior/middle school age range 8–12)*

secondary school list is an extension of this with the addition of the following six topics:

44   **Contraception;**
45   **Parenthood and child care;**
46   **Sexually transmitted diseases;**
47   **Control of body weight;**
48   **Violence on the television screen;**
49   **Cancer.**

Use with adult groups

Parents, teachers, health care professionals (for example school nurses doctors, health visitors, health education officers), and school governors are invited to complete and return the questionnaire. They are specifically asked to have a particular age range in mind as follows:

infant first   (5 to 7 years)
junior/middle   (8 to 12 years)
secondary   (13 to 16 years).

Each person is requested to indicate their view on the level of importance for each topic for inclusion in the school's curriculum. **Figure 27.1** shows the top of the questionnaire for use with parents of junior/middle, eight to 12 year-old children.

Personal Development and Health Education Enquiry   (Parents' Version 4 J/M)

© J. W. Balding 1985   HEC Schools Health Education Unit, Exeter University. Tel. 0392 217532

	Importance for inclusion in the school curriculum for junior/middle school (8–12 year old) children					
Please place ticks in columns to indicate your views – one tick per line						
TOPICS	YES		?	NO		
Titles as listed for the children	Should be included	Useful if time available	Undecided	Not important in this age group	Should be covered outside school	Does more harm than good
1. How my body works						
2. Staying well						
3. Immunisation (injections and drops)						
4. Illness and recovery						
5. Talking with doctors, nurses, dentists						

Figure 27.1 *The headings and the presentation of the first five topics of the 'Just a Tick' questionnaire to parents of children aged 8 to 12 years*

As always with survey methods, great care has to be taken in creating the best atmosphere for collection of information and the approaches to members of each group is conducted with great tact. Parents in particular can become alarmed if they gain the impression that decisions are being taken to include all topics listed in the school programme and wonder if there will be any room for anything else; this is clearly not the intention, but a carefully worded letter from the head teacher is vital in order that the parents can understand clearly that the survey is a method of consultation and represents a genuine attempt on the part of the school to become informed of parental views.

It probably comes as no surprise to readers that different health care professions appear to have different priorities, teachers differ from parents, the male and female view can differ on some topics and from different age groups different topics appear to have greater relevance.

Use with children/students

Questionnaires are completed in the classroom by boys and girls under the supervision of a teacher, preferably who is well known to them and in whom they trust. In primary schools the youngest age group to complete the questionnaire is age seven. For the age range seven to 12 years a very carefully researched set of prompts and method of supervision has been developed (1985 Just a Tick). **Figure 27.2** shows the tops of the Supervisors Guide to List 1–22, which lists the prompts that the teacher is 'allowed to

Supervisor's Guide to List 1–22

Presentation to pupils: "I will read the title, and then I am allowed to read a few more things about it to help you understand it. Do not tick the box until I have finished."

1. How my body works

   This would be about the different parts inside your body and what they do, for example, your muscles, skeleton, heart, lungs and stomach.

2. Staying well

   This would be about how we can look after our health and keep well.

3. Immunisation (injections and drops)

   This would be about how doctors and nurses give us injections or jabs, or drops on sugar lumps, to stop us catching certain illnesses.

4. Illness and recovery

   This would be about what happens to our bodies when we become ill, and how we can help ourselves get better.

5. Talking with doctors, nurses, dentists

   This would be about going to visit the doctor, or nurse or dentist, and knowing what to say.

Figure 27.2 *The supervisor's guide to the presentation of topics numbered 1 to 5, to children aged 7 to 12 years*

read' in order to further clarify the meaning of the topic title for the young children. Secondary school children do not get these additional prompts. All classes are carefully rehearsed in the way of completion of the questionnaire using topics not listed.

Results

Results can be summarized in many ways, the one presented here in **Tables 27.1 and 27.2** is of particular value for examination and clarification at parent teacher meetings. In it the responses from each group have been processed to place each topic in a rank order of **importance** for adult groups and **interest** for children's groups. The rank order placings are themselves interesting and the apparently different priorities portrayed promote attention in debate. The data was collected during the survey of schools from 11 regions in the UK in 1985 as a component of the Health Education Council's (now Health Education Authority) Primary Schools Project, the Exeter University unit provided the survey support work to a project based in Southampton University directed by Trefor Williams. Extensive description and discussion of the results of the surveys is published in two monographs (Balding, 1989a and Balding, 1989b).

Action

In questionnaire design the attempt is made to create each question in such a way that every person responding to it interprets it in the same way. In this particular survey method variations in response would thereafter represent variations in perceived importance of an individual topic. Whilst a vast amount of time, consultation and teamwork have gone into the development of the method with respect to each group surveyed, particularly the boys and girls in the seven to 12 years age range, it is clear that a range of interpretation for several topics exists (Balding, 1988b). Having said this, there is validity in reporting that, for example, 78 per cent of the parents in one primary school using the survey indicated that the topic **How a Baby is Made (human reproduction)** 'should be included' in the curriculum and a further 14 per cent indicated that to include it would be 'useful if time available'.

It is most important that the results gained from the survey should be discussed by people contributing to the survey. Parents' meetings with staff present are particularly valuable to clarify the variation of interpretations amongst responses, this comes out naturally in discussion of the results and does not have to be spelt out as an agenda item. Differences in concept sometimes emerge between parents and teachers often arising from lack of knowledge on the parents' part of current teaching materials or county or national policy. The outcome is towards clarification of vocabulary and experience which enables progress towards meaningful discussion of priorities for the school to be effectively debated. A common outcome of these meetings is the recognition on the parents' part that the social education component of the school's curriculum has been given a lot of serious attention and they find this pleasing, also school policies are often clearer than policies in the home.

The use of the results as an **agenda for debate** cannot be over-emphasized. Examination and comparison of results from different groups all with serious interest in the welfare of the school brings an objectivity to an area of the curriculum that is important to all concerned. This concept of an agenda for debate can be extended to the classroom and provide a realistic resource to stimulate discussion and clarification. Fourth year pupils, aged 14 and 15 years, have vigorously examined the underlying reasons for their own varying points of view, and have been remarkably accurate in predicting parental viewpoints and teachers' viewpoints.

The general health related behaviour surveys

Since 1983 the HEA's schools health education unit in Exeter University has been providing a survey service to schools throughout the United Kingdom. In England, its work is supported by the HEA, and in Scotland, Wales, and Northern Ireland by funds from other statutory bodies. The service enables a school to survey the health behaviour of the boys and girls at different ages. The purpose is to make the planning of programmes in health and social education in the schools more realistic. If teachers and parents have reliable information on levels of behaviour at different ages, appropriate action can be attempted at the right time.

What health behaviour information is gained?

The behaviours measured in the surveys carried out by each school include:

Alcohol consumption	Money
Dental care	Physical activity
Diet	Road use
Drugs	Self-esteem
Homework	Sharing problems
Hygiene	Smoking
Jobs	Social activities
Leisure pursuits	Time to bed/time up
Medication	TV, videos, and suchlike

Do the boys and girls answer honestly?

One essential feature of survey work like this is that the replies to the questions by the boys and girls should be absolutely honest. The method was first used in 1979 and since that time more than one in five comprehensive schools throughout the United Kingdom have used it.

The method of presenting the questionnaire to classes has been under continuous review, and we have established that nearly 100 per cent honesty can be assured when the boys and girls are convinced:

1. Of the value of the exercise to their school and themselves;
2. That their teachers will not read the answers they write down;
3. That the completed questionnaires are completely anonymous.

Our level of confidence in the validity of the data is often questioned, and throughout the ten years of evolution of the questionnaire method the issue of honesty has been continuously addressed. Several characteristics of the survey method are relevant to its validity:

1. Those carrying out the survey pay for the service, and hence in their own interests pay strict attention to the details prescribed to promote validity (for example, the importance to the school and the pupils, its confidentiality, the respondents' anonymity, and so on).

2. Each supervisor completes a form describing any difficulties that arose with individual questions or the procedure. These forms are returned, with each batch of questionnaires to which they relate, to the unit.

3. The completed questionnaires are not inspected at all in school, but are sealed and sent to the unit. The scripts are processed there and summaries are returned to those collecting the data.

4. Many teachers take the data to the respondents as a component of classroom practice. Having the results scrutinized and debated by the boys and girls providing the information, or by their peers, is a unique feature in the methodology. It is a powerful way of checking on the validity of the responses, particularly with respect to honesty and to the levels of comprehension of the questions posed.

5. Systematic work with respondents to examine answers following their completion of the questionnaire is undertaken at intervals by the unit staff and by other experienced interviewers. To date, more than 100 different experienced interviewers have contributed to this most important aspect of validation.

The outcome of all this extensive and painstaking work has been to generate a high level of confidence in the validity of the data gathered from the use of the questionnaire.

The questionnaire content

The preparation of Version 1 of the General Health Related Behaviour Questionnaire in 1978 involved around 50 secondary school teachers in the examination of 30 suggested questions for inclusion. These questions had been taken from an American source and the teachers were asked to comment on the appropriateness of their structure and relevance to inclusion in the questionnaire. Most of the teachers were highly critical and used their 'red ink' freely over the document and then produced proto-types of 'better' questions for inclusion. Around 90 questions were produced from this process, reflecting the views of important health issues for these teachers.

The structure of the questions was refined in consultation with experienced teachers and with trials and interview work with boys and girls in schools. The bank of questions was also reviewed by professional groups other than teachers including road safety officers, school nurses, and health authority personnel (health education officers, district community physicians).

A third process that was applied at this time, that is important to note, was that of circulating the refined list to a number of head and deputy head teachers for their commentary on the sensitivity of inclusion of all the questions. The invitation was to put a red line through any questions, the inclusion of which might cause anxiety amongst some parents and were therefore best excluded. They were not asked for any further information or explanation of any deletions they suggested. This process resulted in the exclusion of all the proposed questions on 'shop-lifting', on 'vandalism', and many of the questions on 'sexual behaviour'.

Over the ten years of its evolution and development the content has been under continuous scrutiny and much revision has taken place. Professions other than teaching have been deliberately drawn in to influence the content, but nonetheless the bias of the content probably still reflects mainly the teachers' concept of health behaviour. Every time that young people are supervised in the completion of the questionnaire the supervisor completes a comments sheet in which difficulties arising, points of interest and suggested amendments are recorded. These comments are a powerful influence in the development and refinement of the method and must further enhance the level of influence of the 'teacher viewpoint' on what are important health issues.

INDIVIDUAL QUESTIONS
Individual questions have been revised to meet particular professional needs, for example the frequency of intake of iron-containing medicines, either prescribed or unprescribed, has been of particular concern and the modification of question 33 (version 11) meets this expressed need.

GROUPS OF QUESTIONS
Groups of questions have been revised similarly in connection with the attention paid to the data derived from their use for example from road safety officers; questions 9, 10, 11 and 12 (version 11) will once again be revised for version 12. The dietary questions probably receive the most criticism and revision of all sections; each expert who has paid attention to them decides that there is room for improvement and change results from their attention. The questions connected with TV viewing have evolved to distinguish between TV programmes, recorded TV programmes on home video, hired video tape viewing, computer games and computer programming, over the past six years in step, or perhaps a little behind, with the changing reported practices of young people.

Another measure that has been applied to the content of the questionnaire is that of the level of use made by the 'consumers' on the return of the summarized data to them. Enquiries reveal that some sections of the questionnaire are much used, for example alcohol, smoking and diet, while others receive little attention. Some sections are receiving more and more use as they become better tailored to meet the needs of the users; the sports and physical activities section is an example of this type of evolution and currently enables a comparison between the provision available in school to be made with the variety of activities and the levels of involvement outside school. Our connections with the Coronary Prevention in Children Project, also based in the Exeter University School of Education, is prompting us to develop indices of physical activity level, to further enhance the use that PE teachers and related organizations may make of either the data returned to schools or available for research purposes in the data banks.

This continuous review depicted above underpins the level of validity of the questions contained in the current version. A planned initiative to focus on the base line statistical needs of health authorities in connection with the health care provision of the age group in question and for young adults is in hand, and to adapt the questionnaire to meet these needs. This could lead to a dilution of the teacher-led view of the important health issues towards a balance between the two professions.

The school survey

The method of sampling within each school year has been carefully researched and tested on several occasions and the guide to supervision has been updated in step with the feedback from so much use over seven years (HEA Schools Health Education Unit, 1987). Completed questionnaires are sent to Exeter University for processing and a bound collection of summarized results together with a guide for action is returned to the school. There are almost always more tables of information than one school manages to make use of but different schools use different components. The sections most commonly used by schools involve **smoking, alcohol and diet,** to a lesser extent **social activities, money** and **sharing problems,** increasing use of the **physical activity** data but very little use of the **road use** statistics.

As mentioned earlier the information fed back to schools is used as a guide to timing of lessons and courses, to the content of lessons and to the selection of appropriate methods and materials to use with the young people. One particular resource in England providing methods and materials on a wide scale for use in schools is Teachers' Advisory Council on Alcohol and Drug Education (TACADE).

	No	Yes	N
1st year (11+ years)	63.8	36.2	80
3rd year (13+ years)	57.1	42.9	105
5th year (15+ years)	59.8	40.2	82
N	160	107	267

Table 27.3 *Percentage responses from boys in one school (aged 11+, 13+ and 15+ years) to the question 'Have you a regular girl friend?'*

	Weeks	1 to 6 months	6 mths to 1 yr	More than 1 year	N
1st year	17.2	31.0	10.3	41.5	29
3rd year	20.0	42.2	15.6	22.2	45
5th year	45.5	36.3		18.2	33
					107

Table 27.4 *Percentage responses from boys in the school represented in Table 27.3 to the question 'If you have a regular girl friend, for how long has this relationship lasted?'*

The method of presentation in 1988 was as shown in **Tables 27.3 and 27.4** which present the summarized answers to two consecutive questions concerning the number of 'girl friends' boys identify. It will be seen that the 107 boys who indicated they had a 'girl friend' are the sample responding to the subsequent questions on the length of time this relationship has lasted. It is clear that the range of questions asked is very broad and, for some, extend beyond their concept of health into other areas.

Annual data banks

The service provided to schools through Exeter University's expertise funded by the HEA has been abundantly used over several years. The first book on one year's statistics was published in 1987 entitled *Young People in 1986* (Balding, 1987). Further year books are in preparation. The data banks lend themselves to the examination of trends in behaviour (Balding, 1988c) and in the relationships between behaviours (Macgregor and Balding, 1987).

References

Balding, J W (1987) *Young People in 1986* Health Education Authority Schools Health Education Unit, University of Exeter, England

Balding, J W (1988c) Teenage smoking: the levels are falling at last! *Education and Health* **6**, 3, 68

Balding, J W (1989a), *Parents and Health Education* Health Education Authority Schools Health Education Unit, University of Exeter, England

Balding, J W (1989b), *Health Education Priorities for the Primary School Curriculum* Health Education Authority Schools Health Education Unit, University of Exeter, England

Coronary Prevention in Children (Director: Neil Armstrong). Project located at the School of Education, University of Exeter, England

Health Education Authority Schools Health Education Unit (1985) *Just A Tick: Health Topic Questionnaire Survey Methods* University of Exeter, England

Health Education Authority Schools Health Education Unit (1987), *Health Related Behaviour Questionnaire (Version 11)* University of Exeter, England

Macgregor, I D M and Balding, J W (1987) Toothbrushing frequency in relation to family size and bedtimes in English schoolchildren *Community Dentistry and Oral Epidemiology* **15**, 181

Teachers' Advisory Council on Alcohol & Drug Education (TACADE), Furness House, Trafford Road, Salford M5 2XJ, England

28. Health education in Scotland – AN OVERVIEW

I Young

Summary: The Scots have a long tradition of innovation. The driving force in Scotland at present is the well organized Scottish Health Education Group (SHEG) formed in April 1980 on the merger between a health education unit and the Scottish Council for Health Education which had been founded in 1943. It is staffed by a multi-disciplinary team. Its work has focused on mass media health promotion including sponsorship of the Scottish Football Cup, marathons, family walks and very substantial work in schools. The mode of the **Health Promoting School** is expanded in detail in this chapter. Recent trends in schools health education are turning towards health related fitness.

Introduction

The Scots have a long tradition of innovation within a system of education that has always attempted to offer educational opportunities to young people irrespective of their social background. For example Scotland in the middle of the nineteenth century offered one university place for every 1,000 of the population. This compared with 1:2,600 in Germany and 1:5,800 in England. Within the United Kingdom the first infant schools, teacher education colleges and university chair in education were pioneered in Scotland.

Scotland today is a country of approximately 5.2 million inhabitants. Central responsibility for health education rests principally with the Scottish Education Department (SED) and the Scottish Home and Health Department (SHHD) of the Scottish Office of Her Majesty's UK Government. The national body for health education is the Scottish Health Education Group (SHEG) and this is a unit within the National Health Service (NHS) in Scotland. Most of the fifteen health boards in Scotland have health education departments which have a recommended establishment of one Health Education Officer (HEO) per 50,000 of the population served. The education authorities in the form of nine regional councils and three island councils have responsibility for the provision of education, including health education, within the schools and colleges under their control.

The SHEG was formed in April 1980 from the merger of the Scottish Health Education Unit and the Scottish Council for Health Education which had been founded in 1943 with the responsibility for organizing training courses. The Group is staffed by a multi-disciplinary team drawn from

medical, nursing, educational, social science, marketing and media backgrounds. SHEG has a budget of approximately £3.25 million (1987/88) to
develop health education in Scotland. In 1982 SHEG was designated a WHO
Collaborating Centre for health education and health promotion research, a
distinction shared with colleagues in Cologne, Dresden and Utrecht. The
work of SHEG includes:

a. the production of health education materials for the public and
   professionals;
b. the promotion of health education in the training of the caring
   professions;
c. the formulation of research proposals for health education activities
   and their evaluation.

SHEG liaises and co-operates with a range of professional groups
including the area health education departments of the health boards. The
majority of HEOs have been drawn from nursing, teaching, community
work or the social sciences. The departments in the health boards are
headed by an Area Health Education Officer (AHEO) who is in turn
responsible to the health board's chief administrative medical officer.

Qualifications and training

Those wishing to specialize in health education have opportunities to
undertake study leading to qualifications such as the Certificate in Health
Education, and the Diploma/Master's Degree course in Health Education.
The certificate course is offered at Queen's College, Glasgow and is
undertaken on a part-time basis over one year by such professionals as
community nurses and by those in the professions allied to medicine. The
Diploma/Master of Science post-graduate qualification is a relatively new
course which commenced in 1988/89 at the University of Edinburgh and this
qualification is taken by a wide range of professionals including health
education officers, medical practitioners, community nurses and social
scientists – over one year full-time study.

The extent to which different professionals have a significant health
education component in their initial professional qualification is variable but
the situation is steadily improving. For example in one of the medical degree
courses in Scotland one week of health education is provided within the
community medicine component and this involves SHEG and HEO staff
contributing in lectures and tutorials. SHEG has been involved in promoting
health education within the basic curriculum of nurses and in increasing the
health education component in teacher education courses, although the
latter is still relatively low (30 hours within a four year degree course for
primary teachers). It is clear that increasing the health education component
in the initial training of a range of professionals is an important area of
expansion for health education in Scotland in the future. Support for this
process has been given by SHEG providing funded lectureships in key
educational establishments and also by the provision of financial support for
individuals to attend courses in health education and community health.

Recent history and trends in mass media health promotion in Scotland

In the 1970s health education in Scotland began to move from a negative problem-based approach addressing those who were considered 'at risk' towards a more positive approach recognizing that, to some extent, people could assume responsibility for their own health. In 1984 the SHEG developed an 'umbrella' theme, Be All You Can Be, which, through a 60-second TV commercial and associated magazine literature portrayed images of physical, social and mental wellbeing. As with all major projects developed by the group, this campaign was tested by the advertising research unit of the University of Strathclyde (Leathar and McNeil, 1984).

The research indicated that the public viewed the campaign as attractive, positive and non-directive. In addition, the concepts that health promotion could be enjoyable and that everyone can take the first steps towards better health were also communicated to the public.

However, the theme Be All You Can Be was considered rather unspecific; therefore it was normally used with a subsidiary message which in the initial launch was Go For Good Health. Since 1984 the campaign Be All You Can Be has been linked with a wide range of SHEG's work including dental health, cigarette smoking, drug education and women's health.

In addition to the use of pre-tested advertisements the SHEG has used sponsorship and public relations techniques to keep health related issued in front of the Scottish public. The group has focused its involvement with sponsorship mainly on sporting personalities and more recently on sporting events and outdoor activities. The sponsor (SHEG) on the payment of the agreed fee is able to associate its name and 'product', good health, with a particular event and its popular heroes. In some cases this offers the advantage of greater media coverage at a significantly lower cost than advertising. The SHEG sponsored the first Glasgow Marathon run which currently has one of the highest participation figures in the world. Recognizing that we do not have to run marathons to enjoy good health and fitness, a campaign entitled Walk About A Bit was developed with the area health boards to encourage participation in family walks.

Since 1982 the SHEG has sponsored the Scottish Football Cup which involved the association of the cup competition, which has a high profile in the mass media, with a range of positive health messages (Young, 1986). The initial research of the cup promotion carried out in 1982 was very positive in several aspects and it allowed the SHEG group to develop the sponsorship further but with a much clearer target group and a more clearly stated objective for the period 1983–86. The young people in the age range 10 to 15 were more able to understand the sponsorship and were not only supportive of the approach but they found the link between football and healthy lifestyles a credible one with which they identified. Although in general adults were very supportive of the sponsorship in some cases they found the link between football and healthy lifestyles less credible.

As a result of the 1983 research the cup sponsorship was targeted at the 10 to 45 age group with a priority sub-group of schoolchildren, particularly in the 10 to 12 age group. The more clearly stated objective for the campaign was to 'improve the image of health through the sponsorship link with football, health being defined in a restricted way for the purpose of this campaign as fitness, non-smoking and moderation in alcohol consumption' (Hastings *et al*, 1985).

The data for school-age boys supported the greater emphasis on positive rather than negative health messages. For example, 77 per cent of the boys felt that the campaign would encourage them and their friends to take up exercise compared to 67 per cent agreeing that it would discourage people their age from starting to smoke.

The main conclusions drawn from the boys' responses to questions relating to general attitudes to health and fitness were twofold. First, they revealed a tendency for the boys to put more emphasis on the social rather than the health drawbacks of smoking and drinking. Second, the more positive sport and fitness issues were considered of greater importance than negative health issues such as smoking and drinking.

The SHEG has attempted to link this mass media health promotion with school health education approached by developing poster competitions for the 10 to 12 and the 12 to 14 age groups which stimulated curricular work on health education within the schools. This has been most successful in primary schools where 'centre of interest' or project work controlled by a single class teacher allowed the integration of health education work related to the sponsorship. Over 800 schools, which represent approximately 33 per cent of the state schools, became involved in the project augmenting their normal health education work and stimulating further interest in health related themes.

School health education

It is clear that the use of mass media techniques has certain advantages but also considerable limitations. The size and scope of the target audience and the reliance on visual images and the spoken word make the broadcast media particularly powerful. However it is recognized that people bring their own beliefs, values and experience to bear on new media information and they frequently select and interpret from new information to reinforce their existing position. It is apparent that more interactive forms of communication are important if we wish to go beyond raising awarness of health issues.

The SHEG has recognized that our schools have a great opportunity to promote good health because they have in theory the potential to develop a planned progressive programme of health education which involves much more than the transmission of information but which actively involves young people in acquiring knowledge and understanding, exploring attitudes and developing new skills. The extent to which schools have fulfilled this potential in Scotland and other countries is limited owing to a complex of constraints which vary from country to country. These issues were explored in a SHEG/WHO Conference in 1986, The Health Promoting School. This event looked beyond the school curriculum to the total life of the school and examined ways in which schools could actively promote the health of all young people (SHEG/WHO, 1986).

The ideas from this symposium have been developed further in a new project which will be published in 1989 in Scotland. This report has developed from a partnership between SHED and the Scottish Consultative Council on the Curriculum which is the secretary of state's advisory body on education. The publication will be entitled *Promoting Good Health* and will focus particularly on the needs of school students between the ages of 10 and 14.

The following issues are reviewed within the report:

Introduction	– The scope of health, health education and health promotion; the importance of the 10 to 14 range
Planning the programme	– Who should initiate the development of health education within the school?
	– What are the responsibilities of the school?
	– Who will teach health education?
	– Who will co-ordinate the programme?
	– What factors will shape policy?
	– What support is available to schools?
	– How can primary and secondary schools collaborate?
The health promoting school	– The nature of health promotion
	– The three elements of the Health Promoting School:
	– The Curriculum
	– The Hidden Curriculum
	– The Health and Caring Services
	– Moving towards the health promoting school
The health education curriculum	– Content, process and method within the health education curriculum
Sexuality and relationships	– An example of an area of the curriculum
Home school relations	– Developing a partnership with parents
Training and staff development	– The training implication of the report

It is not possible to discuss the details of the report but it is perhaps worthwhile to focus on the section that explores the concept of the Health Promoting School. It is suggested that there are three main elements in the health promoting school. Firstly the 'formal' curriculum of the classroom and the guidance and pastoral care of pupils. Secondly, the hidden

curriculum of the school which includes the subtle influences of the inter-
personal relationships in the school, the exemplar role of teachers, the
physical environment of the school and the quality of the home-school
relations. The third component is the role of the health and caring services providing health screening, immunization, first aid and child guidance.

To give a flavour of this section of the report, Table 28.1 extracted from the
report provides 10 key points for school management to consider in moving
from a limited traditional school health education approach towards the
wider concept of the health promoting school.

It is clear that some aspects of traditional health education are essential
and should not be viewed only in negative terms. For example, the
development of good personal hygiene habits and school health service
screening programmes are clearly essential components of health education. However, these traditional elements should be seen within the broader
model of the health promoting school.

Moving from traditional school health education towards the health
promoting school

Traditional Health Education	The Health Promoting School
1. considers health education only in limited classroom terms;	takes a wider view including all aspects of the life of the school and its relationship with the community for example develop- ing the school as a caring community;
2. emphasizes personal hygiene and physical health to the exclusion of wider aspects of health;	is based on a model of health which includes the interaction of the physical, mental and social aspects;
3. concentrates on health instructions and acquisition of facts;	focuses on active pupil participation with a wide range of methods developing pupil skills
4. lacks a coherent, co-ordinated approach which takes account of other influences on pupils;	recognizes the wide range of influences on pupil's health and attempts to take account of pupils' pre-existing beliefs, values and attitudes;
5. tends to respond to a series of perceived problems or crises on a one-off basis;	recognizes that many underlying skills and processes are common to all health issues and that these should be pre-planned as part of the curriculum;
6. takes limited account of psychological fact- ors in relation to health behaviour;	views the development of a positive self image and the individual taking increasing control of his life as central to the promotion of good health

7. recognizes the importance of the school and its environment only to a limited extent;	recognizes the importance of the physical environment of the school in terms of aesthetics and also direct physiological effects on pupils and staff;
8. does not actively consider the health and wellbeing of staff in the school;	views health promotion in the school as relevant to staff wellbeing; recognizes the exemplar role of staff;
9. does not actively involve parents in the development of a health education programme;	considers parental support and co-operation as central to the health promoting school;
10. views the role of school health services purely in terms of health screening and disease prevention;	takes a wider view of the school health services which includes screening and disease prevention but also attempts actively to integrate services within the health education curriculum and helps pupils to become more aware as consumers of health services;

Table 28.1 *The health promoting school model*
10 key points for school management

The report is targeted at policy makers in the education system such as directors of education, advisers and headteachers. In addition a practical size version of the report is being prepared for the busy classroom teacher.

The chapter of the report that gives examples of good work that have been developed to improve communication between the school and the family, is further developed in a separate publication for parents which is being prepared. This popular-style publication attempts to explain the ways in which school health education is changing and encourages parents to become more involved in a partnership with the school. It also attempts to give the parents more understanding of the health and personal development needs of the young person in their family. It is envisaged that this 'user-friendly' publication will be made available to parents at parents' evenings or other channels of communication between the school and home.

A major problem in developing health education in Scottish secondary schools from the third year upwards (age 14/15 plus) is the wide degree of choice and flexibility in the curriculum of each young person. It became increasingly apparent that there was a need to offer flexible courses in health education that could augment the pupils' social education programme or add to the possible contribution of subjects such as biology or physical education. With these thoughts in mind a new series of short courses for 14 to 16 year-old students has been developed within the new standard grade development programme for Scottish schools. These short courses will come under the collective title of Health Studies and they will be internally assessed with external moderation and national certification (Scottish Examination Board, 1988). The courses will be of 20 or 40 hours duration and they will be offered independently or as coherent groups. They will be taught by teachers from a wide range of disciplines and they are designed to complement work carried out in other areas of the curriculum such as drama, English, guidance, home economics, physical education, religious and moral education, science and social education.

In all the short courses pupils will be expected to acquire knowledge and understanding and develop skills such as communication skills, practical skills and decision-making skills. In addition the courses are designed to provide opportunities for pupils to explore in realistic contexts their beliefs and values about important health issues.

The titles of the short courses are:

> What is health?
> Relationships;
> Health and food choices;
> Health and consumers;
> Parenting;
> Healthy risks;
> Health and technology;
> Decision about drugs;
> Health and exercise;
> Stress.

An attempt has been made to explore topics in a novel and a stimulating way. For example safety education has traditionally been seen as a topic related to health education but not quite part of the mainstream of health education. However through the concept of risk taking which is an important aspect of adolescent behaviour, the short course Healthy Risks explores the behavioural aspects of accidents and risk and shows how this is integrated with other health education issues such as the use of alcohol and other drugs.

The Scottish Examination Board issued the health studies course proposals for consultation in May 1988 and it is proposed that teaching materials and staff development materials will be produced in 1988/89 by development officers and teachers for local authorities with support from health education professionals. The first short courses in health studies will probably be offered in Scottish schools in late 1989.

A recent research project in Scotland entitled The Development of Teaching Materials in Health Related Physical Fitness (Ferrally and Green, 1986) indicated a lack of good teaching materials for teachers wishing to promote the health benefits of appropriate physical activity. The important role that exercise has to play in coronary heart disease prevention and the fact that in Scotland coronary heart disease accounts for approximately half of all deaths, were factors supporting the need for action in this area. In addition the other health benefits of exercise such as relaxation, weight control and simply feeling good are well documented. In the last decade there has been a significant improvement in our understanding of fitness and the principles of conditioning. Therefore a co-operative curriculum development project was set up involving SHEG, the Scottish School of Physical Education, the University of St Andrews, Scottish health boards and education authorities. This has resulted in the publication of a pack consisting of a teacher's book and associated computer software (Green *et al*, 1988). This is not intended as a comprehensive review of all aspects of health related physical fitness as the book focuses mainly on one element, aerobic fitness, since this is considered an area of major importance in relation to health. The following issues are covered:

> What is health related physical fitness?
> Principles of aerobic training;
> Teaching health related physical fitness;
> Appropriate fitness tests.

The computer software consists of floppy discs for BBC micro computers each with a set of user instructions that assist the teacher to set up and administer the standard tests associated with this approach – these are on the following themes:

> The six minute run test;
> The 20 meter shuttle run test;
> Aerobic conditioning;
> Body composition.

The pack draws on the Eurofit project which has developed a series of standard tests to measure various aspects of fitness. It is recognized that schools, on a normal time allocation for physical education, cannot make significant improvements in the aerobic fitness of young people unless they build appropriate exercise patterns into their lifestyle and practical suggestions for teachers are built into the teacher's book to promote this. The use of the new materials in schools will be monitored to estimate their effectiveness in influencing the physical education curriculum and this will provide lessons for future curriculum development projects.

References

Farrally, M R and Green, B N (1986) *The Development of Teaching Methods in Health Related Physical Fitness* Jordanhill College of Education, Glasgow

Green, B, Ramsay, I and Young, I (1988) *An Approach to Health Related Physical Fitness* Scottish Health Education Group, Edinburgh

Hastings, G B, Leather, D S and MacAskill, S G (1985) *Scottish Football Cup Sponsorship* Advertising Research Unit 1985, University of Strathclyde, Glasgow

Leather, D S and McNeil, R (1984) *Be All You Can Be pretest* Advertising Research Unit, University of Strathclyde, Glasgow

Scottish Examination Board (1988) *Short Life Working Group Report on Health Studies short courses* Scottish Examination Board, Dalkeith, Edinburgh

Scottish Health Education Group, World Health Organization (Euro) (1986) *The Health Promoting School Symposium 1986*: Scottish Health Education Group, Edinburgh

Young, I (1986) The use of sport sponsorship to raise health issues with schoolchildren *British Journal of Physical Education* **17**, 1

29. Drug education: an integrated strategy in Scotland – A CASE STUDY

M Raymond

Summary: The chapter reviews health education developments in Scotland with particular reference to the work of the Scottish Health Education Group (SHEG) and the school system. The scope of the work of the SHEG is briefly introduced and the nature of training opportunities in health education are explored.

In Scotland the use of mass media has been developed and refined using market research techniques and the methods used to integrate mass media communications with educational approaches in schools are briefly reviewed.

The development of the health education curriculum in Scottish schools is explained, particularly the emphasis in continuity between primary and secondary schools and the need to develop the model of the health promoting school with its emphasis on the total life of the school and greater links with parents. The need to develop a flexible curriculum for pupils in the 14 to 16 age range has resulted in a series of short courses entitled Health Studies being developed within the new standard grade programme in Scotland. These are viewed as complementing the subject-based curriculum and the social education curriculum of the school. The broad aims and content areas of the courses are briefly reviewed.

Specific teaching and learning resources to support health education have been produced in Scotland and a new kit including a teacher's guide and computer software has been produced in 1988 on the subject of health related physical fitness. The research basis and nature of this project are described.

Introduction

Health promotion emphasizes the multi-factorial nature of any strategies to alter health behaviour. Within the range of activities available to health education, the mass media, and television in particular, are regarded with most suspicion. Its effects are difficult to measure and as an essentially passive medium it can shock but rarely challenge.

This paper attempts to indicate the value of the mass media within a multi-dimensional health education strategy. In particular, it will discuss the indirect links which can exist between the use of television and the more immediate and personal style of health education in the classroom or youth club.

Background

In common with many European countries the recorded statistics in the

United Kingdom revealed a sharp upward trend in consumption of illicit drugs from the early 1980s onward. Of particular concern was the use of heroin which had shifted its position in the drug market from a fairly esoteric substance to being easily available and widely used (Home Office 1985).

The United Kingdom trend contained regional variations. In the North West of England, heroin was widely smoked and injecting almost unknown (Parker *et al*, 1986). In Scotland, there was great alarm at the very widespread injecting of heroin (Plant *et al*, 1985). Even before the serious spread of HIV by needle-sharing was noted, hepatitis B and other communicable diseases produced a high mortality rate among drug users (Robertson, 1987). A characteristic of drug users throughout Britain was, and remains the popularity of a wide range of substances with individuals using alcohol, tobacco, cannabis, heroin, solvents and diverted prescribed drugs (Plant *et al*, 1985).

Estimates of the exact rise of the drug problem are difficult to assess. Even in the early and mid-1980s, mortality rates for illicit drug misuse were tiny in comparison to rates associated with alcohol and tobacco use. However, problems are defined in ways other than official statistics, and the press were active in establishing the drugs problem as a scourge likely to blight a whole generation of young people (Kohn, 1987). Certainly, the issue remained a serious problem in the minds of the public throughout this period. In surveys carried out on behalf of SHEG in 1984, 1985 and 1986, respondents to the question 'Which of the following are serious problems in Scotland today?' have picked unemployment, drug misuse and glue sniffing as the three top problems from a list of alternatives. Heart disease, AIDS, violence and other social and health problems have been consistently relegated to minor positions in this league (Plant *et al*, 1985).

With this degree of public concern, the government was fairly quick to react. Recognizing the complexity of the drug trade and drug-taking, departments were drawn together and five broad aims were outlined:

- [ ] reducing supplies from abroad;
- [ ] tightening controls on drugs produced and prescribed here;
- [ ] making policing more effective;
- [ ] strengthening deterrence;
- [ ] improving prevention, treatment and rehabilitation (Home Office, 1985).

The level of collaboration between the various departments pursuing each of these objectives has fluctuated, but in general the degree of co-operation and the extent to which strategy was integrated has been remarkable.

In England and Wales the Department of Health and Social Security (DHSS) and the Central Office of Information (COI) collaborated in 1985 to produce a series of commercials that warned young people of the physical and mental consequences of heroin misuse. The television material was supported by posters and leaflets. In subsequent years this campaign highlighted the social consequences of heroin misuse and latterly, the risks of HIV/AIDS have become central to the television and poster work aimed both at existing drug users and those at risk of becoming involved.

The prevention strategy in England and Wales was complemented by the Department of Education and Science (DES) who supported the three-year appointment of drug education co-ordinators who mainly provided training for a range of professionals working with young people.

The Scottish strategy

In recognition of the separate health, legal and education structures in Scotland and the specific characteristics of the drug problem, a distinctive but related strategy was developed in Scotland. Separate legislation was required to tackle drug traffickers, a separate community-based treatment network developed and the education service responded in a distinctive fashion.

In terms of mass media the SHEG was asked to develop a television campaign aimed at reducing drug misuse among young people.

Mass media

Despite long mass media experience in programmes aimed at reducing alcohol and cigarette use before 1984, the SHEG had restricted its work in drug education to providing support for professionals working with young people through publications and training courses. Careful evaluation of the North American and European literature concerned with drug education was the first step in planning the programme. Two key issues emerged, targeting and message, and it was through discussion of those two considerations that the campaign began to develop.

Targeting

Drug users are notably resilient (sic) to messages aimed at changing their behaviour even in inter-personal communication. Our primary target group was therefore teenagers aged 13–20 years who were either not using drugs or who had perhaps experimented with drugs or were at risk of doing so. It was also recognized that the differing interests and lifestyles of a 13 year-old and a 20 year-old would mean splitting the age group into two sub-targets, 13 to 16 year-olds and 17 to 20 year-olds.

Parents of teenagers were also seen as an important target group not only because they had a significant social influence on their offspring, but because they required balanced, accurate information about drugs to reassure and to equip them for discussion on the subject with young people.

The third target group was the large group of professionals: teachers, youth workers, doctors, nurses, social workers, whose work brought them into contact with young people. Theirs was a key role in both prevention and treatment and the campaign included up-to-date literature and in-service training as a way of supporting their work.

Message

During 1984 the SHEG launched a television commercial under the banner of the slogan Be All You Can Be aimed at promoting positive attitudes to general health. It was important for the SHEG, to maintain this commitment to positive health promotion. Indeed the literature of drug education highlights the ineffectiveness and dangers of emphasizing the medical consequences of drug use and supplying information about drugs without consideration to the social context (Flay and Sobel 1983, Bandy and President 1983). By using the Be All You Can Be approach and avoiding any semblance of shock/horror, the campaign was designed to promote self-esteem and feeling of independence not just by offering alternative sources of satisfaction but by highlighting how young people could achieve a sense of self-identity and enjoy themselves without resorting to drugs.

For parents the rationale was to provide information about drugs in a balanced unsensational way to encourage parents to see drug-taking within the context of social pressures facing young people. Unlike the teenage target group which was best reached through television, it was felt that the need to provide fairly extensive information for parents required a bright glossy magazine-style booklet, distributed through family and women's magazines. To encourage discussion within the family, it was also intended that this 'magazine' would be attractive to and read by young people as well.

The commercials were adapted to refer not to the more extreme medical consequences of drug use, but to indicate the social consequences of drug use, for example, the effects on the family. Innovative video work and contrasting monochrome and colour photography were used to enhance the positive message. The commercial for older teenagers focused on the social interests of this age group, while that aimed at younger adolescents featured credible acceptable alternative activities.

While developing the television commercial and Family Matters, the magazine insert, we were also keen to ensure that politicians and government officials were aware of the direction we were taking. By continually explaining and justifying our approach we were rewarded by support from politicians.

Evaluation

In the months following the launch, the Advertising Research Unit, University of Strathclyde, monitored audience reaction to the television commercials and the magazine insert. The evaluation concentrated on reactions to the materials. There was no attempt to measure attitude or behaviour change. Attitude is only marginally related to behaviour. Many other factors intervene in a young person's decision to become involved in drug misuse. Drug-taking behaviour is notoriously difficult to measure and the techniques required to establish accurate reportage of behaviour were beyond the scope of this study.

The sample incorporated the three target groups: teenagers (13 to 16 yeas), teenagers (17 to 20 years), and parents of 13 to 20 year-olds, of both sexes and from representative class backgrounds. Overall 635 people were interviewed (Advertising Research Unit 1985). Awareness of television material was high, especially among teenagers, at both a spontaneous and prompted level. Thus 67 per cent of 13 to 16 year-olds and 77 per cent of 17 to 20 year-olds were aware, without prompting, of the material targeted at them. These figures rose to over 90 per cent for each age group on prompted recall. Parents too had high levels of awareness, 67 per cent without being prompted and 77 per cent on being shown stills from the commercials. The perceived messages of the campaign were seen as being both positive and negative. For example, among 13 to 16 year-olds 95 per cent agreed that their commercial was telling them of 'things they could do rather than take drugs', while 90 per cent agreed with the more negative 'taking drugs can damage your health'. Given the strong negative associations that are drawn with drugs and drug-taking the positive messages had successfully reached the targeted audience. There was stronger recognition of the material's objectives in establishing that you can enjoy life without drugs rather than its objective of promoting specific alternative activities. At a prompted level, there was considerable agreement that the campaign was liable to promote discussion about drug misuse within the family and between peers. Over a third of respondents had in fact discussed the campaign in this way.

The style of the television materials was seen as being attractive and relevant to the young people targeted. On a more general level, 95 per cent of the sample felt that 'the advertising campaign was a good idea'. However, there was a consistent 20 to 25 per cent of the sample who were critical, feeling that the television materials failed to portray the reality of drug-taking and the realities of the depressed social environment many young people found themselves in. While perceptions of the campaign were in general very positive, for example 90 per cent of each sub-sample felt that it made 'you think that a healthy lifestyle can be fun', around one-third of the sample also felt that it was treating a serious subject 'too lightheartedly'. These reservations were highest among the 17 to 20 year-old group and among the unemployed.

Awareness of the magazine insert was much lower than the television materials. Even with prompts the awareness level only rose to 22 per cent. Further research identified some of the reasons for this. In the light of our philosophy to 'de-sensationalize' the drug issue, the cover gave little indication of the latent subject of the booklet. While there was appreciation of why drugs had been placed within the context of social background and family life, both parents and teenagers were more interested in factual information about drugs. There was also great concern that our totally factual approach which included references to the relative ease with which an individual could pass through heroin withdrawal symptoms did not accord with the public's perceptions of drug-taking based on media coverage. The attractive glossy style coupled with this challenging information reduced the booklet's authority. However, there was considerable support for this type of booklet in principle and a desire for information among both teenagers and parents.

Development and evaluation of 1986 campaign

In terms of audience awareness the 1985 campaign had been successful and the SHEG continued the campaign with a new television commercial aimed at 17 to 20 year-olds, but incorporating enough features to be attractive to the younger age group.

The commercial picked up strengths and weaknesses revealed by the 1985 evaluation and a positive message, 'Choose life, not drugs', was maintained. The treatment focused on the social pressures facing young people. Four factors which could encourage young people to become involved in drugs were featured: media sensationalism, boredom and alienation, family tension and peer group pressure. Within the 40-second format all four scenarios were resolved in a positive way, indicating the potential for young people to make their own decisions in the light of socio-economic constraints. The television commercials were backed by an extensive outdoor poster campaign.

Updated booklets for professionals were also distributed and a new tabloid-style leaflet for parents was developed and distributed door-to-door to households likely to have teenagers living at home.

Evaluation of the 1986 material indicated high levels of awareness, with over 90 per cent of young people being aware of the campaign (Advertising Research Unit 1986). Comprehension of the fairly complex message was at equivalent levels to the 1985 evaluation results and there was a high level of support for the campaign from young people. Indeed, there was particular recognition of the relevance of the social and relationship issues raised in the commercial. While awareness of the tabloid-style leaflet was again disappointing, parents and young people were broadly supportive of the material and it seems to have encouraged discussion with over a third of respondents saying they had spoken about the campaign and its content.

The evaluation confirmed that the level of basic knowledge about drugs and drug-taking runs at a fairly high level among young people, and that they welcome discussion of the wider issues around drug-taking. Despite a recurrent demand from young people for a frightening television treatment, the evaluation showed high levels of identification with the characters and the situations portrayed and strong support for the overall aims of the material.

The 1988 campaign

The limitations of mass media work on health issues have been widely commented on (Advertising Research Unit (1986), Kay (1986)). In a medium which lacks any form of interaction, it is difficult to teach skills, clarify values and discuss the implications of behaviour change. The logical development from the 1985 and 1986 television work was to go beyond a simple acknowledgement of peer group pressure to actually suggesting possible strategies to help adolescents cope with this type of pressure.

The objectives of the 1988 campaign came close to the boundaries of what is realistically possible in social advertising. In portraying reasons for rejecting drugs, and backing that up with demonstrations of how to convey those messages to the peer group, the commercial set the agenda for discussions of lifeskills approaches in school health education. The material's effectiveness was dependent on the realism of the situation portrayed and the relevance of the evasion tactics. Pre-testing also showed it was vital to build self-esteem by conveying the impression that peer group pressure was something which could be broken without damaging valuable relationships. It was also recognized that the peer group could also have a positive role to play in supporting decisions to avoid drug-taking.

Despite a less spectacular visual style than previous commercials, the 1988 campaign achieved very high levels of awareness. More importantly, there was a high level of understanding of the fairly complex messages and a belief in the relevancy of the issues (Advertising Research Unit, 1988).

Education Service

Developments in the education service in Scotland were the responsibility of the Scottish Education Department. However, links between developments in the education service and public education were fostered by a number of key structural factors. Firstly, excellent and regular communication existed between the education department and all other interested government departments both nationally and locally. This enabled the police, for example, to understand the objectives of both the national media campaign and the schools initiatives and to make a strong contribution towards both. Secondly, the role of the SHEG was important. As a health service body with very close links with social work, voluntary agencies and both school and community education, the SHEG is ideally placed to make links between different initiatives. Along with its public education activities in drugs, the SHEG played an important role in virtually all developments in the education service.

Training for teachers and youth workers

Rather than appoint regional drug training co-ordinators, the Scottish Education Department chose to develop a major programme of training in drug education issues for teachers and youth workers.

Separate strategies were developed for the formal and informal sectors. A multi-disciplinary approach was considered but it was felt that in a controversial and challenging area such as drug education, it was important for teachers and youth workers to establish what contribution they could make within their professional sphere before coming together.

A framework was developed in both sectors to allow a balance between central control and regional autonomy. National working parties for the schools and for the community sectors met to develop a series of guidelines for training which could then be implemented by regional authorities. Regions were encouraged to interpret the guidelines in ways which best suited their employees and local conditions. Substantial funding support was provided and guidance provided by bodies like SHEG. Local education authorities were strongly urged to liaise closely with health education, voluntary services, police and social work and those professional groups often contributed to the planning process.

Internal evaluation of the training strategy (National Planning Group, 1987) indicated a high level of support for the courses from participants who saw the relevance of drug education. For many teachers drug-taking was less immediate an issue than problems associated with alcohol. Although the courses focused on illicit drugs they also considered other substances. In addition participants valued the emphasis on skills and educational approaches and recognized their relevance in teaching about other health related issues. The courses placed drug education firmly within the context of health education and the courses had the effect of stimulating interest in integrated curricular approaches to health.

Community education established a national support group, again with SHEG involvement, to provide help for regional community education officers who had the responsibility for developing courses and to collate the formative evaluation. In this way the training strategy has been shaped and developed to cope with expansion into the voluntary youth sector and to meet other health challenges like alcohol and AIDS.

The Guidelines for both school and community placed a premium on the development of skills relevant to health education about drugs and supplied only enough information to give educators the confidence to apply existing and enhanced skills. Most regions opted for a residential setting with two blocks of 2.5 days separated by an assignment period of three months. The assignment directly linked training with practice. In later courses for voluntary organizations, this action element was extended by providing each participant with a small budget to develop a local project.

In terms of content, both courses were shaped by a need to address the day-to-day policy and pastoral problems which drugs might cause for the secondary school or the community centre. It was recognized by organizers and participants alike that no progress could be made in drug-related work unless participants had the opportunity to explore their own prejudices, misconceptions and anxieties about drug use and to explore parallels between the use of illicit and socially acceptable drugs. These issues are commonplace elements in all successful drug training, but for teachers and youth workers alike the emphasis was placed on prevention work with individuals or groups. In the schools courses, particular attention was paid to the possible use of drug education packs and their positioning within a broad health education curriculum.

Teaching materials

The Drugwise 12–14 pack development by the central committee for the curriculum and Strathclyde region was the focus for a great deal of work in the courses. This self-contained pack of teaching materials, designed for the early years of secondary schools, is mainly concerned with the development of good decision-making skills about drugs. Using adequate background knowledge, young people are encouraged to discuss how they would handle peer group pressure. In common with other recently developed United Kingdom drug education material like Drugwise 14–18, this Scottish material places drugs firmly within the problems and opportunities faced by adolescents and goes well beyond a narrow focus on drugs to consider a wide range of social and personal skills. The Drugwise 12–14 pack was partly marketed and piloted through the training programme. Its introduction in schools in Strathclyde and other Scottish regions was carefully evaluated. The findings (Barr and Rand, 1988) revealed high levels of acceptability of this type of approach among pupils and teachers. One lesson involving the police was an excellent example of the structured involvement of a visitor in a longterm educational programme. The skills-based approach was again seen as relevant to both teachers and young people.

Materials specifically designed for youth work are less common than those for schools. However, the community education training again focused on the role of drug education within the youth work curriculum with an emphasis on skills, cultural expectations, managing relationships and understanding personal pressures (National Support Group, 1988). Material developed by a specific project within the Scottish Association of Youth Clubs and supported by SHEG was used in the training as examples of the type of educational work which could take place in a youth club setting.

Conclusion

By placing drug education initiatives in the education sector within the context of wider public education campaigns, the Scottish strategy attempted to establish a consistent approach in terms of both style and content. Only extremely sophisticated and expensive evaluation methodologies would be able to establish the extent to which mass media influenced classroom or youth club activities. The effect on the behaviour of the primary target group would be even more elusive. Certainly the SHEG media campaign made no claims to directly influence behaviour. It is difficult to know whether even intensive classroom activities can have a clear influence on drug-taking.

It seems clear, however, that a confusion of different messages about drugs does not encourage clear thinking and decision making about the issue. In Scotland television, professional training and classroom materials placed a similar emphasis on clarifying opinions, making decisions and putting drug-taking within the context of all the other concerns of adolescence. While it would be wrong to claim that the integrating of mass media with other educational strategies was the result of a fully developed health promotion policy, there was a remarkably high degree of collaboration at national and local levels. Liaison between health, education, enforcement and voluntary agencies was the key to this initiative and offers a useful working model for future development on other health education issues.

References

Advertising Research Unit (1985) *Evaluation of the Scottish Health Education Group's 1985 Drug Education Campaign* University of Strathclyde

Advertising Research Unit (1986) *Evaluation on the Scottish Health Education Group's 1986 Drug Education Campaign* University of Strathclyde

Advertising Research Unit (1987) *Summary Presentation on Tracking SHEG Studies 1985–1987,* University of Strathclyde

Advertising Research Unit (1988) *Evaluation of the Scottish Health Education Group's 1988 Drug Education Campaign* University of Strathclyde

Advisory Council on the Misuse of Drugs (1984) *Prevention* HMSO

Bandy, P and President, P A (1983) Recent literature on drug abuse prevention in the mass media *Journal of Drug Education* **13**, 3

Barr, I M I and Rand, J (1988) *Final Evaluation Report in the Phase 2 piloting of Drugwise 12–14* Consultative Committee on the Curriculum

Flay, B R and Sobel, J L (1983) *The Role of the Mass Media in Preventing Adolescent Substance Abuse* NIDA

Home Office (1985) *Tackling Drug Misuse: a summary of the government's strategy* HMSO

Jaquet, S (1988) *Hey Mister, Got any samples?: the first year of the Fast Forward Project* Youth Clubs Scotland

Kay, L (1986) Prevention charter *Druglink* July/August

Kohn, M (1987) *Narcomania: on heroin* Faber and Faber

National Support Group (1988) *Drug Misuse: a community education approach* SCEC/SHEG

National Planning Group (1987) *Report on Inservice Courses on the Misuse of Drugs*

Parker, H, Bakx, K and Newcombe, R (1986) *Drug Misuse in Wirral* University of Liverpool

Peason, G, Gilman, M, McIver, S (1987) *Young People and Heroin Use in the North of England* Health Education Council

Plant, M A, Peck, D and Samuel, E (1985) *Alcohol, Drugs and School leavers* Tavistock

Plant, M A (1987) *Drugs in Perspective* Hodder and Stoughton

Robertson, R (1987) *Heroin AIDS and Society* Hodder and Stoughton

Bibliography
(Based only on references provided in the papers)

Books and pamphlets

Allen, I (1987) *Education in Sex and Personal Relationships* Research Report No. 665, Policy Studies Institute: London

Anderson, M G and Child, R C (1985) *Systems and Behaviour Change: Health Promotion Objectives in Southern Illinois*. 12th World Conference on Health Education Proceedings, Dublin: Ireland

Balding, J W (1987) *Young People in 1986* HEA Schools Education Unit, University of Exeter: England

Balding, J W (1989) *Parents and Health Education* HEA Schools Health Education Unit, University of Exeter: England

Balding, J W (1989) *Health Education Priorities for the Primary School Curriculum* HEA Schools Health Education Unit, University of Exeter: England

Bandura, A (1971) *Social Learning Theory* General Learning Press: New York

Bandura, A (1986) *Social Foundations of Thought and Action: a Social Cognitive Theory* Prentice-Hall: New York

Bateson, G (1979) *Mind and Nature* Bantam Books

Becker, M H (1974) *The Health Belief Model and Personal Health Behaviour* Health Education Monographs 2

Berkowitz, L ed (1964) *Advances in Experimental Social Psychology I* Academic Press: New York

Berkowitz, L ed (1986) *Advances in Experimental Social Psychology Vol 19* Academic Press: London

Bogatta, E F and Evans, R R eds (1968) *Smoking, Health and Behavior* Aldine: Chicago

Braun, D (1987) *Spon Gate Mums Group: Supporting Mothers of Young Children* CEDC: Coventry

Braun, D and Combes, G (1988) *Working with Parents: A Report of a Teachers' Development Group Working in Birmingham* Distributed by Martineau Education Centre: Birmingham

Brenner, H (1980) *Report on Health Education Second Level Schools* North Western Health Board: Manorhamilton

Cleary, B (unpublished) *The Foroige Personal Effectiveness Model* Foroige: Dublin

Coates, T J, Petersen, A C and Perry, C eds (1988) *Promoting Adolescent Health: A Dialogue on Research and Practice* Academic Press: New York

Combes, G and Craft, A (1989) *Special Health: A Professional Development Programme in Health Education for Teachers of Pupils with Mild or Moderate Learning Difficulties* HEC, Health Education for Slow Learners Project, Health Education Authority: London

De'Ath, E and Pugh, G (1986) *Working with Parents: A Training Resource Pack* National Children's Bureau: London

De Vries, H and Kok, G J (1989) *Adolescent's Beliefs on Smoking: Age and Sex Difference* (in preparation)

De Vries, H, Dijkstra, M and Kok, G J (1989) *Results of the Dutch Smoking Prevention Programme* (in preparation)

Dobert, M T (1984) *Prevención Primaria del Alcoholismo en la Comunidad Chilenda* Iberoamericana de Estudios de los Problemas del Alcohol

Epp, J (1986) *Achieving Health for All: A Framework for Health Promotion* Health and Welfare Canada: Ottawa

Farrally, M R and Green, B N (1988) *The Development of Teaching Methods in Health Studies Short Courses* Scottish Examination Board, Dalkeith: Scotland

Fernandez, O (1986) *Programa de Prevención de Caries Escolares en un Servicio de Salud de Santiage* Monografia 4a Jornada de Salud Publica: Chile

Figueras, T (1984) *Thesis El Programa de Prevencion Primaria del Alcohol desde la perspective del Profesor; un Estudio*

Fishbein, M and Ajzen, I (1975) *Belief, Attitude, Intention and Behaviour: an Introduction to the Theory and Research* Addison Wesley: Reading, Massachusetts

Flay, B R and Sobel, J L (1983) *The Role of the Mass Media in Preventing Adolescent Substance Abuse* NIDA

Freire, P (1972) *Pedagogy of the Oppressed* Penguin: Middlesex

Fry, J ed (1979) *Economy, Class and Social Reality: issues in Contemporary Canadian Society* Butterworth and Co.: Toronto

Gilbert, J J (1976) *Education Handbook* World Health Organization: Geneva

Green, B, Ramsay, I and Young, I (1988) *An approach to Health Related Physical Fitness* Scottish Health Education Group: Edinburgh

Hastings, G B, Leathar, D S and MacAskill, S G (1985) *Scottish Football Cup Sponsorship* Advertising Research Unit, University of Strathclyde: Glasgow

Hetzel, B (1980) *Health in Australian Society* Penguin: Harmondsworth

Hilliard, B (1986) *NWHB Lifeskills Programme for Schools: External Evaluation* Health Education Office: Donegal

Hopson, B and Scally, M (1981) *Lifeskills Teaching* McGraw-Hill: London

Jaquet, S (1988) *Hey Mister, Got any Samples?: The First Year of the Fast Forward Project* Youth Clubs Scotland

Johansson, L (1987) *Kosthold oq Helse* Noras-rapport

Jones, A (1987) *Health Education and the Secondary School Curriculum: A Report for Health Education Council* Health Education Unit: University of Southampton

Kane, P and Ruzicka, L (1987) *Australian Population Trends and Their Social Consequences* Commission for the Future: Melbourne

Kannas, L and Miilunpalo, S eds (1988) *The Yearbook of Health Education* Health Education Series Original Reports 8: National Board of Health: Finland

Kindervatter, S (1979) *Nonformal Education as an Empowering Process* Centre for International Education, Amherst: Mass

King, A J, Robertson, A S and Warren, W K (1985) *Summary Report, Canada Health Attitudes and Behaviour Survey: 9, 12 and 15 year olds* Queen's University, Social Program Evaluation Group, Kingston: Ontario

Koeune, E (1957) *How to Teach Hygiene, Home Nursing and First Aid. A Book for Primary School and Welfare Centres in East Africa* East African Literature Bureau

Kohn, M (1987) *Narcomania: On Heroin* Faber and Faber

Koskela, K (1981) *A Community Based Antismoking Programme as a Part of a Comprehensive Cardiovascular Programme (The North Karelia Project)* Kuopion korkeakoulun jukkaisuja, Kansanterveystiede, Sarja alkuperäistutkimukset

Labonte, R and Penfold, S (1981) *Canadian Perspectives in Health Promotion: A Critique* Queen's University: Social Program Evaluation Group

Lalonde, M (1974) *A New Perspective on the Health of Canadians* Department of Health and Welfare: Canada

Lazes, P M (ed) (1979) *Handbook of Health Education* Aspen Systems Corp: Maryland

Leathar, D S, Hastings, G B and Davies, J K (eds) (1981) *Health Education and the Media* Pergamon: London

Leathar, D S and McNeil, R (1984) *Be All You Can Be* (pretest) Advertising Research Unit, University of Strathclyde: Glasgow

Lindzey, G and Aronson, E eds (1985) *Handbook of Social Psychology Vol 2* Lawrence Erlbaum
    Associates: New York
Long, R (1986) *Developing Parental Involvement in Primary Schools* Macmillans: Basingstoke
Lutwama, J S and Bennett, F J (1969) *Health Education in East Africa: A Challenge to Schools*
    Longmans: Nairobi

McGrath, P J and Firestone, P eds (1983) *Pediatric and Adolescent Behavioural Medicine* Springer:
    New York
McKennel, A C and Thomas, R K (1967) *Adults and Adolescents' Smoking Habits and Attitudes:
    Government Social Survey* Ministry of Health: London
McKeown, T (1976) *The Role of Medicine: Dream, Mirage or Nemesis?* Nuffield Provincial Hospitals
    Trust: London
Mcloone, S and McAuley, B (1985) *the Lifeskills Programme for Schools in the North Western Health
    Board Region* North Western Health Board: Manorhamilton
McMichael, A and Hetzel, B (1987) *The L/S Factor* Penguin: Harmondsworth
McQueen, D (1987) *Research in Health Beahviour, Health Promotion and Public Health* Background
    reading Edinburgh Meeting, Research Unit in Health and Behavioural Change: University
    of Edinburgh
Manuya, S J ( ) *Maarifa Mapya ya Kuelimisha Afya* East African Literature Bureau
Mardones, S F (1984) *Breastfeeding Determinants in Chile* Santiago: Chile
Melchafsky et al (1986) *Programa de Atencion Odontologica Incremental* Monografia 4a Jornada de
    Salud Publica: Chile
Morley, D, Rohde, J and Williams, G (1983) *Practising Health for All* Oxford University Press

Norman-Taylor, W (1956) *A Textbook of Hygiene for Teachers in Africa* Longmans: Nairobi

Oduol, E (1985) *Training Community Health Workers in Southern Sudan: A Field Report* African
    Medical and Research Council

Pallonen, U (1986) *Prevention of Smoking Onset on East Finland Adolescent Population* Health
    Education Series Original Reports 5: National Board of Health: Finland
Parker, H, Bakx, K and Newcombe, R (1986) *Drug Misuse in Wirral* University of Liverpool
Peason, G, Gilman, M and McIver, S (1987) *Young People and Heroin Use in the North of England*
    Health Education Council
Plant, M A (1987) *Drugs in Perspective* Hodder and Stoughton: London
Plant, M A, Peck, D and Samuel, E (1985) *Alcohol, Drugs and School Leavers* Tavistock: London
Pritchard, P ed (1983) *The Practice Nurse and Prevention* Report of Two Study Days for Practice
    Nurses: Oxford Regional Health Authority

Raw, M (1982) *A Brief Guide to the Smoking Treatment Literature* Action on Smoking and Health
    (ASH): London
Robertson, R (1987) *Heroin AIDS and Society* Hodder and Stoughton: London
Robinson, Y K (1987) *Health Education/Promotion in the NHS Post Griffiths* Health Education
    Authority: London
Rodnell, S and Watt, A (1987) *The Politics of Health Education – Raising the Issues* Routledge and
    Kegan Paul: London
Roemer, R (1982) *Legislative Action to Combat the World Smoking Epidemic* WHO: Geneva
Ross, M G and Lappin, B W (1967) *Community Organization: Theory, Principles and Practice* Harper
    and Row: New York
Rubinson, L and Alles, W F (1984) *Health Education: Foundations for the Future* Times Mirror/
    Mosby College Publishers: Toronto

Scotney, N (1976) *Health Education: A Manual for Medical Assistants and Rural Health Workers*
    African Medical Research Foundation
Shaffer, R (1984) *Beyond the Dispensary: On Giving Community Balance to Primary Health Care*
    African Medical and Research Council Report
Shain, M, Suurvali, H and Boutilier, M (1986) *Healthier Workers: Health Promotion and Employee
    Assistance Programs* Lexington Books, D C Heath Co.: Lexington

Ssenyonga, J. Oduol, E and Nzioka, N (1986) *Evaluation of Innovative Projects for Strengthening Community Health Action through Health Education* African Medical and Research Council Report

Stensvold, I et al (1989) *The Effect of Boiled and Filter Coffee on Serum Cholesterol and Triglycerides* (to be published) National Health Screening Service: Oslo

Sutherland, I (1987) *Health Education: Perspectives and Choices* (Chapter 1) National Extension College: Cambridge

Sutherland, I (1988) *Health Education – Half a Policy: The Rise and Fall of the Health Education Council* National Extension College: Cambridge

Tammivuori, T ed (1976) *International Congress of Physical Education* Jyväskylä, Liikuntatieteellisen Seuran Julkaisuja 64: Helsinki

Tones, B K, Tilford, S and Robinson Y K (1988) *Evaluating Health Education: The Meaning of Success* Chapman and Hall (in press) London

Vartiainen, E (1982) *Changes in Cardiovascular Risk Factors during a Two Year Intervention Programme among 13–15 year old Children and Adolescents (The North Karelia Youth Project)* Community Health, Series Original Reports 4: University of Kuopio: Finland

Vicuna, M B (1933) *Los Medicos de Antano en el Reino de Chile* Editorial Ercilla Santiago: Chile

Whitehead, M (1987) *The Health Divide: Inequalities in Health in the 1980s* The Health Education Council: London

Woods, P (1984) *Parents and School* SCDC/ Welsh Consumer Council: Cardiff

Official and corporate publications

Advertising Research Unit (1985) *Evaluation of the Scottish Health Education Group's 1985 Drug Education Campaign* University of Strathclyde

Advertising Research Unit (1986) *Evaluation of the Scottish Health Education Group's 1986 Drug Education Campaign* University of Strathclyde

Advertising Research Unit (1987) *Summary Presentation of Tracking SHEG Studies 1985–1987* University of Strathclyde

Advertising Research Unit (1988) *Evaluation of the Scottish Health Education Group's 1988 Drug Education Campaign* University of Strathclyde

Advisory Council on the Misuse of Drugs (1984) *Prevention* HMSO: London

African Medical and Research Foundation (AMREF) (1977) *Health Behaviour and Education Project Proposal* AMREF

African Medical and Research Foundation (AMREF) (1985) *Folk Media: Communicating for Health Promotion* Kenya Communications Support Project in Turkana District in Kenya, A Concept Paper

Canadian Health Education Society (CHES) (1988) *CHES Ontario Newsletter* Chapter 3 1 March: Ontario

Central Bureau of Statistics of Norway (1985) *Health Survey*

Central Bureau of Statistics of Norway (1987) *Statistical Yearbook*

Cohen Committee (1964) *Health Education* Report of a Joint Committee of the Central and Scottish Health Services Councils, HMSO: London

CONPAN (1979) *Lactancia Materna en Chile* Santiago: Chile

Court Report (1976) *Fit for the Future* HMSO: London

Department of Education and Science (DES) (1968) *A Handbook of Health Education* HMSO: London

Department of Education and Science (DES) (1977) *Curriculum 11–16: Health Education in Secondary School Curriculum* HMSO: London

Department of Education and Science (DES) (1977) *Health Education in Schools* HMSO: London

Department of Education and Science (DES) (1985) *Better Schools* White Paper HMSO: London

Department of Education and Science (DES) (1986) *Education (No. 2) Act* HMSO: London

Department of Education and Science (DES) (1986) *A Health Education from 5 to 16* Curriculum Matters 8. an HMI series, HMSO: London

Department of Education and Science (DES) (1987) *Sex Education at School* Circular No. 11/87 DES: London

Department of Education and Science (DES) *Education Reform Act* HMSO: London

Department of Health (1986) *Health – The Wider Dimensions* Dublin

Department of Health and Social Security (DHSS) (1976) *Prevention and Health: Everybody's Business* HMSO: London

Department of Health and Social Security (DHSS) (1981) *Health Education: The Recruitment, Training and Development of Health Education Officers* Reports of a Working Party of the National Staff Committee for Administrative and Clerical Staff, January, 1988, DHSS: London

Government of Canada (1964) *Royal Commission on Health Services* Vol. 1, Queen's Printer: Ottawa

Government of Canada (1969) *Task Force on the Cost of Health Services in Canada* Department of National Health and Welfare: Ottawa

Government of Canada (1988) *Action on Drug Abuse* Ottawa

Government Publications Office (1970) *Health Act* Government Publications Office: Dublin 2

Hargreaves Report (1984) *Improving Secondary Schools* Inner London LEA

HEA Schools Health Education Unit (1985) *Just a Tick: Health Topic Questionnaire Survey Methods* University of Exeter: England

HEA Schools Health Education Unit (1987) *Health Related Behaviour Questionnaire (Version 11)* University of Exeter: England

Health Education Bureau (1984) *A Value for Effort – Social and Economic Aspects of Health Education/Health Promotion* Proceedings of a conference held in Athlone

Health Education Bureau (1987) *Promoting Health Through Public Policy* Dublin

Health Education Council (HEC) (1987) *Parents, Schools and Community: Working Together in Health Education* Health Education for Slow Learners Project, Distributed by Community Education Development Centre: Coventry

Home Office (1985) *Tackling Drug Misuse: A Summary of the Government's Strategy* HMSO: London

Lincoln Institute of Health Sciences (1983) *Course Accreditation Proposal: PG1 Health Education* Melbourne

Lincoln Institute of Health Sciences (1988) *Course Information Booklet: PG1 Health Education* Melbourne

Ministry of Education (1956) *Health Education* Pamphlet No 31, HMSO: London

Ministry of Health (1972) *The Health Education Division Five Year Plan 1973–1978* Ministry of Health: Kenya

Ministry of Health (1985) *Health Education Strategy in Kenya* Ministry of Health: Kenya

National Council on Smoking and Health (1987) *Supplement to the Norwegian Tobacco Act of 9 March 1973* Draft Act of 18 December 1987

National Consumer Council (NCC) (1986) *The Missing Links between Home and School: A Consumer View* NCC: London

National Planning Group (1987) *Report on Inservice Courses on the Misuse of Drugs*

National Support Group (1988) *Drug Misuse: A Community Education Approach* SCEC/SHEG

Norwegian Coffee Information (1987) *Report 1987*

Norwegian Directorate of Health (1986) *Helseopplysnung i en kommune*

Ontario Ministry of Health (1983) *Health Protection and Promotion Act* Bill 183

Ontario Ministry of Health (1986) *The Role and Functions of the Health Educator in Ontario Boards of Health* March, Public Health Branch

Open University (1982) *Parents and Teenagers* Harper and Row: London

Ottawa Charter (1986) *International Conference on Health Promotion*

PESMIB (1974) *Conocimientos, Actitudes y Practicas de las Madres en Relacion con el Embarazo, Parto y Puerperio* Santiago: Chile

Plowden Report (1967) *Children and their Primary Schools* HMSO: London

Royal College of General Practitioners (RCGP) (1981) *Health and Prevention in Primary Care* Report from General Practice, No 18, RCGP: London

Secretary of Education (1983) *Information* Santiago: Chile

Secretary of Health (1984) *Proyecto Aprender a Ensenar* Santiago: Chile

Secretary of Health (1985) *Monografia 3as Jornadas Nacionales Multidisciplinarias de Educacion para la Salud* Santiago: Chile

Secretary of Health (1988) *Programa Integrado de Salud Materno Infantil* Santiago: Chile

Scottish Examination Board (1988) *Short Life Working Group Report on Health Studies Short Courses* Dalkeith: Edinburgh

Scottish Health Education Group, World Health Organization (Euro) (1986) *The Health Promoting School Symposium* Scottish Health Education Group: Edinburgh

Smoking and Health Foundation (1986) *Annual Report* The Hague

Social Health Office (1988) *Social Health Strategy for South Australia* South Australian Health Commission

Victorian Government (1986) *Ministerial Review of Health Education and Health Promotion: Report to the Minister for Health* Victorian Government Publishing Service: Melbourne

Welsh Heart Programme (1985) *Take Heart* Heartbeat Report No 1

Welsh Heart Programme (1987) *Health Eating Policy for Schools in Wales*

World Health Organization (WHO) (1984) *Health Promotion: A Discussion Document on the Concept and Principles* WHO Euro: Copenhagen

World Health Organization (WHO) (1985) *Targets for All* WHO Euro: Copenhagen

World Health Organization (WHO) (1986) *A Charter for Health Promotion* Report of First International Conference on Health Promotion, Ottawa, WHO Euro: Copenhagen (see also Ottawa Charter)

World Health Organization (WHO) (1987) *Health Promotion: Concept and Principles in Action, A Policy Framework* WHO Euro: Copenhagen

World Health Organization (WHO) (1987) *Report of Regional Workshop on Strengthening the Training of Communication/Education for Health in Health Personnel Training Institutions* Harare, Zimbabwe 6–10 October 1986, WHO Africa: Brazzaville

World Health Organization (WHO) (1987) *Health Promotion: A Discussion Document on the Concept and Principles* WHO: Geneva

World Health Organization (WHO) (1988) *Australian Day. Papers and Workshop* Proceedings 2nd International Conference on Health Promotion, Adelaide, WHO Euro: Copenhagen

World Health Organization (WHO) (1988) *Strategies for Health Public Policy* Report of 2nd International Conference on Health Promotion, Adelaide, WHO Euro: Copenhagen

World Health Organization (WHO) (1988) *Priority Research for Health for All* European Health for All Series 3

Articles, periodicals and working papers

Aaro, L e, Bruland, E, Hauknes, A and Lochsen, P M (1983) Smoking among Norwegian schoolchildren 1975–1980. III. The effect of antismoking campaigns *Scandinavian Journal of Psychology* 24: 277–283

Aaro, L E (1988) Research on health promotion and lifestyles: Some comments about theoretical and practical orientation *in* Kannas, L and Miilunpalo, S

Aaro, L E, Wold, B, Kannas, L and Rimpelä, M (1988) Health Behaviour in schoolchildren. A Who Cross National Survey. A presentation of philosophy, methods and selected results of the first survey *Health Promotion* 1:(1) 17–33

Alanen, L (1985) What can be learned from progress in socialisation research? *in* Anderson, M G and Child, R C

Ashton, J et al (1986) Health cities – World Health Organization's New Public Health Initiative *Health Promotion* 1: 3 319–321

Axelsson, A and Brantmark, B (1975) The anti-smoking effect of chewing-gum with nicotine of high and low bioavailability. In *Proceeding of 3rd World Conference on Smoking and Health*: New York

Badgley, R F (1978) Health promotion and social change in the health of Canadians. Paper presented at Conference on Evaluation of Health Education and Behaviour Modification Programs, Canadian Health Education Society, December

Balding, J W (1988) Teenage smoking: The levels are falling at last! *Education and Health* 6: 3, 68

Bandy, P and President, P A (1983) Recent literature on drug abuse prevention in the mass media *Journal of Drug Education* 13: 3

Barr, I M I and Rand, J (1988) Final evaluation report in the phase 2 piloting of Drugwise 12–14 Consultative Committee on the Curriculum

Baum, F and Brown, V A (1988) Healthy cities (Australia) project: From vision to reality. In *Proceedings, 2nd International Conference on Health Promotion*, Adelaide: World Health Organization: Geneva

Bauman, K E and Chenoweth, R L (1984) The relationship between the consequences adolescents expect from smoking and their behaviour: A factor analysis with panel data *Journal of Applied Social Psychology* 14: 28–41

Beazley, R and Belzer Jr, E G (1984) The professionalization of health education in Canada *CHES Technical Publications* Canadian Health Education Society 7, Fall

Best, J A, Flay, B R, Towson, S M J, Ryan, K B, Perry, C L, Brown, K S, Kersell, M W and D'Avernas, J (1984) Smoking prevention and the concept of risk *Journal of Applied Social Psychology* 14: 257–273

Best, J A, Thomson, S J, Santi, S M, Smith, E A and Brown, K S (1988) Preventing cigarette smoking among schoolchildren *Annual Review of Public Health* 9: 161–201

Biglan, A, Severson, H, Bavry, J and McConnel, S (1983) Social influence and adolescent smoking: A first look behind the barn *Health Education* 14–18

Bolaria, S (1979) Self-care and lifestyles: Ideological and policy implications *in* Fry (1979)

Botvin, G J and Eng, A (1982) The efficacy of a multicomponent approach to the prevention of cigarette smoking *Preventive Medicine* 11: 199–211

Braun, D and Combes, G (1987) Parental involvement: What are we preparing teachers to do? *Community Education Journal* 6 (2): 24–28

Broadhead, P (1985) Social status and morbidity in Australia *Community Health Studies* 14: 2 87–97

Brown, V A (1981) From sickness to health: An altered focus for health care research *Social Science and Medicine* 15A: 195–201

Brown, V A (1985) Social health in a small city. In *Proceedings 3rd International Conference on Health Education*, Dublin

Cameron, H (1987) Status and trends in school health education in Canada. Paper presented to School of Physical and Health Education and Recreation: Dalhousie University, November

Clavell, F and Benhamor, S (1984) Desintoxication tabagique. Comparison de l'efficacite de differentes methodes. Resultats intermediares d'une etude comparitive Prres. Medic 13: 975–977

Collishaw, N (1986) Healthstyles: Final results. Presentations at 77th annual meeting of the Canadian Public Health Association, Vancouver: British Columbia, June

Combes, G (1986) Transcript of discussions with the 'Out of the House Group' Birmingham (unpublished)

Combes, G and Lloyd, J (1988) Working with teachers *Community Education Network* 8 (7): 4

De Vries, H and Kok, G J (1986) From determinants of smoking behaviour to the implications for a prevention programme *Health Education Research* 1: 85–94

De Vries, H, Dijkstra, M and Kuhlman, P (1988) Self-efficacy: the third Factor besides attitude and subjective norm as a predictor of behavioural intentions *Health Education Research* (3) (in press)

Evans, R I (1976) Smoking in children: developing a social psychological strategy of deterrence *Journal of Preventive Medicine* 5: 122–127

Evans, R I, Rozelle, R M, Mittelmark, M B, Hansen, W B, Bane, A L and Havis, J (1978) Deterring the onset of smoking in children: knowledge of immediate physiological effects and coping with peer pressure, media pressure and parent modeling *Journal of Applied Social Psychology* 8: 126–135

Fisher, K F, Howat, P A, Binns, C W and Liveris (1986) Health education and health promotion: An Australian perspective *Health Education Journal* 45: 95–98

Flay, B R, D'Avernas, J R, Best, J A, Kersell, M W and Ryan, K B (1983) Cigarette smoking: why young people do it and ways of preventing it *in* McGrath and Firestone (1983)

Fowler, G (1983) The opportunity for preventive medicine in general practice *in* Leathar et al (1981)

French, J and Adams, L (1986) From analysis to synthesis: Theories of health education *Health Education Journal* Vol 45: No 2: 71–74

Friedman, L S, Lichtenstein, E and Bigland, A (1985) Smoking onset among teens: an empirical analysis of initial situations *Addictive Behaviors* 10: 1–3

Fry, D (1982) Frameworks in health education. A paper presented at the 11th International Conference on Health Education: Hobart

Geirnaert, M (1984) Parents' involvement in health education in primary schools. Paper presented at a National Conference on Health Education and Youth: Southampton University 24–29 September 1984

Goodstadt, M (1982) An evaluation of two school based alcohol education programs *Journal of Studies on Alcohol* 43: 3

Goodstadt, M (1986) Factors associated with cannabis non-use and cessation of use: Between and within survey replications of findings *Addictive Behaviors* 11

Griffiths, J (1987) The health promoting school organization and policy developing in Welsh secondary schools *Health Education Journal* 46: 3

Hancock, T (1986) Promoting health in the urban context. Working paper for healthy cities symposium, Lisbon: World Health Organization

Health and Public Policy Committee: American College of Physicians (1986) Methods for stopping cigarette smoking *An. Int. Med.* 105: 281–291

Health and Welfare Canada (1982) Perspectives of the past: Twenty years of health education in Canada, an interview of Michael Palko by Frances Sgro *Health Education* 21: 1 Summer

Hirschman, R S, Leventhal, H and Glynn, K (1984) The development of smoking behavior: conceptualization and supportive cross-sectional survey data *Journal of Applied Social Psychology* 14: 184–206

Horning, E C, Horning, M G, Caroll, D I, Stillwell, R N and Dzidic, I (1973) Nicotine in smokers, non-smokers and room air *Life Science* 13: 1331–1346

Hurd, P D, Johnson, C A, Pechacek, T, Bast, L P, Jacobs, P R and Luepker, R V (1980) Prevention of cigarette smoking in seventh grade students *Journal of Behavioral Medicine* 3: 15–28

Jessor, R (1982) Critical issues in research on adolescent health promotion *in* Coates, T J, Petersen, A C and Perry, C

Jowett, S and Baginsky, M (1988) Parents and education: A survey of their involvement and a discussion of some issues *Education Research* 30 (1): 36–45

Kannas, L (1981) The dimensions of health behavior among young men in Finland *International Journal of Health Education* 24: 146–155

Kannas, L (1988) Role and development of smoking prevention programmes in schools *Hygie* VII: 18–21

Kannas, L, Tynjala, J, Aaro, L and Wold, B (1988) Leisure time physical activity and health related behaviour in four European countries *International Review for the Sociology of Sport* (in press)

Kay, L (1986) Prevention charter *Druglink* July/August

Kickbusch, I (1986) Health promotion: A global perspective *Canadian Journal of Public Health* Autumn

Klepp, K I, Halper, A and Perry, C L (1986) The efficacy of peerleaders in drug abuse prevention *Journal of School Health* 56: 407–411

Labonte, R (1985) Social inequality and healthy public policy. A paper presented at the 12th World Conference on Health Education: Dublin
Leventhal, H and Cleary, P D (1980) The smoking problem: a review of the research and theory in behavioral risk modification *Psychological Bulletin* 88: 370–405
Loken, B (1982) Heavy smokers', light smokers' and non-smokers' beliefs about cigarette smoking *Journal of Applied Psychology* 67: 616–622

McAlister, A L, Perry, C and Maccoby, N (1979) Adolescent smoking: onset and prevention *Pediatrics* 63: 650–658
Macgregor, I D M and Balding, J W (1987) Toothbrushing frequency in relation to family size and bedtime in English schoolchildren *Community Dentistry and Oral Epidemiology* 15:181
McGuire, W J (1964) Inducing resistance to persuasion *in* Berkowitz, L (1964)
McGuire, W J (1985) Attitudes and attitude change *in* Lindzey, G (1985)
McMichael, A (1985) Social class and mortality in Australian males in the 1970s *Community Health Studies* 9: 3 220–230
Marmot, M G et al (1984) Inequalities in death – specific explanations of a general pattern? *The Lancet* i, 1003–1006
Milio, N (1988) Making healthy public policy: developing the science by observing the art: An ecological framework for policy studies *Health Promotion* 2: 3
Mittelmark, M B, Murray, D M, Luepker, R V and Pechacek, T F (1982) Cigarette smoking among adolescents: is the rate declining: *Preventive Medicine* 11: 708–712
Murray, D M, Johnson, C A, Luepker, R V and Mittelmark, M B (1984) The prevention of cigarette smoking in children: a comparison of four strategies *Journal of Applied Social Psychology* 14: 274–288
Mutter, G (1988) Education and training unit: School Health Component, mimeo
Mutter, G (1988) Using research results as a health promotion strategy: A five year case study in Canada (unpublished paper) Health and Welfare Canada, March.

Newman, I M and Martin G L (1982) Attitudinal and normative factors associated with adolescent cigarette smoking in Australia and the United States of America: a methodology to assist health education planning *Community Health Studies* 6: 47–56

Oduol, E (1988) Health education for diarrhoea control in children under five years: a challenge for health workers. Paper presented at the Kenya Paediatric Association Annual Scientific Conference, March

Page, R M and Gold, R S (1983) Assessing gender differences in college cigarette smoking: intenders and non-intenders *Journal of School Health* 53: 531–535
Petty, R E and Cacioppo, J R (1986) The elaboration likelihood model of persuasion *in* Berkowitz, L (1986)
Puska, P, Koskela, K, McAlister, A and Pallonen, U (1979) A comprehensive television smoking cessation programme in Finland *International Journal of Health Education* 22: 4 Supplement
Puska, P, Nissinen, A and Salonen, J (1985) The community based strategy to prevent coronary heart disease: conclusions from the ten years of the North Karelia project *Annual Review of Public Health* 6: 147–193

Raw, M and Hellier, J (1983) Smokers' clinics in Britain: A descriptive survey. In *Proceedings of the 5th World Conference on Smoking and Health*: Winnipeg
Raw, M (1985) Does nicotine chewing-gum work? *British Medical Journal* 290: 1231–1232
Read, M (1957) *Social and cultural background for planning public health programmes in Africa*. A paper presented at WHO seminar on Health Education in Africa: Dakar
Russell, M A H, Raw, M and Jarvis, M J (1980) Clinical use of nicotine chewing gum *British Medical Journal* 280: 1599–1602

Salber, E J, Freeman, H E and Abelin, T (1968) Needed research on smoking: Lessons from the Newton study *in* Borgatta, E F and Evans, R R (1968)

Salvador, T, Marin, D, Gonzalez, J et al (1986) Trantamiento del taboquismo: Comparacion entra una terapia de soporte y una terapia utilizan do soporte, chicle de nicotina y refuerzo del comportamiento *Rev. Med. Clin.* 87: 403–406

Schinke, S P, Gilchrist, L D and Snow, W H (1985) Skills intervention to prevent cigarette smoking among adolescents *American Journal of Public Health* 76: 665–667

Scotney, N (1979) Development of health education programmes. A paper presented to the royal College of Obstreticians and Gynaecologists Study Group on 'Maternity Services in the Developing World: What the community needs': London

Shufflebeam, D L (1976) Evaluating the context, input, process and product of education *in* Tammivuori, T

Stenmarck, S (1988) The role of non-governmental organizations in mobilization for a healthy public policy. Paper presented at 2nd International Conference on Health Promotion: Adelaide

Super, D E (1975) Vocational guidance: Emergent decision making in a changing society *Bulletin of the International Association for Education and Vocational Guidance* No 29

Tannahill, A (1986) What is health promotion? *Health Education Journal* 44: 167–168

Telch, M J, Kilen, J D, McAlister, A L, Perry, C L and Maccoby, N (1982) Long-term follow-up of a pilot project on smoking prevention with adolescents *Journal of Behavioral Medicine* 5: 1–7

Tones, B K (1981) Health education: Prevention or subversion? *Royal Society of Health Journal* March 1981: 114–117

Tones, B K (1981) The use and abuse of mass media in health promotion *in* Leathar et al (1981)

Tones, B K (1986) Preventing drug misuse: The case for breadth, balance and coherence *Health Education Journal* Vol 45: No 4: 223–230

Tones, B K (1986) Health education and the ideology of health promotion: A review of alternative approaches *Health Education Research* 1: 3–12

Tones, B K (1987) Promoting health: The contribution of education. Paper presented at WHO Consultation on Co-ordination Infrastructure for Health Education, WHO: Copenhagen

Tones, B K (1988) The role of the school in health promotion: The primacy of personal and social education *Westminster Studies in Education* (forthcoming)

Tones, B K (1988) Selecting indicators of success in health education, the importance of theory and philosopohy *in* Kannas, L and Miilunpalo, S

Torkington, K (1986) Involving parents in the primary curriculum *Perspectives* 24: 12–20

Urberg, K and Robbins, R (1984) Perceived vulnerability in adolescents to the health consequences of cigarette smoking *Preventive Smoking* 13: 367–376

Waaler, H T (1982) Tuberculosis and socio-economic development *Bulletin of the International Union Against Tuberculosis* Vol 57

Young, I (1986) The use of sport sponsorship to raise health issues with schoolchildren *British Journal of Physical Education* Vol 17, No 1

Biographical notes on editors and contributors

John Acham (Chapter 17) is currently acting chief health education officer of the division of health education within the Ministry of Health, Kenya. He has wide experience in the practice of health education in Kenya through working as a district public health education officer, 1964–1967, a provincial health education officer in charge of Nyanza and the Western Province, 1967–1975 and also as a senior mass media officer, 1975–1987. He holds several qualifications; a certificate of senior management, a diploma for meat and other foods, a diploma in public health, a diploma for public health officers for overseas appointment and a BSc in community health from California State University. He led the national maternal and child health/family planning programme – part of a plan for an expanded information and education programme for the World Bank 1977–1979.

Z A Ademuwagun (Chapter 19) is Professor of public health education in the department of preventive and social medicine at the University College Hospital, Ibadan, Nigeria. He is also a Director of the African Regional Health Education Centre which is based at the University of Ibadan.

Kenneth Allison (Chapter 13) is a research scientist in the workplace, school and family section of the prevention studies department at the Addiction Research Foundation in Toronto, Canada. He is also an assistant professor in the department of behavioural science, division of community health, faculty of medicine at the University of Toronto. After completing undergraduate degrees in both education and physical and health education, he worked in the field of physical fitness counselling and administration for several years. He then completed a MHSc degree, specializing in health promotion, and MSc and PhD degrees in community health at the University of Toronto. A past chairman of the Canadian Health Education Society, Ontario Chapter, he is currently involved in research on the individual and environmental influences on drug use, and teaches in the health promotion programme at the University of Toronto.

Mercedes Baez Cruz (Chapter 9) is a professional health educator. She holds a Master's degree from the school of public health in the University of Chile and is professor of health community programmes in the Faculty of Medicine in there. She is head of the health education in health service, metropolitan region, and since 1979 has worked on a national level in the Ministry of Health. She was executive co-ordinator of a sexual education project, which was aimed at health teams, teachers, parents (1969–1973), and was responsible for the learn to teach project which was targeted at all health professionals involved in primary health assistance. She was responsible for the *National Journal of Health Education* from 1983 to 1988 and is assessor and temporary consultant of the Pan American Health Organization for Latin American countries. She is consultant in Health Education for non-governmental organizations such as the Peace Corps and the Red Cross. She is co-author of the book *Norms of School Health*.

John Balding (Introduction and Chapter 26 and co-editor of the Yearbook) has a wide background in teaching in science and health education, together with earlier interests in physical education. At one stage during his career, for a period of about ten years, he was substantially involved in group work skills and counselling. He is a senior lecturer in education, and for the past seven years, he has also been the director of the Health Education Authority Schools Health Education Unit within the University of Exeter. The work of the unit has evolved around the curriculum planning methods he has originated and refined in the areas of attitudes to health topics and of surveying health related behaviour among young people. An indication of the scope of these methods and of related published work are present in his chapter within this text. He is the managing editor of the journal *Education and Health* published from the University of Exeter five times a year with a circulation of 16,000, many copies of which are sent to colleagues in other countries.

Richard Beazley (Chapter 14) is an associate professor of health education at Dalhousie University at Halifax, Nova Scotia, Canada. He has had a long-standing commitment to the development of health education in Canada, and in 1983 completed a national study of the role of community, patient and school health educators. At present he is on a leave-of-absence at Queen's University where he is co-director of the 'Canada Youth and AIDS Study – 1988'. He is the recipient of a national AIDS scholar award for 1988–89'.

J Bobes Garcia (Chapter 8) is Professor of Psychiatry in Oviedo University, Spain.

Annelise Bredholt (Chapter 4) is a trained teacher of domestic science. Since 1962 she has been employed by the Danish government Home Economics Council (now reorganized under the name: The National Consumer Agency of Denmark), where has has been in charge of consumer information and nutritional information. Since 1973, she has been the manager of the information department.

Valerie Brown (Chapter 15) is currently director of Health Advancement Services in Canberra, Australia. She has distinguished herself in both the academic and administrative aspects of her career. A recent and exciting emphasis within her work is in connection with the concept of 'health cities'.

N O Bwibo (Chapter 17) is currently Professor of Paediatrics and Principal of the College of Health Sciences, University of Nairobi. He is a graduate of Makerere Medical School and has carried out graduate training in the Universities of California, Washington, Seattle, London and Copenhagen. His academic qualifications include an MBChb, an MPH and Boards in Paediatrics of the American Academy of Paediatrics, and he also holds an MRCP of the University of London. His dual training in public health, particularly in maternal and child health and clinical paediatrics, places him in a good position to apply his experience in the practice and teaching of paediatrics. His other role is as chief administrator and principal of a busy institution which offers training in various health disciplines at university level. He has published several articles in learned medical journals and chapters in textbooks on a wide range of topics, particularly, in infectious diseases malnutrition, medical education and accidents. He has held various honorary posts in professional societies in Kenya.

Gill Combes (Chapter 26) formerly worked on the Health Education Council's health education for slow learners project at Bath University in the UK, where part of her work was to consider how parents and the wider community can become involved in health education. She now works as schools health education adviser for the Central Birmingham Health Authority, where she has run in-service training for teachers, and worked with individual schools on developing parental involvement.

B de la Torre Arrarte (Chapter 8) works in the school of nursing, Oviedo, Spain.

Hein de Vries (Chapter 2) started the Dutch smoking prevention project in September 1984 at the University of Limburg, The Netherlands. In 1989, he will be the senior invesigator and projecting leader of a new large project on primary prevention of cancer (the ABC project). Besides incorporating Dutch Smoking Prevention Project, the ABC Project also includes projects on smoking cessation, cancer prevention by a community approach, smoking cessation at the workplace, alcohol, and health promotion and information processing.

Margo Dijkstra (Chapter 2) has been involved with the Dutch smoking prevention project since 1986. She is also directing a second project on smoking prevention (1986–1990) comparing different kinds of interventions. This project is also funded by the Dutch Cancer Foundation.

Eugene Donoghue (Chapter 5) is a senior official in the Health Promotion Unit, Department of Health, Eire. Formerly, he was manager of programmes, including education and training, in the Irish Health Education Bureau. He is currently actively involved on a committee to organize a European schools initiative in health education, jointly sponsored by the European Community, World Health Organization and the Council of Europe. He graduated with a BA from University College Cork, received a Higher Diploma in education from Maynooth University and an MA in educational psychology from Manhattan College, New York. He is a part-time lecturer in health education in the department of education, University College, Dublin.

Eli Endresen (Chapter 21) is currently a research worker in the 'Pregnancy and Work' programme at the department of preventive medicine, University of Oslo. She is a graduate of the Sydsvenska Gymnastik Institutet, Lund, Sweden. Eli has held several posts related to obstetrical physiotherapy and pedagogy, psychosomatic physiotherapy and health education and promotion. She has published numerous articles about pregnancy, childbirth and parenting.

John Griffiths (Chapter 23) is a graduate of the University of Wales and trained to be a teacher of biology at Avery Hill College, Eltham, London. He has taught in comprehensive schools in London and Cardiff in the UK. In 1986, he was seconded to 'Heartbeat Wales' as education adviser, where he now works as senior health promotion adviser (secondary education) in the Health Promotion Authority for Wales. He represents the Health Promotion Authority on the national 'No-Smoking Day' committee and the cancer education co-ordination group.

Hans Hagendorn (Chapter 1) studied political sciences at Amsterdam University and specialized in mass communication. During his career he has worked in several organizations for health education, involved with family planning, sexual education and mental health. Since 1984, he has been the director of the Dutch Health Education Centre, a World Health Organization collaborating centre. He is vice-president for Europe of the International Union for Health Education.

Anna-May Harkin (Chapter 5) works in the Health Promotion Unit in the Department of Health in Dublin. She holds a master's degree in sociology and a postgraduate in psychology. She was formerly a research officer with the Health Education Bureau and has lectured in behavioural science and communications to third level students in a Regional Technical College.

Duncan Harris (Series editor) graduated in physics at bachelor level and by research at master's level at Nottingham University. His doctorate was in education from the University of Bath.

After being an instructor officer in the Royal Navy, and a teacher in schools, he became lecturer in education and then senior lecturer in education at the University of Bath. He is currently Professor and Head of Education at Brunel, the University of West London. His current interests include educational technology, assessment and evaluation. He has written and edited several books including a *Dictionary of Instructional Technology* (with H Ellington) and *Evaluating and Assessing for Learning* (with C Bell).

Helen Howson (Chapter 24) took her first degree in Nutrition and Food Science at Cardiff University in 1979. This was followed by a postgraduate degree in Nutrition at Queen Elizabeth College, London, UK. Helen taught in a secondary school in Wales for three years before joining the Health Promotion Unit in South Glamorgan in Wales. Here she was mainly responsible for the development and implementation of the Food and Health Policy, but also had responsibility for primary school health education, liaison with industry and dental health education. In early 1986 Helen joined 'Heartbeat Wales' as the nutritionist and was responsible for the development of the nutrition strategy. This involved developments primarily at macro level. Since the reorganization of the Health Promotion Authority for Wales, Helen's remit has been extended and she now has a responsibility to oversee the strategy for industry and commerce, as well as the on-going nutrition programme:

Chris James (Introduction and co-editor of the Yearbook) worked as a research physiologist at the University of Keele for six years before entering teaching. He taught science and health education in two comphrensive schools before moving to the University of Bath where he is currently a lecturer in the School of Education. He was co-director of the Health Education Council's health education for slow learners project from 1984 to 1987, and his research interests include health education and the organization and management of schools.

Alan King (Chapter 14) is the director of the social program evaluation group at Queen's University and Professor of Sociology of Education. His research projects have been mainly concerned with the health of Canadian youth. Recent major studies include: *Canada Health Knowledge Survey: 9, 12 and 15 year-olds – 1982–83; Canada Health Attitudes and Behaviours Survey: 9, 12 and 15 year-olds – 1984–85; Canada Youth and AIDS Study – 1988;* and *The Adolescent Experience.*

Maria Luisa Lopez (Chapter 8) is a doctor of medicine. Her doctoral thesis was on school health, and she has been head of service in health education and health promotion for ten years with the autonomous government in the North of Spain. In addition to several articles and papers in international journals and presented at conferences, she has published the *First and Second Book of Child Health* and two books about dental health education and smoking prevention, for all the schools of the autonomous government territory. At present she is a Professor of Public Health at Oviedo University, where she mainly works in research on health education.

Catherine Lyttle (Chapter 11) is the director of the Bureau of Health Education, Ministry of Health, Jamaica and a graduate of the University of the West Indies' diploma programme in community health. She worked as a school nurse and a family planning education officer in rural Jamaica prior to joining the Bureau of Health Education staff in 1974.

Ivy McGhie (Chapter 11) is a lecturer and health education specialist in the department of social and preventive medicine, faculty of medical sciences at the University of the West Indies. Her academic qualifications include a BSc and an MPH in public health. At present Mrs McGhie is engaged in a special project for training first line health educators for the Caribbean region. She has been working in the field of health education for thirty years, and was head of the Bureau of Health Education in the Ministry of Health, Jamaica, during the period 1958 to 1971. Mrs McGhie served as a member of the World Health Organization (WHO) expert advisory panel on health education 1971–81 and has been a temporary advisor and short-term consultant to PAHO and WHO within the Caribbean on a number of occasions. She worked as area secretary for the Caribbean Americas and Europe in the overseas division of the British Methodist Church in London from 1980 to 1987.

Brian McAuley (Chapter 6) has been project manager of the schools' programme for the North Western Health Board in Eire since its inception in 1981. He has a primary teacher's diploma from Marino Training College and took his primary degree at University College, Dublin. Having wide experience of educational work with young people in school and in the community, he has taught in primary schools and in secondary level schools, both in Ireland and in Africa. Between 1982 and 1984 he was national chairman of *For'oige*, a national youth development organization. In recent years he has worked as a guidance counsellor, having a Dip. ASEd (guidance and counselling) and an MA in educational psychology from the University of Ulster. He is currently engaged in research on community health promotion strategies.

Jens Mathiesen (Chapter 3) has been director of the Danish Committee for Health Education since 1984. He graduated in medicine from the University of Copenhagen in 1967 and worked as a lecturer from 1968 to 1984 at the Institute of Social Medicine, University of Copenhagen. He has written booklets on drug misuse and alcohol and is a member of the National Prevention Council in Denmark. The Danish Committee for Health Education is a non-governmental organization working closely with government institutions and local authorities.

Archangela Mongelli (Chapter 20) is a public health nurse manager. She qualified as a general nurse and later as a public health nurse in the Italian Red Cross schools in Rome. She qualified as nurse manager at the La Sapienza University in Rome and is currently employed at the Health Ministry in the Direzione Generale dei Servizi di Medicina Sociale. She has recently been engaged in planning and carrying out a research project concerned with nursing care problems in Italian hospitals for the government commission on AIDS. She teaches a course on the principles and methodology of health education in the Italian Red Cross school for public health nurses in Rome. She is also engaged in preparing and organizing courses on health education for nurses in all fields of activity, in keeping with the aims of primary health care. She has published several papers, articles and books on various aspects of Health Education.

Pilar Najera (Chapter 7) is a technical adviser on health education in the 'Carlos III' National Institute of Health in Madrid and a lecturer in health education at the National School of Public Health of Spain. She was formerly head of the Health Education Service of the Ministry of Health and Consumer Affairs. She qualified as a medical doctor and specialized in public health, health services administration and health education. She was editor of the *Revista de Sanidad e Higiene Pública* for 12 years and she has published papers and contributed to several books in the fields of health services administration and health education. In 1987, she was the secretary of the European Conference on Health Education of the International Union for Health Education and was the editor of the conference proceedings.

David Nyamwaya (Chapter 18) is the director of the health behaviour and education department of the African Medical and Research Foundation, Nairobi, Kenya.

Elly Oduol (Chapter 18) is a health education officer working with the African Medical and Research Foundation, Nairobi, Kenya.

Martin Raymond (Chapter 29) has been senior educationist with the Scottish Health Education Group since 1984. Apart from a general interest in health education within community education, he has been responsible for the group's work in the fields of drug misuse and HIV/ AIDS, where he has been involved in all aspects of these topics from in-service training to mass media campaigns. Before joining SHEG he taught in a community school in Aberdeenshire in Scotland.

Marilyn Reid (Chapter 12) is a physician, and the senior medical officer for the metropolitan area of Kingston and St Andrew. A graduate of the Universities of Glasgow and the West Indies where she received the MB, ChB and Diploma in Public Health respectively, Dr Reid worked as a medical officer both in Jamaica and in Kent, England. She was the medical officer for the parish of St Catherine, Jamaica before transferring to Kingston.

Nilda Segura Cid (Chapter 10) is a social worker and health educator. She holds a Master's Degree from the School of Public Health at the University of Chile. As a social worker, she has taken part in community work projects in urban and rural regions. She has been a health educator worker in the Nuble Health Service since 1980 and is director of the Health Education committee, the principal organization for the co-ordination and supervision of the region's educational activities. She is the author of the book *Community Participation*.

Keith Tones (Chapter 25) is a reader in health education at Leeds Polytechnic in the UK, where he directs the Health Education Unit in the department of health and community studies. He started his professional career in teaching after studying modern languages and psychology at Cambridge University. After working in a secondary modern school he lectured for some years in teacher training establishments. He joined Leeds Polytechnic in 1970 and launched a postgraduate diploma course in health education there in 1972. The Unit currently offers a postgraduate Diploma/MSc course in health education and health promotion and a diploma course for students from developing countries. He has acted in a consultative capacity for the World Health Organization and was a council member of the Health Education Council prior to its demise. Recent writings and research activities have included the role of the health education specialist, health education in schools, breast-feeding and evaluation in health education.

Jean Tulloch-Reid (Chapters 11 and 12) has been a lecturer/health education specialist in the department of social and preventive medicine, faculty of medical sciences at the University of the West Indies since 1980. Her main responsibility is to provide training in health education at a variety of levels, including undergraduate and postgraduate programmes. She began her work in health education with the Bureau of Health Education, Ministry of Health Jamaica. After a short stay with the National Family Planning Board as assistant director of education and information, she joined the University in 1973 as tutor in family life education within the department of extra mural studies. After completing the certificate in social work at the University of the West Indies she pursued a BA in sociology and Masters degree in public health programmes at the University of Minnesota.

Harri Vertio (Chapter 22) has been senior medical officer at the National Board of Health, Department of Health Promotion, Finland for the last ten years. He graduated from Helsinki University in medicine in 1972 and worked for two years in health centres and hospitals. He was then assigned to the headquarters of the Finnish Defence Force to plan and implement the health education of recruits. He worked there for three years and as a result produced a dissertation on the health behaviour of conscripts in 1984. His work is concerned with the development of health promotion, including the co-ordination of the World Health Organization 'healthy cities' project in Finland.

Rodney Wellard (Chapter 16) is chairman of the department of health in La Trobe University, Carlton, Australia. He leads and co-ordinates a team of approximately 20 staff from diverse backgrounds. He has wide experience in administration, teaching and research in the health field and is frequently used as a consultant.

Beverley Walker (Chapter 16) is currently researching the use of computers in secondary education in the context of social relationships and beliefs about the social world. She is a senior lecturer in health education and promotion in La Trobe University, Carlton, Australia.

Christopher Wood (Chapter 18) is the Director General of the African Medical and Research Foundation, Nairobi, Kenya.

Ian Young (Chapter 28) is educational adviser to the Scottish Health Education Group (SHEG) in Scotland. He taught biology for ten years and had a special interest in health education and environmental education. Prior to working at the SHEG he was an adviser in science education in Strathclyde Region Education Department. Since 1983, he has been responsible for the education section at the SHEG. As part of SHEG's role as a World Health Organization (Euro) collaborating centre for health education, Ian has acted as an adviser to the World Health Organization (WHO) at several international meetings which were related to school health education and education for safety. He is a member of the EC/Council of Europe/WHO working group which is preparing a teacher education manual in health education.

Index